# THE FUNDAMENTALS OF BRAIN DEVELOPMENT

# THE FUNDAMENTALS OF
# BRAIN DEVELOPMENT

## INTEGRATING NATURE AND NURTURE

❖ ❖ ❖

Joan Stiles

**HARVARD UNIVERSITY PRESS**

Cambridge, Massachusetts, and London, England

2008

Original and adapted illustrations by Matthew S. Davis

*Library of Congress Cataloging-in-Publication Data*

Stiles, Joan.
The fundamentals of brain development : integrating nature and nurture / Joan Stiles.
p. ; cm.
Includes bibliographical references and index.
ISBN-13: 978-0-674-02674-2 (alk. paper)
ISBN-10: 0-674-02674-8 (alk. paper)
1. Brain—Growth.   2. Nature and nurture.   I. Title.
[DNLM: 1. Brain—embryology.   2. Brain—growth & development.   3. Mental Disorders—
etiology.   4. Neurons—physiology.   5. Neuropsychology. WL 300 S856f 2008]
QP376.S815   2008
612.8'2—dc22          2007023464

*To Nik,*

*for his love and support through this long
but very rewarding process,
and to my children, Anne and Matthew,
whose development has been both a joy
and a wonderful education*

# Contents

# Preface

OVER THE PAST several decades, significant advances have been made in our understanding of the basic stages and mechanisms of mammalian brain development. While very little of this work has been—indeed, *could* have been—carried out on humans, it has, nonetheless, greatly informed our understanding of human brain development. Studies elucidating the neurobiology of brain development span the levels of neural organization from the macroanatomic to the cellular to the molecular. Together this large body of work provides a picture of brain development as the product of a complex series of dynamic and adaptive processes operating within a highly constrained, genetically organized but constantly changing context (Morange 2001; Waddington 1939). The view of brain development that has emerged from the developmental neurobiology literature presents challenges and opportunities to psychologists seeking to understand the fundamental processes that underlie social and cognitive development and the neural systems that mediate them.

For decades the central debate in the field of developmental psychology has centered on the very old, and I would argue outmoded, dichotomy of nature versus nurture. While proponents of both positions in this debate acknowledge the role of nature and nurture in development, from each side the concession to the other view is more often perfunctory than substantive. The intellectual divide in this debate is clearly drawn, and there is little room for reconciling the two positions. Proponents of strongly nativist views see no alternative to the positing of innate constraints on cognitive development, while proponents of a more nurture-based view see no evidence for the biological plausibility of such constraints. Constructivist views, such as the one originally espoused by Piaget, argue for adaptive interaction. However, within the field of developmental psychology, there are little actual data on the interaction between experience and biological development. Indeed, for decades, the central arguments that underlie the various elaborations of the nature-nurture debate have unfolded in the absence of substantive information about the nature and process of brain development. Thus it is in some sense strange that the central debate in developmental psychology should revolve so centrally around claims about *either* what is innate *or* how experience shapes brain and mind.

However, while the case for interaction is difficult to make from the behavioral data of the developmental psychologists, a compelling and coherent case for the fundamental importance of interaction has begun to emerge from the growing body of data in developmental neurobiology. From the very first stages of embryonic brain development to the experience-mediated organizational changes in the adolescent brain, the evidence of interaction and the capacity for adaptive change abounds. This evidence points to what Nelson (1999) has called "the subtle but orchestrated dance that occurs between the brain and the environment; specifically, it is the ability of the brain to be shaped by experience and, in turn, for this newly remolded brain to facilitate the embrace of new experiences, which lead to further neural changes, *ad infinitum*" (p. 42). These data are critical to addressing the very important questions posed by those who seek to understand the origins of human thought and social interaction. They argue strongly for the need for psychologists to fundamentally rethink the constructs of interaction and adaptation and their essential role in human development.

Ultimately, the goal of developmental neuropsychology will be to link the major milestones of cognitive and social development with changes in the neural substrate that mediates those functions. But this is a field that is still in its infancy, and we are far from achieving this goal. At this point, an attempt at a synthesis or even a complete summary of the links between behavioral and neural development is premature. There is just too much that we do not know to tell a coherent story about brain and cognitive development. However, it is not too early to attempt to provide a framework for exchange in the form of books designed to bridge disciplinary divides. This volume was designed to provide one part of this interdisciplinary bridge. It provides an overview of the fundamentals of brain development from conception through adolescence. It emphasizes recent work in developmental neurobiology that points to the dynamic nature of brain development and the importance of interaction between events that are genetically specified and those that are the product of the organism's experience of the world.

The preparation and writing of this book has been a remarkable and rewarding adventure. Many people have contributed in different ways to the final product, and I deeply appreciate all of the help I have received. I am grateful to the students in my graduate and undergraduate classes for their patience and feedback in working with and, I hope, learning from earlier drafts of the chapters. I want to thank my graduate students, Sarah Noonan, Silvia Paparello, Tami Harrison, and especially Brianna Paul, for their careful reading and invaluable comments on the manuscript. I am also deeply indebted to my biology colleagues for their input, insight, and advice. Ralph Greenspan provided expert advice and comments on both the scientific and the historical aspects of the genetics chapter. Nick Spitzer's review of the neuron development chapters was extremely helpful. My greatest debt of thanks goes to Harry Uylings of the Netherlands Brain Research Institute, who critically reviewed the entire book, offering invaluable advice and input on everything from genetics to embryology to postnatal experience on brain development. Harry and I met several years ago in Dubrovnik at a FENS/IBRO workshop on human brain development. The conference was excellent but demanding in that the topics ranged from molecules to behavior. One very notable feature of the conference was the questions from a very distinguished Dutch gentleman, Harry Uylings, who asked direct and on-point questions of every speaker regardless of topic. Two years later, I met Harry again at a second FENS/IBRO conference. I had begun work on the book and understood how valuable Harry's input would be in shaping the final product. He very kindly agreed to take on the task of reviewing the entire manuscript. His comments were thorough and comprehensive. I cannot overstate the importance of his contributions to the depth, the accuracy, and the completeness of the final book.

Finally, writing a book is one thing; producing it is quite another. I am particularly indebted to two people for their help in actually generating the finished product. The first is my son, Matthew Davis, who took on the job of illustrating the book. When I began this project, Matthew's credentials as an artist/scientist had recently been confirmed in his graduation from UC Berkeley with degrees in physics and visual art. I asked if he would be interested in taking on a more biological art project—the illustrations for my book. I was pleased when he agreed but delighted when the finished products were complete. His work has contributed greatly to both the clarity and the aesthetics of the book. Finally, I am deeply indebted to Janet Shin, my laboratory manager, for the tremendous effort she has put into the completion of this book. Janet worked literally hundreds of hours to produce the finished product. She approaches every task with care, concern, and professionalism, and her work on the book was no exception. Her discerning eye, focus on detail, high professional standards, and tireless effort in many ways made this book possible.

## References

Morange, M. 2001. *The misunderstood gene.* Cambridge, MA: Harvard University Press.

Nelson, C. A. 1999. "Neural plasticity and human development." *Current Directions in Psychological Science,* 8: 42–45.

Waddington, C. H. 1939. *An introduction to modern genetics.* New York: Macmillan.

THE FUNDAMENTALS OF BRAIN DEVELOPMENT

# ONE

# The Central Questions about Psychological and Biological Development

THE CENTRAL DEBATE in the field of developmental psychology has centered for decades on the very old and somewhat fluidly defined dichotomy between nature and nurture. The unifying questions of the psychological debate concern the origins of knowledge and action. That is, how do children come to know and understand the world and their place in it? To what extent are humans innately prepared to interpret the world, and to what extent do they rely on learning? The central ideas and core premises of each side in the psychological debate find their roots in the much older ideas of the rationalist and empiricist philosophers, which in turn date back to the writings of ancient Greeks. In the tradition of their predecessors, nativists stress the availability, universality, and continuity of core knowledge across human populations. Within the modern psychological discussion, the classical empiricist view has been largely supplanted by information-processing and constructivist views, both of which argue that even children's earliest knowledge derives from their engagement with the world. Although proponents of both positions in this debate acknowledge the importance of both nature and nurture in development, the heart of the debate centers around the issue of whether there is a critical set of innate, nonlearned core concepts that form the foundation for later learning, or whether complex concepts can emerge from more primitive and presumably innately endowed sensory and motor abilities.

The intellectual divide in this debate is clearly drawn, and there is little room for reconciliation. Proponents of strongly nativist views see no alternative to positing innate constraints on cognitive development. To support their claims of innate knowledge, they point to evidence suggesting that young infants exhibit understanding of core concepts in the absence of direct experience. By contrast, proponents of a more nurture-based view argue that the availability of basic learning mechanisms and sensorimotor primitives, coupled with the child's active engagement with the world, are sufficient to support knowledge acquisition. They challenge both the necessity of and the evidence for the innate concepts.

One question that has received very little attention in the psychological literature is how claims from either side of the debate might be instantiated biologically. What does it mean for a concept or a learning mechanism to be innate? Indeed, some proponents of nativism have argued that since concepts are psychological constructs, the question of biological implementation is not relevant to the central nativist claims (Samuels 1998, 2002; Spelke 1998). From the constructivist side, theorists beginning with Piaget have argued for adaptive interaction. However, there are few actual data that provide a plausible account of the nature of interaction between experience and biological development, that is, of how experience can influence the development of a biological system in ways that support meaningful psychological development. Thus it is in some sense strange that the central debate in developmental psychology should revolve around claims about either what is innate and thus presumably part of the biological endowment of the organism or how experience shapes brain and mind. From both sides of the theoretical aisle, the central arguments that underlie the various elaborations of the nature-nurture debate have unfolded in the absence of substantive information about the nature and process of developmental change in the biological system that mediates all social and cognitive development—the brain.

Over the past several decades, significant advances have been made in our understanding of the basic stages and mechanisms of mammalian brain development. Although very little of this work has been—indeed, could have been—carried out on humans, the animal studies have nonetheless greatly informed our understanding of human brain development. Studies elucidating the neurobiology of brain development span the levels of neural organization and function from the macroanatomic to the cellular to the molecular. This large body of work provides a picture of brain development as the product of a complex series of dynamic and adaptive processes operating within highly constrained but constantly changing biological and environmental contexts (Morange 2001; Waddington 1939). The view of brain development that has emerged from the developmental neurobiology literature presents both challenges and opportunities to psychologists who seek to understand the fundamental processes that underlie social and cognitive development and the neural systems that mediate them.

The remainder of this chapter will explore key questions posed by the nature-versus-nurture debate from the perspectives of both psychology and biology. It will also describe in greater detail the major issues and controversies within the field of developmental psychology concerning the origins of knowledge.

## Nature versus Nurture: The Psychological Debate

The debate over the origins of knowledge centers on a number of key issues. Table 1.1 presents five of the major points of controversy about the origins of knowledge and summarizes the major arguments from the two sides in the nature-nurture controversy for each.

## The Role of Experience in Concept Formation

The first and most central issue of the nature-versus-nurture debate is the question of whether there exists a set of innate concepts that underpin and structure early conceptual development. A concept, whether innate or acquired, is "the mental representation that encapsulates the commonalities and structure that exist among items within categories" (Oakes and Rakison 2003, p. 3) of objects or events. In that sense, concepts are abstractions that define the relationships among objects and events in the world. "The meaningfulness we ascribe to objects and events is due to our conceptual interpretation of them . . . The [infant's] concept of animal . . . is the infant's *interpretation* of the dog it is observing" (Mandler 2003, p. 104). While concepts often involve the categorization of objects into meaningful groupings (animals, furniture, things that move), conceptualization extends beyond object categories to other domains, such as space, time, or quantity.

Table 1.1  Major issues in the nature-versus-nurture debate

| Question/Issue | Nature | Nurture |
| --- | --- | --- |
| The role of experience: core concepts versus acquired concepts | Core concepts constitute a small but essential subset of concepts. Core concepts are acquired in the absence of direct experience. | Concepts develop from the interaction of basic sensory and motor abilities and experience in the world. |
| Domain specific–domain general (innate versus acquired modularity) | Core concepts are domain specific and encapsulated from other information sources (i.e., they are modular). | Domain-general learning mechanisms underlie conceptual development. Modularity is the product of development. |
| Invariance | One mark of a core concept is that it is constant over the span of development. | Because knowledge is emergent and constructed by the child, change is evident across development. |
| Universality | Core concepts are universal, constant across cultures. | Ubiquity does not necessarily reflect innate origins. Adaptation to universal conditions can produce common constructs. |
| Triggering versus induction | Environmental inputs serve to "trigger" the availability of core concepts. | Concepts are acquired through induction, that is, through hypothesis formulation and testing. |

For example, it has been shown that "infants younger than one year of age can form categorical representations for spatial relations such as above, below, and between" (Quinn 2003, p. 70).

It is generally agreed that most concepts are acquired. However, proponents of the nativist view assert that there is a small set of fundamental concepts that provide the foundation for conceptual development. These concepts are often referred to as core knowledge, core domains, or core concepts (Carey and Markman 1999; Gelman 2000; Spelke 2000). According to the nativist account, core concepts are distinguished from acquired knowledge in that they are available to the child in the absence of any prior direct experience of the concept. As summarized by Elizabeth Spelke, a prominent and highly regarded nativist theorist, "The nativist-empiricist dialogue is . . . about whether knowledge of things in the external world develops on [the] basis of encounters with those things" (Spelke 1998, p. 192).

Indeed, a major debate in the field of developmental psychology involves the interpretation of findings from studies that purport to present evidence of core knowledge in the absence of prior experience. The literature from this active area of investigation is much too large to review here, but one example will serve to illustrate the controversy. A number of investigators have used preferential-looking methodologies to determine whether young infants have knowledge of rudimentary arithmetic operations, such as simple addition or subtraction (e.g., Simon, Hespos, and Rochat 1995; Wynn 1992, 1993). For example, in a typical study, an infant might be shown a stagelike display containing one doll. A screen rotates up, blocking the infant's view of the display area and the doll. Next, the child sees a hand holding a second doll go behind the screen and then return empty (this example illustrates addition, but comparable studies have examined subtraction). At test, the screen is lowered, revealing either one or two dolls. The finding that infants look longer on test trials presenting a single doll than on those presenting two dolls has been interpreted as evidence that the child's expectation that the display should contain two dolls has been violated. The investigators argue that to have this expectation, the child must be able to compute very basic arithmetic operations. Thus, according to the nativist interpretation, infants have "an ability to determine the results of simple arithmetical operations. The fact that these abilities are evident . . . at a very early age in human infancy suggests that we are innately equipped with such knowledge, rather than learning it through induction over experience" (Wynn 1993, p. 222). However, studies by other investigators have challenged the interpretation of these findings and raised methodological questions. Specifically, studies designed to control for baseline perceptual cues and looking preferences suggest that infants' responses may reflect sensitivity to more general perceptual attributes of the display (Clearfield and Mix 1999; Cohen and Marks 2002; Simon 1997). In line with this view, constructivists have argued that detailed examination of the development of concept acquisition reveals that postulation of "innate core knowledge ... may be unnecessary or even misleading ... [infants develop] their knowledge about the world by way of a continuous interplay between a set of domain-general learning mechanisms and changing environmental experiences" (Cohen, Chaput, and Cashon 2002, p. 1324).

## Domain-Specific and Domain-General Knowledge

Innate concepts are characterized as both domain specific and modular (Fodor 1986; Spelke 2000). Nativists have argued that the encapsulated, domain-specific character of core knowledge systems serves to constrain and direct learning while retaining each system's integrity as a special-purpose processor. "Domain-specific structures encourage attention to inputs that have a privileged status because they have the potential to nurture learning about that domain; they help learners find inputs that are relevant for knowledge acquisition and problem solving within that domain" (Gelman 2000, p. 854). In contrast, nonnativists contend that domain specificity is the product of development rather than the starting point (Bates 1999; Karmiloff-Smith 1991). They argue that specialized higher cognitive functions derive from marshalling more elementary domain-general functions. Constructivists suggest that an alternative to nativist claims about the priority of domain-specific knowledge is "that domain-specific knowledge can be acquired and processed by domain-general mechanisms ... The cognitive machinery that makes us human can be viewed as a new machine constructed out of old parts" (Bates 1999, pp. 236–237).

## Universality and Invariance of Concepts

Core knowledge is claimed to be found universally among human populations and is described as present in an invariant form across development (Gelman 2000). Evidence of similarities in fundamental aspects of cognitive and affective processing in diverse and geographically remote cultures and populations is taken as evidence of innate constraints on knowledge acquisition. Nonnativists counter these claims by arguing that neither universality nor invariance of a concept need arise from its status as an innate construct. Regularities both in the world and in basic human perceptual, attentional, and stochastic learning mechanisms can, in principle, interact to yield consistent and predictable conceptual structures.

"Universality will be found amid the correlations and statistical regularities that are grounded in perception, the structure of the world, and in concrete lexical categories" (Smith, Colunga, and Yoshida 2003, p. 300).

## Availability of Concepts: Triggering versus Induction

One final question about innate concepts concerns their availability. Stated more precisely, how does core knowledge become available to the child? It is important to note that environmental factors are postulated to play an important role in nativist accounts of concept acquisition for both innate and learned concepts. However, the mechanism of acquisition for innate concepts differs from that described for concepts acquired via inductive learning. Specifically, concept-specific inputs are postulated to act as "triggers" to the availability of innate concepts. Unlike concepts acquired through inductive learning, there is no "rational relation" between the innate concepts and the cause of their acquisition; rather, the relation has been characterized as "brute-cause" (Fodor 1981). Thus, by this view, the child's experience of the trigger is both necessary and sufficient for the acquisition of innate concepts (Chomsky 1995; Cowie 1999; Fodor 1981). By contrast, in constructivist accounts experience is a necessary part of the developmental equation but a single encounter with a stimulus is usually not sufficient for learning or concept acquisition. Constructivists emphasize the central role of domain-general, or at least domain-relevant (Karmiloff-Smith 2002), learning mechanisms (Newcombe 2002). They focus on the possibility of gradual acquisition and the possibility of having partial knowledge of a concept (Elman et al. 1996; Haith and Benson 1998) and they stress, most centrally, the importance of understanding the developmental processes that underlie knowledge acquisition.

As this brief and greatly simplified sketch of the major arguments within the mainstream psychological debate over nature versus nurture suggests, proponents from both sides of the theoretical aisle pose well-articulated, if opposing, arguments on key questions concerning the origins of knowledge. Notably, the arguments from both sides contain the same basic elements. Both acknowledge the importance of innate structures, both recognize that most knowledge is the product of learning, and both articulate a central role for the environment in the development of the organism. The central dispute revolves around the status of a limited but important set of concepts, defined as core knowledge by the nativists. At the heart of the debate is the question of whether a meaningful account of development requires the postulation of some innate concepts, or whether early concepts can be constructed from the organism's interaction with the world via innate biological learning mechanisms acting in concert with basic sensory, motor, and perceptual processes. Importantly, although both the construct of innateness and that of the interaction between biological structures and experience are intricately woven into the fabric of arguments on both sides, the focus of debate has been over what is innate rather than what it means for something to be innate. Innateness and, more specifically, claims about the biological feasibility of innate structures or functions have not been a central focus of the psychological debate. A set of candidate characteristics (present without learning, universal, invariant, part of the biological endowment of the organism, and so on) often stands as a proxy for a definition of innateness. It is important to ask how proponents from each side in the debate articulate and defend their definition of the construct that is at the heart of the psychological debate: the concept of innateness.

## Definitions of Innateness

The question of what it means for something to be innate is not new. The philosophical antecedents of the question date back thousands of years. However, in the modern psychological recasting, the question has become a scientific one involving evidentiary threads from both psychology and biology. The issue of specifying biologically feasible mechanisms that can account for the acquisition of psychological constructs is well recognized as a deep and difficult problem. What is the nature of information contributed by the genes, cells, or cell assemblies; what is contributed by the environment; and most important, how do these sources of information interact? Responses from psychologists to the question of what it means for something to be innate have been interestingly diverse.

## Levels of Inquiry and Nativist Arguments

A common argument from the nativist side of the debate regarding the question of biological feasibility of innate concepts is that the question is ill posed within the context of the psychological debate. A number of investigators have argued that information about the development of biological structures and functions is not central to the psychological questions about the origins of knowledge (Chomsky 1995; Samuels 2002; Spelke et al. 1992). Spelke, for example, suggests, "The nativist-empiricist dialogue is not about the interaction of genes and their environment, but about whether knowledge of things in the external world develops on [the] basis of encounters with those things . . . These questions are not addressed by research on interactions between genes and gene products but by research on the emerging and changing capacities of children in interaction with their surroundings" (Spelke 1998, p. 192). Innate concepts are those concepts that emerge in the absence of learning. The relevant data, they argue, come from the answer to the question of whether knowledge will follow a prescribed developmental course regardless of the context in which the child is placed. Indeed, it has been argued that questions about innate knowledge cannot be addressed through the methods and means of scientific inquiry (Chomsky 1995). In response to the challenge to provide a more specific account of how an innate concept might be represented biologically, nativists have suggested that their agenda may simply address a different level of inquiry. By this view, nativists may be "pursuing a different project altogether . . . that of simply unearthing the extent to which . . . learning is visibly constrained in ways that promote the acquisition of specific items or types of knowledge. Such a project may be deliberately noncommittal concerning the precise way in which . . . [it] is achieved" (Clark 1998, p. 573). By this view, the necessary and sufficient evidence for an innate concept can be found within the context in which it emerges, that is, from behavioral evidence that the concept emerges in the absence of learning. Further, although the question of biological instantiation is important in its own right, it is not an essential part of the psychological debate. Questions about biological mechanisms of innateness are the purview of a different discipline (Spelke 1998).

It is important to note that although proponents of nativism define the behavior of the organism as the appropriate level of evidence in the psychological debate over innateness, the biological system plays a critical role in their view of development. Spelke and Newport (1998) have argued specifically that the "striking continuity of the core abilities . . . suggests that biology plays a strong role in the growth of knowledge" (p. 321). The central issue from their perspective is that of defining the differential roles of biology and experience in the development of knowledge. They suggest that central to the nature-nurture dialogue is the "thesis that human knowledge is rooted partly in biology and partly in experience, and . . . that successful explanations of the development of knowledge will come from attempts to tease these influences apart" (p. 323). Acquisition of innate concepts is described as the product of an "intrinsic growth process" (Spelke 1998) presumably anchored in the internal biological processes of the organism. Although they do not specify the nature of those intrinsic processes, proponents of nativist views clearly distinguish between genetic determinism and nativism (Spelke 1999). They reject what they view as attributions of preformationism by theorists on the other side of the nature-versus-nurture debate (Spelke 1999) and assert that nativism makes no specific claims about programming at the genetic or cellular level (Marcus 1998). Nativist arguments typically embrace the importance of the biological system in development but take no specific stand on the biological mechanisms that would serve to instantiate an innate psychological concept.

## Levels of Constraint and Constructivist Arguments

Constructivist arguments about early conceptual development typically focus on the question of interaction between biological systems and the experience of the organism (Cohen, Chaput, and Cashon 2002; Johnson 2003; Newcombe 2002). By this view, development is initially directed by the biological systems that implement basic learning and memory mechanisms and support attention allocation and perceptual and motor exchange with the world. Perhaps the most comprehensive statement of what it means for something to be innate within the context of a constructivist model comes from a book by Elman, Bates, Johnson, Karmiloff-Smith, Parisi, and Plunkett (1996) titled *Rethinking Innateness*. The authors begin by placing innate processes within the context of organism-environment interactions. They distinguish between organism-internal and organism-external environments and define innate functions as those that are internal to the organism, "interactions between the genes and their molecular and cellular environments without recourse to information from outside the organism" (Elman et al. 1996, p. 22). Having anchored their definition of innateness in the distinction between organism-internal and organism-external factors, they then propose a framework for thinking about the different "ways that things can be innate." In their model, they consider which aspects or levels of the neurobiological system might feasibly support or constrain the processing of different kinds of information and whether the development of different levels of neurocognitive organization could plausibly occur on the basis of organism-internal factors alone.

According to the model proposed by Elman and colleagues, for a neurocognitive outcome to be considered innate, it must be constrained at one or more of three hypothesized levels: representational, architectural, or chronotopic.[1] Representational constraints are implemented within the complex circuitry of the cerebral cortex. The cortical circuitry is considered necessary for the storage and processing of abstract knowledge representations. Elman and colleagues suggest that the definition of innateness proposed by proponents of the nativist view is captured in the first level of constraint, that of representational innateness. They argue that if children were born with innate concepts, that information would, of necessity, be hardwired in the cortical microcircuitry. They contend that representational constraints are the least plausible model of innateness, finding little support in the neurobiological data.

Architectural constraints have three forms within the model, representing different levels of granularity: the neural unit, local circuits, and macrolevel circuits. Unit architecture constraints are imposed by properties of neurons, such as cell type, response characteristics, or neurotransmitter type, all of which define the most basic level of computation in the brain. Local architecture constraints arise from the structure and function of local networks and include such features as cortical layering, neuronal packing density, or excitatory/inhibitory connectivity, all of which contribute to the areal parcellation of the cortex. Global architectural constraints arise from the macrolevel cir-

---

1. Elman et al. provide examples from both computational and neurobiological models in defining the levels of innate constraints. For brevity, this discussion will focus on the proposed levels of the neurobiological system.

cuitry that connects different regions of the brain. The architectural constraints operate at multiple levels of brain circuitry, including input/output pathways that serve to establish primary sensory and motor areas, intra-areal networks that establish local processing centers, and interareal connections that set up neural networks. These constraints are good candidates for implementing the neurobiologically documented patterns of intrinsic and extrinsic signaling that serve initially to set up the basic sensory and motor areas and later to establish higher-order association areas. However, the relationship between the architectural constraints and knowledge systems is less obvious than the relationship between representational constraints and knowledge. The functioning of the architectural constraints is more likely embedded in developmental processes required for concept acquisition than in the representation of concepts per se.

Finally, chronotopic constraints are imposed by the temporal unfolding of events across the course of development. These bear the least direct relationship to knowledge systems because they act to constrain and modulate change in developing brain and cognitive systems through time. Chronotopic constraints capture the idea that development is a temporally bound event that progressively incorporates the developmental history of the organism.

## Can Developmental Neurobiology Contribute to the Ongoing Dialogue in Psychology?

Both sides in the psychological debate over nature versus nurture recognize the importance of the developing neural system to our understanding of the origins of knowledge. Although nativists emphasize that the proper focus of psychological inquiry lies in the behavior of the organism, they also stress the importance of distinguishing and carefully defining the biological and psychological influences on development. Recent constructivist arguments have also embraced the task of defining the biological sources of innate structures and processes. The interaction between intrinsic and extrinsic processes is central to the constructivist argument, and a key element in their agenda is the explication of how experience can influence the development of a biological system.

## Inseparability of Biological Inheritance and Environment

Recent progress in developmental neurobiology has begun to demonstrate that central questions of defining innateness and interaction are, from the side of biology, tractable. From a biological perspective, the concept of innateness has historically been closely linked to questions of biological inheritance, that is, to those things that are transmitted from one generation to the next. As will be discussed at length in Chapter 2, the concept of biological inheritance is one that has evolved over many years and has in the past century been closely tied to the emerging concept of the gene. One of the most important aspects of the modern view of innateness from the perspective of biology is the inseparability of biological inheritance and environmental influence. "We can see how absurd it is to try to separate what is . . . *innate* . . . from what is . . . due to the environment, although unfortunately this is often attempted. Everything is innate, *and* everything is acquired. The most we can say is that what is innate makes it possible to select from the environment what will be . . . taken into account in the development program" (Danchin 2002, pp. 270–271). At first glance, this description appears to accommodate either the psychological nativist position or the constructivist view. However, closer examination of this idea of inseparability within the biological context suggests something fundamentally different from either the notion of a "triggering" event postulated by the psychological nativists or the operation of a biologically based learning mechanism. Within the neurobiological literature, the inseparability of inherited and environmental factors is fundamental, and it drives development itself. The construct of "environment" is multiply construed as encompassing both influences external to the organism and local, internal organismic states. Throughout the lifespan, and most particularly during early development, local environmental cues organize and control the complex molecular and cellular interactions that direct the development of the organism. Further, local cues are themselves influenced by both external cues and other local cues, some of which are created by the very molecular and cellular interactions directed by the original local cue. In this vein, Gottlieb (2002) has argued for the construct of "probabilistic epigenesis," which maintains that psychobiological development depends upon bidirectional influence at all levels of the neurobehavioral system, from the molecular to the cellular to the organismic to the external environment. He suggests that "the cause of development—what makes development happen—is the relationship of the two components [genes and environment], not the components themselves. Genes in themselves cannot cause development any more than stimulation in itself can cause development" (Gottlieb 2002, p. 38). Development occurs because of the dynamic and ongoing interactions among the inherited genes and cellular machinery, local-environment cues and events, and organism-external factors.

## What Is Inherited?

Within this model, brain development is a process that relies on inherited factors functioning within specific contexts to produce the constantly changing and emerging structure of the developing brain. The inherited factors include the genes and the cellular mechanisms that make it possible to make use of the information coded in the genes. The information contained in a gene is a template for generating proteins, which are the molecules that play active roles in biological signaling. The contexts, or environments, are multifaceted and constantly expanding over the course of development. They range from the internal environment of the cell to collections or assemblies of cells, to signaling pathways, to input coming from the outside world through either sensory or molecular mechanisms. Development is the set of biological processes put in motion by the contextually constrained interactions among innate factors. These interactions result in signaling cascades that direct a diverse range of developmental processes from specification of cell type to axon guidance to synapse stabilization.

## Inheritance, Environment, and Development

It is important to note that the model proposed here considers the role of inherited factors and environmental context in directing the developmental processes that give rise to neural structures and functions. It is within this specifically developmental model that the notion of inseparability is critical. Developmental processes rely on inherited factors that operate within specific but constantly changing contexts, and in that sense inherited factors and environment are inseparable. But the construct of inheritance, or inherited factors, refers quite specifically to gene products and cellular machinery and should not be confused with the more general construct of heritability. Heritability refers to the proportion of phenotypic variance that can be accounted for by genetic variance. It is a population statistic that looks at the relative influence of inherited factors on the prevalence of traits within the range of environments in which the phenomena are studied. As such, it is a very different level of analysis that examines the statistical probabilities of the differential, and hence separate, contributions of inherited and environmental factors on the prevalence of a trait. These analyses are very useful in describing trait frequencies across populations, but assessment of the heritability of a trait cannot specify the causal relationship between a particular inherited factor (gene) and its prevalence in a population, nor can it specify the function of the inherited factor in the organism. The specific causal role of a gene product in a biological process requires assessment at the molecular level, and at that level it is the interaction of inherited factors operating within specific contexts that ultimately defines a gene's function or functions and its role in development (see Chapter 2 for further discussion of Moss's constructs of the Gene-P and the Gene-D.)

The biological model of development presents a very different perspective on key questions raised in the nature-nurture debate. It is a perspective that may be usefully applied to theories of psychological development. By this view, the emerging structures and functions of the brain are the product of the developmental processes created by the interaction of inherited and contextual factors. Developmental processes, and the structures and functions that derive from them, rely upon but are distinct from the inherited and contextual factors that interact to create them. This is a very different way of thinking about what it means for something to be innate. Because developmental processes rely equally on inherited and contextual information, the attempt to categorize the origins of a brain structure as the product of nature or nurture is misdirected. This model shifts the focus of inquiry to the question of development itself. Specifically, what set of developmental processes gives rise to a particular biological structure or neural mechanism, and what are the constraints on those developmental processes that lead, in most cases, to the typical trajectory of brain development?

The burgeoning body of data from developmental neurobiology illustrates and defines in elegant detail these ideas of developmental
process and the inseparability of biological inheritance and environmental influence. Therefore, the study of brain development has the
potential to make significant contributions to the conversation about
the development of psychological processes. Information about the
basics of brain development is important for developmental psychologists both because it can at once constrain and expand the range and
content of the discussion of developmental mechanisms, and because
it can much more rigorously define the biological constructs that are
central to, but underdefined in, the psychological debate.

To be clear, knowledge of the details of brain development by itself
will not answer the fundamental questions about the relationship between brain and behavioral development that are a core interest of
psychology. The study of neurocognitive/social development is still in
its infancy, and although considerable progress has been made in the
past decade, we are still many years away from a comprehensive account of the origins of brain-behavior relations. But ultimately such an
account will require the integration of data from brain and behavioral
sciences. Thus the bridge between behavioral and brain sciences is an
important one that requires exchange across both sides of the interdisciplinary aisle. However, the rate of progress over the past decade in
our understanding of the basic principles of brain development presents a challenge to investigators trained principally in behavioral sciences. The field of developmental neurobiology is technical, and as
the technology has advanced, the important content of the field has
gradually become less accessible to nonexperts. This growing divide
presents a challenge to both biologists and psychologists. This book attempts to distill the fundamental principles of brain development into
a form that is both rigorous and accessible to the nonexpert, with the
goal of fostering the important interdisciplinary exchange that will be
essential to a full understanding of how children come to know about
the world. A complete account of social and cognitive development is
inseparably and reciprocally linked to our understanding of brain development. Thus knowledge of brain development is critical for
understanding psychological development, and cross-disciplinary exchange will be critical for solving the complex riddle of knowledge
acquisition.

## Plan of This Book

The study of neuropsychological development is a very large, highly multidisciplinary enterprise that requires expertise from diverse fields, each with very different vocabularies, methodologies, and questions. The goal of understanding brain and behavioral development requires the bridging of core disciplines. However, the pieces of the bridge that will eventually provide a unified theory of neurobehavioral development are often found in specialized books and journals that do not easily transfer across disciplines. The purpose of this book is to provide nonexperts with an overview of the fundamentals of mammalian brain development. It is particularly directed to students and investigators working in the behavioral sciences who wish to understand the biological underpinnings of the complex changes observed in perceptual, cognitive, affective, and social development. Therefore, material provided in this book is intended to inform key arguments about the biological feasibility of the core assumptions that are at the heart of the psychological debate over nature versus nurture. The goal is not—cannot be—to resolve the debate but rather to provide basic information from an important, related discipline that may constrain or elaborate the psychological theories. The substance of the book draws from several decades of work in the field of developmental neurobiology. Within that field, tremendous progress has been made in understanding both the intrinsic and the extrinsic factors that contribute to the development of the human brain. Although the biological model of brain development is far from complete, basic principles of gene action have begun to emerge in tandem with growing specification of the mechanisms by which experience can influence biological development. The chapters that follow provide a basic overview of the major steps in brain development from conception through adolescence. Each chapter focuses on a different aspect or period of development and discusses the major intrinsic and extrinsic factors that influence and direct the observed changes. The remainder of this section will provide a brief overview of the content and major themes of each chapter.

An important part of interdisciplinary exchange is the consideration of possible parallels across disciplines in the major theoretical debates that have shaped each field. This chapter has focused on the central role of the nature-versus-nurture debate in developmental psychology.

Interestingly, within the biological sciences there has been a centuries-long debate over the origins and nature of inherited factors that parallels the debate over nature versus nurture within the psychological sciences. These arguments are most clearly articulated in the long history of thought about what Johannsen (1911) first termed the "gene." Chapter 2 presents a brief summary of this debate, highlighting the central arguments about constancy and variability of inheritance and the material nature of the gene.[2] Included in Chapter 2 are short sections intended to introduce the nonexpert reader to some basic concepts about genes and gene expression that will be important for understanding the discussion of gene effects in later chapters.

Chapters 3 through 5 focus on the embryological period of development, which in humans encompasses the first eight weeks postconception. During this important period of development, the basic structures and fundamental organization of the brain and the central nervous system are established. Chapter 3 examines the very earliest steps in neural development, focusing on the initial differentiation of the cell lines that will give rise to the central nervous system. Specifically, it examines the process of gastrulation, which occurs during the third week postconception in humans. By the end of gastrulation, the embryo has three well-defined cell layers. Further, the basic spatial dimensions are established such that the embryo has clearly defined front-back (anterior-posterior), right-left, and top-bottom (dorsal-ventral) axes. Chapter 4 concentrates on the emergence of the first discernible neural structure, the neural tube. The formation of the neural tube occurs during the fourth week postconception in hu-

---

2. The question of inheritance is central to the history of thought and scientific discovery in biology. Debate about the nature and mechanisms of inheritance has extended over centuries and has involved the contributions of many investigators from different disciplines. Because of space limitations, Chapter 2 provides only the most cursory overview of this complex and interesting debate, highlighting major shifts in theory and thought and citing the work of only a fraction of the many scientists who have contributed to advances in this field. For more details on the history of this debate, the reader is referred to some of the many books and edited volumes on this topic, for example, Allen 1975; Beurton, Falk, and Rheinberger 2000; Carlson 1966; Creath and Maienschein 2000; Danchin 2002; Gilbert 1991; Horder, Witkowski, and Wylie 1986; Keller 1995, 2000; Lewontin 2001; Morange 2001; Moss 2003; Oyama, Griffiths, and Gray 2001; and Portugal and Cohen 1977.

mans. This critical embryonic structure will give rise to the brain and the spinal column. Chapter 5 considers more elaborated patterning within the embryonic nervous system. It examines the initial ballooning of the most anterior regions of the neural tube that will become the brain, as well as the emerging organization within both anterior and more posterior regions. By the end of the embryonic period, the primitive neocortex is established, and its basic organization is specified.

Chapters 6 and 7 take a more microscopic look at early neural development, examining the production and development of the basic information-processing cells in the brain, the neurons. Chapter 6 summarizes the production of neurons. Neuron production begins soon after the formation of the neural tube and continues until midgestation, about four and a half months in humans. Chapter 6 also considers the production and function of the other major class of cells that comprise the brain, the glial cells. Chapter 7 considers what happens after neurons are born. Neurons are generated in the major proliferative zones deep within the developing brain. They must then migrate away from the proliferative region and identify their appropriate location in the developing cortex. Once they arrive at their cortical destination, they must generate the cellular processes and molecular substances necessary for communicating with other neurons.

Chapter 8 begins with a topic of historical debate (now largely resolved) within the field of developmental neurobiology. Specifically, it reviews the debate over the extent to which intrinsic, that is, largely genetic factors determine early brain organization and the extent to which neural organization is determined by input from the environment. These two perspectives are captured by the protomap and protocortex models of development, respectively. Two related topics are also considered in this chapter. They are the major "subtractive" events that are critical for normal brain development: programmed neuronal cell death and synaptic exuberance and pruning. Both neurons and connections between neurons (the synapses) are massively overproduced early in development and then later removed or retracted by these two well-defined subtractive processes. Most programmed cell death occurs in the late fetal and early postnatal periods. Synaptic exuberance and pruning are largely postnatal events that extend in selected brain regions at least through adolescence.

Chapter 9 considers the structural changes in the developing brain in the late fetal and postnatal periods. It begins with a consideration of the emergence of gyral and sulcal patterning, that is, the characteristic enfolding of the surface of the cortex. It then considers the formation of myelin, the sheath of fatty substance that surrounds the axons of neurons and facilitates rapid and efficient communication between neurons. Finally, a review of postnatal change in the patterns of gray and white matter will be presented.

Chapter 10 considers the effects of postnatal experience on the development of brain organization. There is substantial evidence that specific types of experience are necessary for the emergence of typical patterns of brain organization, and that experience can alter the initial patterning established during the embryonic and fetal periods. Experience-dependent changes in brain organization are thought to reflect the essential plasticity of the developing brain, which is considered the basis for normal development and for the capacity of the developing brain to adapt to both insult and abnormal experience.

Chapter 11 returns to the questions raised in Chapters 1 and 2 and asks how knowledge of the fundamental processes of brain development can inform basic questions about the nature of inheritance and the role of experience in development. It uses examples from earlier chapters to illustrate how the basic processes of progressive differentiation and progressive commitment can guide the orderly development of the organism without the requirement to build in specific a priori structures or functions. It argues that development is a process that unfolds over time, and that temporal constraints are an essential component of the developmental dynamic. At each moment of development, the organism has both a state and a history that define its current level of development, and constrain and direct its future developmental course.

Finally, the book includes two features that are designed to assist the reader with material that may be unfamiliar. The first is a glossary of the major terms used in the book. The glossary is arranged alphabetically and can be found at the end of the book. Second, most chapters contain at least one clinical correlation. Each clinical correlation describes the consequences of interfering with the developmental event described in the chapter. For example, the chapter on neuronal migration considers the effects of ethanol exposure during the peak period of migration. The clinical correlations are designed to provide a concrete link between the somewhat abstract developmental events described in each chapter and the consequences of interruptions to those events in the real-life history of the developing child.

## Nomenclature and Notation Systems

As is the case in most complex fields of inquiry, biologists have developed conventions for representing various ideas and concepts. Although they provide a convenient and systematic shorthand for experts, these notational systems are often not transparent to nonexperts. Three categories of notational conventions are particularly important for the discussion of brain development. The first concerns notational systems for specifying age during the prenatal period. The second relates to nomenclature for genes and their transcription products. The third concerns the terminology used to designate the spatial dimensions of the organism at different points in development.

## Age Conventions in the Prenatal Period

At different stages of life, age is denoted by different units of time. New parents describe the age of their newborns in days (even hours), but by the end of the first year, months are the convention. Toddler lives are partitioned into half years, and it is not until the school-age period that the full-year designation becomes adequate. By the end of the lifespan, whole decades are often the acceptable unit, as in the case of octogenarians or nonagenarians. There are age conventions for the period before birth as well. One is the sometimes confusing designation of weeks of pregnancy, which is calibrated from the timing of the last menstrual period, thus introducing the odd circumstance that one may not be pregnant at all during the first two weeks of pregnancy. (Perhaps that is when one is just a little pregnant!) Scientific convention needs greater precision, and the terminology that has emerged refers to age in terms of the day postconception, or embryonic day (E). Thus the start of "gastrulation," an important set of events that results in the establishment of neural progenitor cells and begins 14 days after conception, is denoted E14.

It is important to note, however, that the ages cited in the text are only approximate. For the period of embryonic development, which includes the first eight weeks postconception, the estimates for humans are based on the data from a large collection of human embryos in the Carnegie Collection of the Human Developmental Anatomy Center, which is part of the U.S. National Museum of Health and Medicine. The Carnegie Stages describe a series of 23 separate anatomical descriptions that capture the major developmental changes in human embryos. Carnegie staging was developed in the early 1900s by the then director of the Carnegie Collection, George Streeter. In the Carnegie Staging system, which has become the standard in the field, estimates of development are based on the presence of stage-specific anatomical structures rather than a simple measure of age. As is the case with development at any stage of life, there are individual differences in the timing of when particular embryos reach particular levels of development. Approximate estimates of age (in days) are provided for the Carnegie Stages, but the exact timing is variable. Throughout this book, the designation in E reflects the estimates based on the Carnegie Staging system.

A second question about specification of the timing of developmental events concerns the species with which the experimental study was run. For some of the basic milestones in brain development beyond the embryonic period human data are available. However, as suggested earlier, there is some variability in estimates of timing across sources that reflects, in part, individual variability in early development. For consistency, references to the timing of events during human fetal development will be based on two sources, *Langman's Medical Embryology* (Sadler 2006) and *Human Embryology* (Larsen 2001). However, much of our knowledge about human brain development is extrapolated from studies of nonhuman species, and much of what is reported about brain development in this book relies on animal studies. There are marked and obvious differences in developmental timing across species, and specifying correspondences for any single event is a challenge. Fortunately, there have been several recent attempts to compile cross-species correspondence data specifically for events in neural development. Clancy, Darlington, and Finlay (2001) have provided a particularly scholarly and comprehensive estimate of developmental correspondences that includes data from nine mammalian species (including humans) on the emergence of 95 brain structures or events. Throughout this book, when data from animal studies are reported, as a notational convention and for completeness, the primary designation will refer to the species under study. Corresponding times for humans are based on the Clancy, Darlington, and Finlay estimates.

## Names for Genes and Gene Products

As will be discussed in Chapter 2, genes are the sequences of molecules that make up deoxyribonucleic acid (DNA). They are sequestered within the nucleus of the cells. Gene expression involves the copying of the original sequence via a process called transcription; transport of the copied sequence out of the nucleus and into the cytoplasm of the cells; and, finally, translation of the copied sequence into a new molecular sequence that is typically a protein. The active agents in all cell biological processes are the gene products, the proteins, rather than the genes themselves. This complex process of transcription and translation introduces the potential for confusion in terminology. Biologists recognized the potential for confusion between genes and their products and thus developed conventional notation systems involving use of upper- and lowercase letters, italics, and name length. With the accelerating pace of gene discovery, the conventions have become more complicated and they are not always applied uniformly. To complicate things further, scientists working with different species have developed somewhat different notational systems. Thus the rules for mouse, rat, and chicken differ from those for humans. For clarity a simplified notational system, based on the basic guidelines and general recommendations for human and animal gene naming, will be adopted for this book. For humans the notational system will include the following:

- The full name of a gene is spelled out in lowercase letters and is not italicized: sonic hedgehog.
- The name of the gene symbol (the most common way of referencing a gene) is in capital letters and italicized: *SHH*.
- The name of the gene product is the same as the name of the gene symbol, but it is not italicized: SHH.

These conventions are based upon guidelines from the Human Gene Nomenclature Committee (HGNC), which is authorized by the Human

Genome Organization (HUGO) and funded by a number of U.S. government agencies, including the National Institutes of Health.

This book includes references to many animal studies, and those studies include a wide range of species from mouse to rat to amphibian to fly to primate. Unfortunately, the notational conventions differ across species with regard to capitalization and italicizing. For most of the animal species discussed in this book, the notational conventions are as follows:

- The full name of a gene is spelled out in lowercase letters and is not italicized: sonic hedgehog.
- For the name of the gene symbol, only the first letter is capitalized and the name is italicized: *Shh*.
- For the name of the gene product, only the first letter is capitalized and the name is not italicized: Shh.

These conventions are based upon guidelines from the International Committee on Standardized Genetic Nomenclature for Mice and the Mouse Genomic Nomenclature Committee.

## Spatial Dimensions of the Organism

Within the mature organism, the conventions for describing the spatial axes are well defined. For mammals, the dimensions usually refer to the characteristic orientation of a quadruped and thus must be transformed for bipedal species such as human. Figure 1.1A shows the characteristic designations for the body axes in both the prone and upright positions. The rostral and caudal dimensions refer to the head-to-tail axis; dorsal and ventral refer to the back and stomach axis; right and left are conventional and from the perspective of the organism. Figure 1.1B indicates the conventional dimensions for the brain. Anterior and posterior refer to the front and back of the brain, designated by the frontal lobe and the occipital lobe, respectively. Superior and inferior refer to the top-to-bottom dimension. Right and left are from the perspective of the organism. Figure 1.1C indicates spatial dimensions for the early embryonic stages of development. The figures show the shape of the embryo during gastrulation. The spatial dimensions are indicated in the figure.

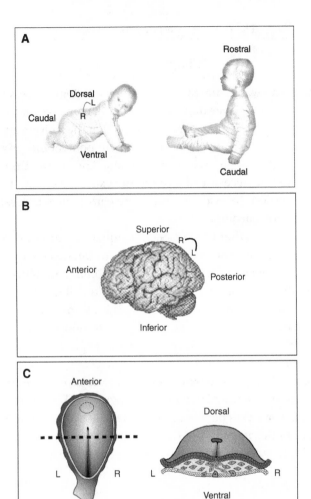

Figure 1.1. Spatial axes for different organisms and structures. A. The characteristic designations for the human-body axes in both the prone and upright positions. B. The conventional terms for the major spatial axes of the mature human brain. C. Spatial dimensions of the embryo during gastrulation. The figure on the left shows the top of the embryo, with a view looking down on the dorsal surface; the anterior end of the embryo is at the top of the figure. The figure on the right shows a cross section of the embryo taken from the point indicated by the dotted line in the figure on the left. In cross section, the position of the dorsal and ventral surfaces of the embryo can be appreciated. (B from DeArmond, Fusco, and Dewey 1989. Adapted with the permission of Oxford University Press.)

## Chapter Summary

- The nature-versus-nurture debate in psychology centers on the question of whether there is a core set of concepts that are available without learning. Nativists argue that the universality and invariance of such concepts across human populations provide support for their status as innately available knowledge. Constructivists question the necessity of positing the existence of core knowledge and question the evidence that these early concepts develop in the absence of learning.

- One question that has not been adequately addressed concerns the biological feasibility of claims about innate concepts and learning mechanisms. Data from developmental neurobiology have the potential to make significant contributions to the conversation about psychological processes. Knowledge of the basics of brain development is important for developmental psychologists because it can both constrain and expand the range and content of this discussion.

- The psychological debate over nature versus nurture finds a parallel in the historical debate in biology over the nature of inheritance. The next chapter will consider the evolution of the concept of inheritance from early naturalist concepts of essence or vital force through the modern concept of the gene.

## References

Allen, G. E. 1975. *Life science in the twentieth century*. New York: Wiley.

Bates, E. 1999. "Plasticity, localization, and language development." In *The changing nervous system: Neurobehavioral consequences of early brain disorders*, ed. S. H. Broman and J. M. Fletcher, 214–253. New York: Oxford University Press.

Beurton, P. J., R. Falk, and H.-J. Rheinberger, eds. 2000. *The concept of the gene in development and evolution: Historical and epistemological perspectives*. Cambridge: Cambridge University Press.

Carey, S., and E. M. Markman. 1999. "Cognitive development." In *Cognitive science: Handbook of perception and cognition*, 2nd ed., ed. B. M. Bly and D. E. Rumelhart, 201–254. San Diego, CA: Academic Press.

Carlson, E. A. 1966. *The gene: A critical history*. Philadelphia: W. B. Saunders Company.

Chomsky, N. 1995. "Language and nature." *Mind,* 104: 1–61.

Clancy, B., R. B. Darlington, and B. L. Finlay. 2001. "Translating developmental time across mammalian species." *Neuroscience,* 105: 7–17.

Clark, A. 1998. "What's knowledge anyway?" *Mind and Language,* 13: 571–575.

Clearfield, M. W., and K. S. Mix. 1999. "Number versus contour length in infants' discrimination of small visual sets." *Psychological Science,* 10: 408–411.

Cohen, L. B., H. H. Chaput, and C. H. Cashon. 2002. "A constructivist model of infant cognition." In "Constructivism today." Special issue, *Cognitive Development,* 17: 1323–1343.

Cohen, L. B., and K. S. Marks. 2002. "How infants process addition and subtraction events." *Developmental Science,* 5: 186–201.

Cowie, F. 1999. *What's within? Nativism reconsidered.* New York: Oxford University Press.

Creath, R., and J. Maienschein, eds. 2000. *Biology and epistemology.* Cambridge: Cambridge University Press.

Danchin, A. 2002. *The Delphic boat: What genomes tell us.* Cambridge, MA: Harvard University Press.

DeArmond, S. J., M. M. Fusco, and M. M. Dewey. 1989. *Structure of the human brain: A photographic atlas.* 3rd ed. New York: Oxford University Press.

Elman, J. L., E. A. Bates, M. H. Johnson, A. Karmiloff-Smith, D. Parisi, and K. Plunkett. 1996. *Rethinking innateness: A connectionist perspective on development.* Cambridge, MA: MIT Press.

Fodor, J. 1981. "The present status of the innateness controversy." In *Representations: Philosophical essays on the foundations of cognitive science,* 257–316. Cambridge, MA: MIT Press.

———. 1986. "The modularity of mind." In *Meaning and cognitive structure: Issues in the computational theory of mind,* ed. Z. W. Pylyshyn and W. Demopoulos, 3–18. Norwood, NJ: Ablex Publishing.

Gelman, R. 2000. "Domain specificity and variability in cognitive development." *Child Development,* 71: 854–856; discussion, 860–861.

Gilbert, S. F., ed. 1991. *A conceptual history of modern embryology.* New York: Plenum Press.

Gottlieb, G. 2002. "From gene to organism: The developing individual as an emergent, interactional, hierarchical system." In *Brain development and cognition: A reader,* ed. M. H. Johnson, Y. Munakata, and R. O. Gilmore, 36–49. Malden, MA: Blackwell Publishers.

Haith, M. M., and J. B. Benson. 1998. "Infant cognition." In *Handbook of child psychology,* vol. 2, *Cognition, perception, and language,* ed. D. Kuhn and R. S. Siegler, 199–254. New York: Wiley.

Horder, T. J., J. A. Witkowski, and C. C. Wylie, eds. 1986. *A history of embryology*. Cambridge: Cambridge University Press.

Johannsen, W. 1911. "The genotype conception of heredity." *American Naturalist*, 45: 129–159.

Johnson, S. P. 2003. "The nature of cognitive development." *Trends in Cognitive Sciences*, 7: 102–104.

Karmiloff-Smith, A. 1991. "Beyond modularity: Innate constraints and developmental change." In *The epigenesis of mind: Essays on biology and cognition*, ed. S. Carey and R. Gelman, 171–197. Hillsdale, NJ: Lawrence Erlbaum Associates.

———. 2002. "Development itself is the key to understanding developmental disorders." In *Brain development and cognition: A reader*, ed. M. H. Johnson, Y. Munakata, and R. O. Gilmore, 375–391. Malden, MA: Blackwell Publishers.

Keller, E. F. 1995. *Refiguring life: Metaphors of twentieth-century biology*. New York: Columbia University Press.

———. 2000. *The century of the gene*. Cambridge, MA: Harvard University Press.

Larsen, W. J. 2001. *Human embryology*. 3rd ed. New York: Churchill Livingstone.

Lewontin, R. C. 2001. "Gene, organism and environment." In *Cycles of contingency: Developmental systems and evolution*, ed. S. Oyama, P. E. Griffiths, and R. D. Gray, 59–66. Cambridge, MA: MIT Press.

Mandler, J. M. 2003. "Conceptual categorization." In *Early category and concept development: Making sense of the blooming, buzzing confusion*, ed. D. H. Rakison and L. M. Oakes, 103–131. New York: Oxford University Press.

Marcus, G. F. 1998. "Can connectionism save constructivism?" *Cognition*, 66: 153–182.

Morange, M. 2001. *The misunderstood gene*. Cambridge, MA: Harvard University Press.

Moss, L. 2003. *What genes can't do*. Cambridge, MA: MIT Press.

Newcombe, N. S. 2002. "The nativist-empiricist controversy in the context of recent research on spatial and quantitative development." *Psychological Science*, 13: 395–401.

Oakes, L. M., and D. H. Rakison. 2003. "Issues in the early development of concepts and categories: An introduction." In *Early category and concept development: Making sense of the blooming, buzzing confusion*, ed. D. H. Rakison and L. M. Oakes, 3–23. New York: Oxford University Press.

Oyama, S., P. E. Griffiths, and R. D. Gray, eds. 2001. *Cycles of contingency: Developmental systems and evolution*. Cambridge, MA: MIT Press.

Portugal, F. H., and J. S. Cohen. 1977. *A century of DNA*. Cambridge, MA: MIT Press.

Quinn, P. C. 2003. "Concepts are not just for objects: Categorization of spatial relation information by infants." In *Early category and concept development: Making sense of the blooming, buzzing confusion,* ed. D. H. Rakison and L. M. Oakes, 50–76. New York: Oxford University Press.

Sadler, T. W. 2006. *Langman's medical embryology.* 10th ed. Philadelphia: Lippincott Williams & Wilkins.

Samuels, R. 1998. "What brains won't tell us about the mind: A critique of the neurobiological argument against representational nativism." *Mind and Language,* 13: 548–570.

———. 2002. "Nativism in cognitive science." *Mind and Language,* 17: 233–265.

Simon, T. J. 1997. "Reconceptualizing the origins of number knowledge: A 'non-numerical' account." *Cognitive Development,* 12: 349–372.

Simon, T. J., S. J. Hespos, and P. Rochat. 1995. "Do infants understand simple arithmetic? A replication of Wynn (1992)." *Cognitive Development,* 10: 253–269.

Smith, L. B., E. Colunga, and H. Yoshida. 2003. "Making an ontology: Cross-linguistic evidence." In *Early category and concept development: Making sense of the blooming, buzzing confusion,* ed. D. H. Rakison and L. M. Oakes, 275–302. New York: Oxford University Press.

Spelke, E. S. 1998. "Nativism, empiricism, and the origins of knowledge." *Infant Behavior and Development,* 21: 181–200.

———. 1999. "Innateness, learning and the development of object representation." *Developmental Science,* 2: 145–148.

———. 2000. "Core knowledge." *American Psychologist,* 55: 1233–1243.

Spelke, E. S., K. Breinlinger, J. Macomber, and K. Jacobson. 1992. "Origins of knowledge." *Psychological Review,* 99: 605–632.

Spelke, E. S., and E. L. Newport. 1998. "Nativism, empiricism, and the development of knowledge." In *Handbook of child psychology,* vol. 1, *Theoretical models of human development,* ed. R. M. Lerner, 275–340. New York: Wiley.

Waddington, C. H. 1939. *An introduction to modern genetics.* New York: Macmillan.

Wynn, K. 1992. "Addition and subtraction by human infants." *Nature,* 358: 749–750.

———. 1993. "Evidence against empiricist accounts of the origins of numerical knowledge." In *Readings in philosophy and cognitive science,* ed. A. I. Goldman, 209–227. Cambridge, MA: MIT Press.

# TWO

✦ ✦ ✦

# The Gene:
# Evolution of a Concept

FOR MORE THAN three centuries, biologists have been working to describe and explain the mechanisms of intergenerational inheritance. Central to this work is the long-standing conundrum introduced by the observation that any viable theory of inheritance must account for both intergenerational constancy and individual variation. The debates of the late nineteenth and twentieth centuries reflect the struggle that occurred within the biological community to formulate a theory that could incorporate both constancy and variation as aspects of inheritance. In this regard, the biological approach to the questions of inheritance stands in contrast to the key issues articulated in the psychological debate over innateness. Within the psychological debate, the constructs of constancy and variation, as they pertain to core and acquired knowledge, are attributed to different factors. The markers of innate knowledge are such things as universality, domain specificity, and invariance, all of which reference intergenerational constancy. Variability, by contrast, is the index of experience and learning. The psychological debate recognizes individual variation is in skills and abilities that are likely attributable to some combination of biological factors and experience. However, the central debate rests on the issue of how core knowledge is transmitted, and on that question there is a decoupling of constancy and variation. Core knowledge is a constant that is universally transmitted; variation in knowledge arises from the experience of the individual. In attempting to formulate a unified account of intergenerational inheritance that incorporates both constancy and variation, the biological perspective provides a very different approach to thinking about what it means for something to be innate. The struggle to account for both constancy and variation at the level of inheritance is at the heart of the story of the evolving concept of the gene. The solution in biology, which ultimately did incorporate both constancy and variation in models of inheritance, led to a very different view of the contributions of inherited factors to the development of the organism.

This chapter provides an overview of the debates that occurred within biology as scientific advances shaped and constrained possible accounts of what is inherited and how. These debates all centered on the definition of what eventually came to be known as the gene. The historical course of the biological debate is important to consider because it captures the evolution of a concept and highlights the impact of a particular definition on contemporary scientific thought. In the nineteenth century, the emergence of the idea that inherited factors may be particulate and thus material and subject to direct investigation fundamentally changed the course of scientific inquiry. In the first part of the twentieth century, the fact that factors external to the organism could affect gene structure and function began to be appreciated. Later work suggested that there may be specific associations between individual genes and particular functions. The later part of the twentieth century up through today has presented much more complex and challenging accounts of gene structure and function that have led to a very different perspective within biology on the relationship between inherited and experiential factors and on their role in development. The contemporary definition of what a gene is and how it functions within the organism has led to the view that from the very beginning of biological development, inherited factors and experience act in concert to influence and direct the biological processes that drive development. This perspective has important implications for the psychological debate over nature versus nurture.

## Historical Perspectives on Biological Inheritance

The modern concept of the gene has a rich and complex history that spans centuries and incorporates ideas from a range of philosophical and scientific traditions. Seventeenth- and eighteenth-century reformulations of more ancient preformationist and epigenetic ideas provided the intellectual context for scientific thought of the early-nineteenth-century naturalists. During the late nineteenth and twentieth centuries, different threads of the evolving story of the gene can be traced through dialogue and debate involving at least four modern scientific disciplines and their historical antecedents: evolutionary biology, which finds its roots in the theories of Darwin; population and quantitative genetics, which traces its origins to the studies of Galton; the study of hereditary transmission, originating with Mendel; and developmental biology, which finds its basis in the study of embryology. Each discipline provided a different perspective on the question of inheritance, and during the late nineteenth and the early twentieth centuries, each provided unique contributions to the evolving concept of the gene as the material, physical unit of intergenerational inheritance. Evolutionary biology focuses on the origins of species and species change over time. Population genetics takes a quantitative approach, asking about frequencies and distributions of characteristics and traits within and across generations. The study of hereditary transmission focuses on single genes and allelic variation. Developmental biology involves the study of the individual organism as it passes from larva to pupa or from embryo to fetus.

The very brief history that follows touches on only a small sample of the ideas and discoveries that have contributed to the modern concept of the gene. Indeed, as will be clear, it is a concept that continues to change and evolve. The gene as it was first defined by Johannsen in 1911 is not the gene that Watson and Crick described in 1953, and the gene that Watson and Crick described is not the gene of modern developmental geneticists. There are many threads to the story of the gene and many themes that could be emphasized. The account that follows will focus on three. The first is the overarching issue of accounting for both the constancy and the variability of biological inheritance. It is the most ancient and the most persistent question and it is at the heart of the attempt to define the concept of a gene. The second theme concerns the level of scientific inquiry, because the perception of what a gene is can be influenced by the question the investigator has chosen to ask. An investigator who wishes to understand the source of a trait's frequency and distribution in a population poses a different question than an investigator who seeks to account for individual variants or one who asks about developmental origins. The third theme focuses on defining the material nature of the gene. Ideas about what is inherited have changed dramatically over the years. They range from the abstract sixteenth-century notion of a vital force to seventeenth-century preformationist ideas of the homunculus, to the early conceptualization of the material gene, such as Darwin's gemmules or Mendel's unit factors, to Avery's identification of the chemical structure of genes as deoxyribonucleic acid (DNA), to Watson and Crick's characterization of the double helix, and recent discoveries of repeated, overlapping, and nested genes.

An important part of this brief history will be the introduction of key concepts that have defined the modern ideas of what genes are, how they are expressed, and how they function. These ideas will be critical for understanding the role of genes in brain development. Presented within the context of their historical discovery, basic information about gene structure and function will be introduced. This will include descriptions of the composition of genes, the basic processes of gene transcription and translation, and the role of enhancers and promoters in gene transcription, as well as basic information on some of the complex variations in patterns of gene expression, including editing, alternative splicing, overlapping genes, and nested genes. In addition, a summary of major classes of gene products, focusing primarily on the special transcription factors and secreted molecules that play a critical role in the regulation of development, will be provided.

## Philosophical Roots: Preformationism and Epigenesis

Early attempts to explain the constancy and the variability of inheritance were anchored in the much-older constructs of preformationism and epigenesis. The central tenet of preformationism is that the form of the individual is predetermined and inherent in the organism. This idea can be traced as far back as Plato, who stressed form and constancy over process and change. The concept of epigenesis (Van Speybroeck, De Waele, and Van de Vijver 2002) can be traced to the Aristotelian idea that form arises through gradual elaboration. During the seventeenth century, mechanistic views of natural phenomena began to replace classical vitalist philosophy. Natural phenomena became viewed as tractable objects of study that could be understood through observation, rather than products of a hidden, unknowable force. The idea of nature as a well-functioning machine led to the search for underlying mechanisms (Van Speybroeck, De Waele, and Van de Vijver 2002), and preformationism fit well within the new paradigm. Seventeenth-century preformationist theory held that the fully formed adult organism was contained in miniature inside every egg, or germ cell. The miniature adult organism, in turn, contained another germ cell that contained another miniature adult and so forth in a kind of "Russian doll" arrangement that was referred to as emboitement or encapsulation. Development, by this view, was equated with the simple growth, or enlargement, of the fully formed organism. The ascendancy of preformationism during this time rendered epigenesist views largely irrelevant.

By the eighteenth century, natural science, now well anchored in observational methodologies, had advanced considerably, and the focus in embryology shifted to the study of emergent form and the revival of epigenetic theories. There was ample evidence that embryonic forms not only differed from the mature forms but also underwent systematic change with development. These data forced the abandonment of simplistic versions of preformationism, but the need to account for intergenerational constancy remained. What emerged was a formulation of something more akin to an inherent form or essence. The notion of an immutable abstract essence provided a means of reconciling the disparate observations of constancy of species type despite developmental change in form (Van Speybroeck, De Waele, and Van de Vijver 2002). The changing views of the relationship between sources of constancy and variation also introduced the idea that change in the form of the organism could be derived from external factors. Both Lamarckian ideas of acquired inheritance and primitive ideas about long-term effects of small, early variation were introduced. The twin themes of stability and variation permeated these early debates and set the stage for the scientific advances and debates of the nineteenth and twentieth centuries.

## The Early Nineteenth Century: Darwin and Mendel

In the early part of the nineteenth century, experimental approaches to embryology began to supplant earlier descriptive methodologies. Older beliefs about inherent essence gave way to a search for the identity of what is contained within the organism that provides for the heritable stability of structures and traits. Although Mendel's work remained largely undiscovered until the end of the nineteenth century, his studies of hybridization in peas led to the formulation of his rules of inheritance, which were associated with what he referred to as the "unit factors" of the organism. Mendel's rules define the conditions for transmission of material hereditary factors and constitute the first attempt to define the organism as the product of specifically defined, hereditary determiners that are discrete and particulate in nature (Portin 1993). The unit factors were what accounted for both the stability of trait transmission and individual variation.

The nineteenth century also saw the introduction of Darwin's ideas about evolution, fitness, and adaptation, which represented a major shift in thinking about the problem of origins. His descriptions of species variation, coupled with his observations about selection by the environment, constituted a revolutionary formulation. Lewontin (2000) has suggested that a critical contribution of this work was Darwin's separation of internal and external factors. According to Darwin's theory of pangenesis, the internal factors, or gemmules, are inherited from the organism's parents but are also the source of variability within the organism. He believed that variation in internal factors could arise either from external environmental events acting on the reproductive organs and thus indirectly affecting the offspring, or by direct effects on the organism itself, affecting both parent and offspring. He also believed that the environment acts to select those individuals whose unique attributes, acquired via inheritance and variation, are best suited to the demands of the environment. Thus Darwin's theory of evolution both retains elements of preformationism in the form of inherited elements and specifies a role for the environment in inducing heritable variation, and more critically in adaptation and selection (Gayon 2000). Darwin's theory predicted slow incremental change, with natural selection acting as the primary determiner. By his view, patterns of inheritance provide the source of organismic stability, but environmental factors both induce variation and set boundaries for selection.

## The Late Nineteenth and Early Twentieth Centuries

Throughout the nineteenth century, the idea of providing a unified account of stability and change was beginning to emerge in the work of other scientists. The threads of the old debates over nature versus nurture continued, but the arguments began to shift as both sides confronted the task of accounting for the mounting evidence not easily reconciled by strong forms of either position. As William Morton Wheeler suggested in 1899, "The pronounced 'epigenesist' of to-day who postulates little or no predetermination in the germ must gird himself to perform Herculean labors in explaining how the complex heterogeneity of the adult organism can arise from chemical enzymes, while the pronounced 'preformationist' of to-day is bound to elucidate the elaborate morphological structure which he insists must be present in the germ. Both tendencies will find their correctives in investigation" (Wheeler 1899, p. 284).

In the 1890s, redefinition and elaboration of key questions within the field of embryology began to emerge. Until this time, embryology had been essentially a subdiscipline within the study of evolutionary phylogeny (Gilbert 1978). Its emergence as a separate field of study under the name developmental mechanics brought a shift in the focus of scientific inquiry to questions about cellular organization during the very earliest points in development. Biologist C. O. Whitman felt that the answer to the central question in the debate over preformationism and epigenesis must lie in the study of the very earliest stages of development. He reasoned that the degree of stability or variability in the beginning of embryonic development should either reflect an inherited organization or suggest epigenetic change (Maienschein 1985). However, work by investigators such as Roux and Driesch, examining the effects of experimental manipulations introduced at the earliest point in development, yielded conflicting results and interpretations.

Roux's "mosaic" theory of early embryonic development derived from studies in which he destroyed one of the two cells produced after the first cell division in frog embryos. This manipulation consistently produced malformed embryos. Roux reasoned that distribution of genetic material must change with each new cell division, and that the specific material acquired by each cell determined its fate. Early destruction of one cell thus destroyed half the embryo's genetic material and disrupted the developmental process. However, contemporary work by Driesch challenged this interpretation. Driesch conducted a series of studies that were conceptually similar to Roux's but differed methodologically. The critical difference involved the method for isolating the early embryonic cells. Rather than destroying one of the original cells, Driesch instead agitated the cells to separate them. In contrast to Roux, Driesch found that both cells developed normally. From these findings he concluded that Roux's mosaic theory of genetic predetermination was incorrect. Rather than progressive partitioning and distribution of heritable material with each new cell division, he found that in the initial stage of development, dividing cells retained all the information necessary for the normal development of the embryo. He introduced the idea of "harmonious equipotentiality" of a system governed by "external environmental influences, and progressive interactions of the developing parts" (Moss 1992, p. 337).

### The Cellular Locus of Heritable Material

One line of debate that would prove critical for the later conceptualization of the gene concerned the location of the hereditary material within the cell. By the later half of the nineteenth century, the cell had been identified as the carrier of inherited material, but debate continued over the locus of heritable material within the cell. The central question was whether the nucleus or the cytoplasm contains the inherited material and thus controls heredity and development (Gilbert 1978). Debate and ultimate resolution of this question would prove critical for later conceptualization of the gene.

The debate over the cellular locus of inheritance arose within the context of two important sets of discoveries. First, in 1900, three independent scientists, Correns, Von Tschermak, and de Vries, published papers reporting on the "rediscovery" of Mendel's rules of inheritance (Allen 1975). Working on plant-breeding studies similar to those of Mendel, each scientist reported findings that conformed closely to those of Mendel. The "rediscovery" of Mendel's laws provided support for a modern variant of a preformationist model in which the material units of inheritance were contained within the cells. The rules of inheritance provided a mechanism for accounting for both constancy and systematic intergenerational variation.

A second major discovery came in 1903 with independent reports from both Sutton and Boveri positing chromosomal theories of inheritance. Boveri's studies of fertilization in sea urchins led him to assert the existence of chromosomes and to link them to Mendelian factors (Gilbert 1978). During this same period, work by McClung (1902) provided evidence of the existence of distinct sex chromosomes, which was soon confirmed and extended in studies by Stevens (1905) and Wilson (1905). Together these findings provided converging evidence of a tangible and specifically defined locus of heritable material within the nucleus of the cell.

One prominent opponent of the chromosomal theory of inheritance was the young embryologist T. H. Morgan (Allen 1975). Early in his career, Morgan criticized the growing emphasis in the field of embryology on the "rediscovered" principles of Mendel, which he viewed as an unwelcome return to preformationist principles. "The nature of present Mendelian interpretation and description inextricably commits to the 'doctrine of particles' in the germ . . . It is essentially a morphological conception with but a trace of functional feature . . . With an eye seeing only *particles* . . . there is no such thing as the study of *process* possible . . . Mendelian description . . . has strayed very wide of the facts . . . it has declared a discontinuity where there is now proved continuity; it has postulated preformationism where there is now evident epigenesis" (Morgan 1909, pp. 509–510). Morgan was also critical of work suggesting that the locus of inheritance was in the chromatin of the cell nucleus, and in his studies of mutation in *Drosophila* (fruit fly) he sought to demonstrate that development was controlled by factors in the cytoplasm (Gilbert 2006). His initial studies manipulating the amount of cytoplasm in eggs with fully intact nuclei led him to conclude that the essential form of the embryo was determined by factors in the cytoplasm (Gilbert 1978).

Morgan's views conflicted with those of his friend E. B. Wilson. Wilson was a proponent of the nuclear-origin view of inheritance. He was convinced that chromatin, which is found in the cell nucleus (and is now known to consist of DNA attached to a protein structure base), "is the most essential element in development" (Wilson 1896, p. 262). "[It] is known to be closely similar . . . with a substance known as nuclein . . . a nucleic acid . . . and albumin" (Wilson 1895, p. 4). Support for his view came from his own work and that of other investigators, including Boveri, McClung, and Stevens.

The ongoing debate between Morgan and Wilson over the question of the cellular locus of inheritance prompted Morgan to initiate a series of studies that would ultimately convince him that his own ideas were wrong. Cross-breeding studies of *Drosophila* conducted in Morgan's laboratory produced unexpected variants that could not be explained by cytoplasmic factors. L. V. Morgan, T. H. Morgan's wife and collaborator, first noted the presence of a white-eyed male in a population of red-eyed flies. Systematic breeding of the white-eyed variant revealed that the white-eyed trait was both sex linked and followed the patterns predicted by the Mendelian rules of inheritance (Morgan 1910). Subsequent work documented a variety of other sex-linked mutations with the *Drosophila* population. These studies ultimately convinced Morgan that the critical material of inheritance must be the chromosome, and that this material must indeed conform to something like Mendel's unit factors. This work provided critical data on the emerging concept of the gene.

*"Genes," "Genotype," and "Phenotype": Johannsen's Ahistoric Approach*
Around the time that Morgan published his first *Drosophila* studies, the Danish geneticist Wilhelm Johannsen published a seminal article that introduced the terms *gene, genotype,* and *phenotype.* "The 'gene' is nothing but a very applicable little word . . . It may be useful as an expression for the 'unit-factors,' 'elements' or 'allelomorphs' in the gametes . . . A 'genotype' is the sum total of all the 'genes'" (Johannsen 1911, pp. 132–133). "The genotype-conception is thus . . . 'ahistoric'" (Johannsen 1911, p. 139). With this article, Johannsen consolidated the emerging particulate view of inheritance. He insisted that the proper focus of science was on the relationship between genes and the genotype, not other factors such as traits and the phenotype. He argued that traits or characters are the product of the developmental history of the individual organism, while genes are the fundamental units of inheritance that are transmited to the offspring at the moment of conception. In making this critical distinction, Johanssen separated the question of inheritance from the question of development (Moss 2003). "The genotype-conception is thus an 'ahistoric' view of the reactions of living beings . . . This view is an analog to the chemical view . . . $H_2O$ is always $H_2O$, and reacts always in the same manner, whatsoever may be the 'history' of its formation or the earlier states of its elements" (Johannsen 1911, p. 139). "The talk of 'genes for any particular character' ought to be omitted" (Johannsen 1911, p. 147).

Johannsen's redefinition of the construct of heredity had a marked effect on Morgan's already-shifting view of the science of heredity. Johannsen's formulation provided a framework within which Morgan could pursue a more narrowly defined concept of genetic inheritance without completely abandoning his commitment to development. Morgan's work during the 1920s and 1930s, for which he won a Nobel Prize, took a markedly different theoretical turn. His own studies documenting factors that were well described by the new ahistoric concept of the gene led him toward a more mechanistic view that was aligned with the more rigorously defined version of a "particulate" view of inheritance and increasingly distanced from notions of development and epigenesis (Allen 1986). His work on chromosome theory provided a more concrete, material basis for the otherwise abstract notions of "unit factors" and ultimately led to his embrace of key constructs from Mendelian theory.

### *Altering the Structure of Genes: Early Studies of Mutation*

By the late nineteenth and early twentieth centuries, considerable progress had been made in defining the gene as a unit of inheritance that could account for intergeneration constancy. During this same period, studies of mutagenic processes, which focus on alterations of inherited material, made significant contributions to the understanding of intergenerational variation. In 1889, de Vries published a theory of inheritance that incorporated his ideas about specific mutagenic processes, which were based on his cross-breeding studies of the evening primrose. This work showed that large-scale, discontinuous variations could emerge in a single generation. These findings contrasted with the gradual change predicted by Darwin's process of natural selection, and de Vries attributed these large-scale changes to what he termed *mutagenic processes* (Allen 1975). De Vries proposed that the hereditary material of the organism, which he called the pangens, is initially located in the nucleus of each cell in an inactive, or latent, state. A subset of the pangens passes from the nucleus into the cytoplasm of the cell where it becomes metabolically active; pangens can also return to the nucleus and resume a latent state (Stamhuis, Meijer, and Zevenhuizen 1999). De Vries proposed that movement of hereditary material induces change in the organism, which he characterized as reflecting three types of mutation: progressive, digressive, and retrogressive. Progressive mutation referred to the emergence of new species characters that arise from actual changes in the pangens. Digressive mutation referred to the activation of a latent character that had previously been

active, while retrogressive mutation is observed when a previously active character becomes latent.

Prior to beginning his studies of genetic variation in *Drosophila,*
Morgan had visited de Vries in 1903 and was impressed with his work
on discontinuous variation in plants (Portugal and Cohen 1977). In
1908, Morgan began his cross-breeding studies in *Drosophila.* In addition to the question of the cellular locus of heritable material, an important aspect of that work was the test of de Vries's theory of mutation. Specifically, Morgan wanted to determine whether large-scale,
discontinuous variation could be observed in an animal species. Although he did not find evidence of species-level change, his observation of change in eye color in *Drosophila* provided evidence of within-
species change. Morgan attributed this spontaneous change to
changes in the X chromosome (Allen 1975).

Over the next decade, work by Morgan and his students, Sturtevant
and Mueller, provided significant insight into processes of recombination and mutation. The view of chromosomal organization that
emerged from Sturtevant and Morgan's work envisioned genes as linearly arranged along the chromosome. This structural organization led
Morgan to hypothesize a specific mechanism of discontinuous variation, recombination. In recombination, the two chromosomal strands
become intertwined during meiosis, resulting in a systematic exchange
of genetic material (Figure 2.1A). The linear arrangement of genes on
the chromosome was postulated to account for a range of correlated
variations observed in the *Drosophila* studies. Building upon Morgan's
ideas, Sturtevant provided evidence for patterns consistent with another, more complex type of variation, the double crossover (Figure
2.1B). The double crossover provided a mechanism for accounting for
the appearance of trait combinations that could not be accounted for
by the simpler mechanism of crossover.

Mueller's subsequent work on X-radiation-induced mutations
proved critical for finally establishing genes as a material element of
inheritance. His demonstrations that an external factor (X-radiation)
could alter the structure and function of hereditary particles confirmed
the material, particulate nature of genes. Further, the mutations were
found to be stable over generations and thus transmissible. Mueller con-
ceptualized genes as microscopic particles of inheritance. He asserted
that they must exhibit three properties that defined their structure,

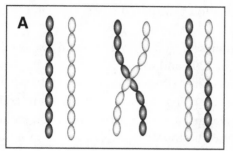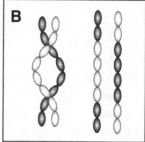

Figure 2.1. Examples of recombination of genetic material. A. Exchange of genetic material through crossover recombination. B. Double crossover is a more complex form of recombination.

function, and capacity for mutation: (1) they had to have internal structure and the capacity to self-reproduce, (2) they must give rise to all the other products that are necessary for the development of the organism, and (3) they had to be capable of reproducing their own mutations (Falk 2000). Mueller's formulation of these three fundamental properties further elaborated the particulate nature of the gene.

## The Mid-Twentieth Century: Defining the Structure and Function of the Particulate Gene

By the 1940s, considerable progress had been made in defining more specifically both the function and the structure of the gene. George Beadle, in collaboration with Boris Ephrussi and Edward Tatum, pursued a course of study aimed at understanding how genes direct the function of living systems (Portin 1993; Portugal and Cohen 1977). Their work was initially influenced by the work of another of Morgan's students, Sturtevant, whose studies of eye-color mutations in *Drosophila* hinted at the importance of interactions between cells and pointed to the involvement of some type of diffusible factor as a mediator of that interaction. Sturtevant's work suggested that the appropriate focus of research should be on understanding the "chains of reactions," that is, on the study of gene action (Keller 1995). On the basis of their own studies of eye-color mutations in *Drosophila*, Beadle and Ephrussi proposed that the appearance of different mutants reflected a series of specific biochemical changes in the organism, each mediated by the action of a specific gene. However, they also reasoned that the actions of an individual gene had to be mediated by a specific enzyme (Carlson 1966). This "one-gene–one-enzyme" proposal was verified by their later work with a simple fungus, *Neurospora*. In this work, they demonstrated that although wild types (forms obtained in their natural, unaltered state) of the fungus were capable of growing in a simple medium (a basic nutrient solution in which cells are grown in the laboratory), they failed to do so when irradiated. Beadle and Tatum identified the loci of mutation in different irradiated strains and were able to demonstrate that each strain would grow on a medium that was supplemented with a specific nutrient (in these experiments, usually components of vitamins). These findings suggested that irradiation resulted in the loss of a specific gene function involved in the synthesis of some required nutrient (Portugal and Cohen 1977). The fungi that could not synthesize the nutrient failed to grow unless an external source of the nutrient was added to the growth medium. Because their studies documented effects on vitamin synthesis, which was known to be under enzymatic control, Beadle and Tatum's original proposal of a one-gene–one-enzyme relationship was confirmed (Carlson 1966).

Work focused on understanding gene structure advanced in parallel with studies of function. Specification of the chemical structure of genes came with the work of Avery, MacLeod, and McCarthy (1944). Their studies were based upon earlier work by Frederick Griffith (1928), who had demonstrated that a living, nonvirulent strain of bacteria could be transformed into a living, virulent strain by exposure to the heat-killed remains of the same virulent bacterial strain. Griffith reasoned that something in the dead bacterial material acted to transform the living nonvirulent bacteria into a virulent strain. Although Griffith's work did not identify the "transforming agent," Avery and colleagues were able to demonstrate that the transforming agent was deoxyribonucleic acid (DNA). Although the details of their procedure are beyond the scope of this review, it is sufficient to say that through a long, ordered series of experiments the investigators were able to exclude, one by one, different molecules as potential candidates for the active, transforming agent. Ultimately this process of elimination led to the identification of one molecule as the "transforming substance" of inheritance, and defined DNA as the chemical substance of genes (Portugal and Cohen 1977). Although the initial response to Avery,

MacLeod, and McCarthy's work was mixed, their findings were later confirmed by Hershey and Chase (1952; Portin 1993). Thus by the middle of the twentieth century, the material nature of genes was well established, and the molecular substance was defined as DNA.

The work of Morgan, Mueller, Avery, Beadle, and Tatum together represented a major shift in the concept of the gene in the first half of the twentieth century. The material nature and indeed the chemical substance of genes had been established, and functional associations were captured in the one-gene–one-enzyme construct. The modern concept of the gene that was emerging was consistent with Mueller's conceptualization of a cohesive entity defined as a single unit of structure, function, and mutation. But there were also dissenting voices, theorists who disagreed with the emerging picture of gene structure and function. Wright, and later Dobzhansky, suggested that gene function might be more complex than suggested by proposals such as the one-gene–one-enzyme model. Rather, they proposed that individual gene function is dependent upon and arises from a gene's interactions with other genes in a complex context-dependent way (Beurton 2000).

### The Double Helix

In 1953, James Watson and Francis Crick published what would become a watershed article in which they described the basic structure of the DNA molecule. The article described the DNA molecule as a right-turning double helix in which two well-defined nucleotide strands are linked together along their length and coiled into a spiral (Figure 2.2A). Nucleotides are the basic molecular unit of the DNA molecule. Each contains a base that in combination with the bases of adjacent nucleotides defines the coding sequences of the genes contained within the DNA. Watson and Crick's critical insight into the structure of the DNA molecule provided an essential clue to understanding gene expression. The formulation of their idea drew from work by a number of different investigators, most notably Chargaff's work identifying the association between concentrations of base-pair compounds and Rosalind Franklin and Maurice Wilkins's X-ray-diffraction studies of the organization of the components of the DNA molecule (Snustad and Simmons 2003). The double-helix model proved crucial for addressing what became known as the coding problem, that is, the problem of translating the "information" in sequences of the nucleotides that make up the genes within DNA into the relevant protein sequences that define and support biological structure, function, and development.

### The Structure of DNA

On the basis of these early insights and later studies, the structure of DNA is now well described. The DNA molecule is composed of two strands of nucleotides joined in an orderly fashion. The two strands of nucleotides coil around each other to form a double-helix structure (see Figure 2.2A). Each nucleotide consists of a sugar-phosphate group to which a base is attached (see Figure 2.2B). Four different bases

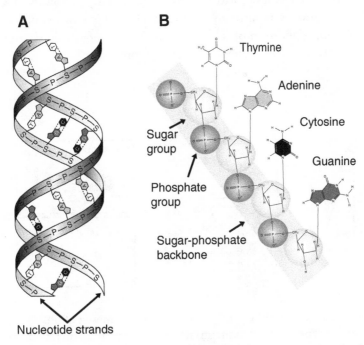

**A**

**B**

Thymine

Adenine

Cytosine

Sugar
group

Guanine

Phosphate
group

Sugar-phosphate
backbone

Nucleotide strands

Figure 2.2. A. The structure of the DNA molecule is a right-turning double helix in which two nucleotide strands coil around each other. The two strands are linked together by chemical bonds (dotted lines) between the bases (denoted by T, A, C, G) of nucleotides. B. The basic unit of DNA is the nucleotide. Each nucleotide consists of a sugar-phosphate group to which a base is attached. The sugar-phosphate groups are linked together (broken lines) to form the backbone of each strand of DNA. There are four bases: thymine, adenine, cytosine, and guanine.

distinguish four different nucleotide types. The four nucleotide bases in DNA are adenine (A), guanine (G), thymine (T), and cytosine (C). Two nucleotide bases, adenine and guanine, have a double-ring chemical structure and are called purines; and two, thymine and cytosine, have single-ring chemical structures and are called pyrimidines (see Figure 2.2B).

Within each strand, the sugar-phosphate group of each nucleotide is linked to the sugar-phosphate groups of adjacent nucleotides to form the backbone of the DNA strand (Figure 2.2B). The sugar-phosphate backbones of the two nucleotide strands are "antiparallel," or reversed, in their bonding structure such that one strand has what is referred to as a 5'-to-3' chemical polarity and the other a 3'-to-5' polarity (Figure 2.3A). The reverse polarity of the two nucleotide strands is important for accurate replication of the genes within the nucleotide strands because DNA transcription always proceeds from 5' to 3'.

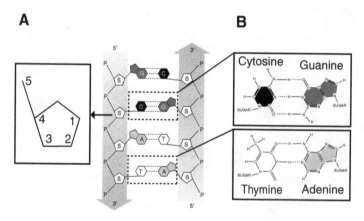

Figure 2.3. A. The individual strands of DNA are composed of linked nucleotides. The two nucleotide strands are "antiparallel" such that one strand has a 5'-to-3' chemical polarity and the other a 3'-to-5' polarity. The numbers refer to the binding sites of the five carbon-sugar rings. The numbering and order of the binding sites on the sugar rings are shown in the enlarged figure to the left of the strands. On one DNA strand, the bonding sites are ordered from 5' to 3' and in the other from 3' to 5'. B. The two DNA strands are joined together by bonds between complementary base pairs. Adenine and thymine, and guanine and cytosine, always form base pairs.

The two nucleotide strands are joined together by the complementary bonding of the bases of nucleotide pairs (Figure 2.3B). Each nucleotide in one strand of DNA is paired and bonded with a complementary nucleotide in the second strand. Nucleotide bases form specific, complementary pairs such that A and T always form base pairs, and G and C always form base pairs. Thus, although each base pair contains a purine and a pyrimidine, the purine A never pairs with the pyrimidine C, and the purine G never pairs with the pyrimidine T. Thus the two nucleotide strands that make up the DNA molecule are both complementary in the pairing of their bases and reversed in polarity along the longitudinal axis of the DNA strand.

Genes are sequences of nucleotides within the DNA. The sequences of bases along each strand of DNA provide the templates for gene expression. Gene expression occurs through the processes of DNA transcription and RNA translation. The primary product of gene expression is the formation of proteins.

### The Central Dogma

The implications of the double-helix structure of DNA as the basis for implementing gene expression were quickly recognized. The linear organization of the nucleotides along the DNA strands provided support for a template model of gene expression (Gamow, Rich, and Ycas 1956). In 1958, Crick proposed a model of gene expression that involved two hypotheses, the Sequence Hypothesis and an idea that he referred to as the Central Dogma of biology. The Sequence Hypothesis suggested that the sequences of bases within the DNA molecules serve as a template for coding of the amino-acid sequences that make up proteins. Amino acids are a class of organic molecules that can combine linearly to form proteins; proteins are the principal constituents of cells and are the primary product of gene expression. The Central Dogma proposed that "once 'information' has passed into protein *it cannot get out again*" (Crick 1958, p. 153). Information is defined here as the exact sequence of nucleotides in the DNA. The key tenet of the Central Dogma is that information can pass from DNA to protein, but transfer of sequence information from one protein to another protein or from a protein back to DNA is not possible.

Earlier work defining DNA as the vehicle for inheritance had also documented its location within the nucleus of the cell. If, as Watson and Crick postulated, the initial step in gene expression involved transcription of the DNA nucleotide sequence, it must occur within the nucleus of the cell. However, it was also clear that most protein synthesis occurs in the cytoplasm of the cell rather than in the cell nucleus. This physical separation of the processes of DNA transcription and protein synthesis suggested that an additional set of molecules must participate in the replication process. The candidate molecule was thought to be ribonucleic acid, or RNA. RNA is very similar in structure to DNA, with two main differences. First, the two molecules differ in the sugar that makes up the backbone of the molecule: DNA contains 2-deoxyribose, while RNA contains ribose. Second, RNA contains the pyrimidine base uracil instead of thymine; and uracil pairs with adenine. Two major discoveries concerning RNA were published in 1961. First, direct evidence that RNA codes for specific amino acids was published by Nirenberg and Matthaei (1961). Second, Brenner, Jacob, and Metelson (1961) published a landmark article demonstrating the role of RNA in DNA transcription. This work established a particular form of RNA called messenger RNA as the critical intermediary involved in gene expression, confirming earlier suggestions by Volkin and Astrachan (1956). As discussed in greater detail later, the messenger RNA (mRNA) is a molecule that carries a complementary transcript of the DNA nucleotide sequence from the nucleus of the cell to the cytoplasm, where it is then translated into the amino-acid sequence of proteins. The gathering evidence on the important role of RNA in these critical processes led Jacob and Monod (1961) to hypothesize their one-gene–one-messenger RNA model. Over the next decade, basic elements of DNA synthesis, specifically, DNA transcription and mRNA translation, were verified.

### DNA Transcription and RNA Translation

Genes are nucleotide sequences embedded within DNA. DNA is contained within the chromatin of the cell nucleus. Chromatin is a complex of DNA and a set of proteins called histone proteins that support the structure of the DNA molecule. The basic unit of chromatin, called the nucleosome, consists of 146 base pairs of DNA wrapped around a histone core (Figure 2.4). The histone core is composed of two copies each of four histone proteins (H2A, H2B, H3, H4). The organization and primary function of the histone proteins in chromatin are to stabilize the DNA structure and limit gene transcription (Gilbert 2006; Snustad and Simmons 2003).

At the onset of DNA transcription, a section of the DNA molecule uncoils, and the nucleotide base pairs in the unfolded section separate exposing a single-stranded DNA nucleotide template (Figure 2.5A). During DNA transcription a complementary copy of the nucleotide sequence in the exposed section of DNA is produced in a strand of RNA. The formation of the RNA strand, which is referred to as RNA synthesis, involves the linear transcription of the information coded in the exposed section of DNA. Nucleotides are added, one at a time, in a linear sequence (in the 5' to 3' direction on the DNA template) to the growing RNA strand. Each nucleotide that is added to the RNA strand contains a base that is the complement of the base in the nucleotide of the DNA template (Figure 2.3B). The complementary pairing of bases during RNA synthesis mirrors the pairing observed between the two DNA strands, except that uracil, rather than thymine, pairs with adenine in the RNA. Once the RNA transcript, or copy, of the DNA nucleotide sequence is complete, the transcript is transported out of the cell nucleus through small openings in the nuclear membrane called neural pores and enters the cytoplasm of the cell as mRNA.

RNA translation involves the conversion of the information in the mRNA into the amino-acid sequences of proteins (Figure 2.5B). The formation of proteins is called protein synthesis. It is carried out at

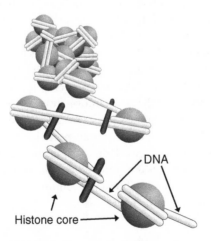

Figure 2.4. Structure of chromatin.

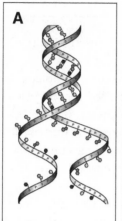

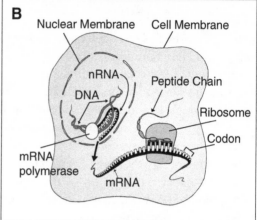

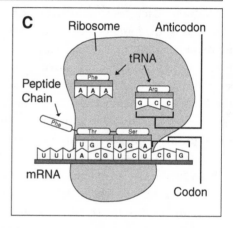

Figure 2.5. DNA transcription and RNA translation result in protein synthesis. A. When the DNA strand uncoils and separates, a segment of the nucleotide sequence is exposed. The exposed segment serves as a template for DNA transcription. B. DNA transcription occurs in the cell nucleus and results in the formation of an mRNA transcript. The mRNA transcript leaves the nucleus and enters the cytoplasm. Protein synthesis occurs at the ribosomes and involves translation of information in the mRNA into amino acid sequences. The basic coding units of mRNA are nucleotide triplets called codons. C. The amino acids are transported to the ribosome by tRNA. Each tRNA consists of a nucleotide triplet and an amino acid. Each tRNA triplet, or anticodon, is the complement of a codon in the mRNA. When the codon and anticodon bond, the amino acid is released and incorporated into the protein chain.

structures in the cell cytoplasm called ribosomes. Ribosomes have been described as factories for assembling amino-acid sequences in that they physically support the mRNA and other molecules involved in protein synthesis, and they aid in the formation of bonds between amino acids in the emerging protein (Snustad and Simmons 2003). Just as the nucleotides in DNA served as a template during RNA synthesis, the nucleotide sequence in the mRNA serves as the template for specifying the complementary nucleotide sequences during protein synthesis. Nucleotide triplets, or codons, within the mRNA serve to specify the amino-acid sequences in the emerging protein strand. The amino acids that will make up the protein are transported to the ribosome by another class of small RNA molecules called transfer RNA (tRNA). Each tRNA is composed of three nucleotides, called an anticodon, that is the complement of a codon in the mRNA. Each tRNA molecule carries one amino acid to the ribosome (Figure 2.5C). During translation, the mRNA codon attracts the anticodon of the tRNA, following the principle of complementary pairing. When the codon and anticodon triplets join, the associated amino acid is released by the tRNA and incorporated into the growing protein chain. The translation of information from mRNA to the protein product completes the process of gene expression. The proteins then go on to participate in a wide range of functions within the organism.

Identification of the structure of DNA and specification of the mechanism for its transcription crystallized the concept of the material unit of inheritance into the modern construct of the nuclear gene. By the early 1960s, the term *gene* had become synonymous with the DNA template of nucleotide sequences located in fixed positions within the larger strand of chromosomal DNA. By this definition, all the genetic information necessary for the development and functioning of the organism is contained in sequences of nucleotides that make up the DNA. However, it was also discovered that the information contained in the nuclear gene is not used directly. Genes do not, as de Vries and other early scientists suggested, leave the nucleus of the cell. Rather, the information contained in the genes is made available through the complementary processes of DNA transcription by RNA synthesis and translation of the mRNA transcripts into protein sequences. It is not the genes themselves, but rather the proteins, which are the products of gene expression, that play an active role in biological development and function.

## Modern Views of the Gene

The gene of the early 1960s provided a well-defined and tangible mechanism for understanding the problem of inheritance. Individual nuclear genes had specific structures that were well defined by their sequence of nucleotides. That sequence was copied and used to create
the active agents in biological development, proteins. However, the
story of the gene as a straightforward template of material inheritance
began to change almost as soon as it emerged. This section will consider subsequent work that showed that gene expression is considerably
more complex than envisioned in the early 1960s. At a structural level,
it became clear that the associations between sequences of DNA and
proteins are often indirect or altered by processes that intervene between the creation of the initial transcript and the coding of the protein. It has now been shown that the same sequence of DNA can, in
some cases, generate dozens of different specific proteins. Further,
there appear to be large segments of noncoding DNA, that is, segments
that do not participate in the generation of proteins. Thus at a structural level, the simple model of the gene as a straightforward, relatively
independent template for protein coding has given way to a much
more complicated model involving multiple, interacting, and overlapping components.

At a functional level, it has become clear that a considerable portion
of DNA codes for what have been termed regulatory rather than structural proteins. Regulatory genes code for proteins that modulate the
expression of other genes. Indeed, many regulatory genes are themselves controlled and modulated by the expression of yet other genes,
within a system of complex signaling cascades that direct and shape development and function. The effects of gene expression are often dependent upon specific concentrations and/or distributional patterns
of expression, alterations of which can dramatically change the organization of a system or alter the functional role of the gene product. Thus
an important aspect of gene expression is the regulation of gene expression itself. Furthermore, it is now well documented that the same
gene can play multiple roles in the development and functioning of an
organism. Some genes are expressed at several different times across
development, others are expressed in multiple organ systems. This
property of genes, which is termed *pleiotropy*, is observed for many of the

most important genes involved in brain development. In addition, it has become clear that there is remarkable conservation of genes across species. The same gene can serve similar functions in species as diverse as human and fly. Finally, very recent work has suggested that inheritance can involve nongenetic factors. Studies of a phenomenon referred to as epigenetic inheritance have shown that non-DNA modulators of gene expression, as well as the genes themselves, can be transmitted across generations.

Thus, as elegant as the early ideas that the problem of inheritance might be solved by simple one-gene–one-enzyme or one-gene–one-mRNA schemes may have been, they very quickly gave way to much more complicated models that continue to change and to be elaborated. Although a complete account of this emerging story of the gene is far too large and complex to review here, a few of the major findings that have modified the simple story of gene transcription and translation will be considered.

## Complexities of Gene Structure: Editing the Nuclear RNA Transcript

By the late 1970s, it had become clear that the RNA transcript that is first generated from the DNA nucleotide sequence is not the same as the mRNA transcript used to code proteins in the cytoplasm of the cell (Portin 1993). Rather, the first transcript is the nuclear RNA (nRNA). Critically, it was found that nRNA transcripts are typically many times longer than the mRNA transcripts, suggesting that the original nRNA transcripts must undergo significant editing before translation in the cell cytoplasm. Subsequent work showed that the nRNA transcripts contain both protein-coding elements, called exons, and noncoding elements, called introns (Figure 2.6A). Before transport out of the nucleus, the nRNA transcripts are altered to remove the noncoding intron segments. The removal of noncoding segments is accomplished by special complexes called spliceosomes that consist of small nuclear RNA (snRNA) and a number of proteins, called splicing factors. After completion of the initial nRNA transcript, different subsets of cell-specific splicing factors accumulate at splicing sites located at both the 5' and 3' ends of the intron that is targeted for removal from the transcript. When enough of the splicing factors have accumulated at the two ends of the intron, they make contact and form the spliceosome. The spliceosome acts to excise the intron and to join the two flanking exons (Figure 2.6B), creating the edited RNA transcript.

Studies of nRNA editing have shown that the patterns of splicing can vary greatly and are not confined to simple editing out of noncoding introns. Alternative splicing of the same initial transcript can yield a range of mRNA transcripts that in turn produce varying protein products called protein isoforms (Snustad and Simmons 2003; Figure 2.6B). In some cases, only the introns are excised. In other cases, alternative splicing may include excision of exon sequences in addition to introns, yielding an mRNA transcript that will produce a different protein than one produced from the full complement of exons. Finer variations in protein products can be generated by more subtle differences in nRNA editing that involve partial excision of exon segments (Gilbert 2006). It is important to note that although alternative splicing can selectively eliminate segments of nucleotides, the sequence of the exons that remain in the edited transcripts retains colinearity with the original DNA sequence (Snustad and Simmons 2003). That is, the order of nucleotides

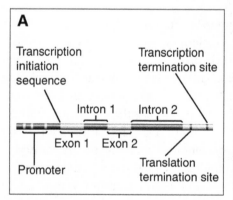
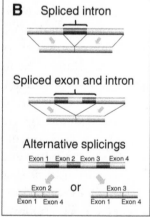

Figure 2.6. Editing the DNA transcript. A. Genes contain both coding sequences called exons and noncoding sequences called introns. B. DNA transcripts are edited before leaving the nucleus. The noncoding intron segments are eliminated and the remaining exon segments are respliced. Alternative patterns of splicing involving elimination of both exons and introns can give rise to a range of different transcripts from the same gene.

in the final transcript is the same as that in the original DNA sequence. Nonetheless, alternative splicing can result in the production of dozens of structurally and functionally different proteins from the same initial RNA transcript. These variations in patterns of alternative splicing appear to be specific to both developmental stage and tissue type (Portin 1993).

## DNA Transcription: Where and When to Start?

One important question concerns the signals that initiate and terminate gene expression. The signals that initiate gene transcription derive from a number of sources and involve elements of the gene itself. Genes are composed of a number of distinct subunits (Figure 2.6A). Gene expression always begins at the 5' end of the nucleotide sequence and proceeds toward the 3' end. The 5' end of the gene contains a promoter region, which is the site on the gene where the enzyme necessary for the synthesis of RNA, RNA polymerase, binds to initiate gene transcription. However, RNA polymerase cannot bind to DNA or initiate transcription by itself. It requires the assistance of at least six accessory proteins called basal transcription factors. These transcription factors (TFs) are proteins that are produced in all cells and are necessary for gene expression. The basal TFs act in concert to identify the DNA binding site (called a TATA box after its nucleotide base sequence), initiate the uncoiling of the DNA strand, and align and stabilize the RNA polymerase on the promoter site (Snustad and Simmons 2003). However, the binding and stabilization of the RNA polymerase on the promoter site are often not sufficient to induce gene expression at the transcription initiation site. Most genes also require the activity of special transcription factors that bind to other regions of the gene called enhancer sites (Gilbert 2006). The special TFs interact with the basal TFs to regulate gene expression, and they can act to either increase or suppress expression rates. Many genes have multiple enhancer sites that can bind different special TFs, and the multiple special TFs can interact in control of gene expression. The enhancers may also be specific to certain types of cells such that the expression of the same gene is modulated differently in different parts of the body. For example, the gene *Pax6* plays an important role in the development of the pancreas, the lens and cornea, the retina, and the embryonic nervous system.

*Pax6* has four distinct enhancer regions, each of which controls gene expression for a different body system (Gilbert 2006). Genes also contain regions that control the termination of transcription and translation. These are located near the 3' end of the gene. The transcription termination site serves as a stop signal for DNA transcription (Figure 2.6A). The translation termination site is coded during gene transcription and becomes part of the RNA transcript.

The question of where and when transcription is initiated was further complicated by the discovery of overlapping and nested genes. Overlapping genes are nucleotide sequences within the DNA that are used to code different nRNA transcripts. Common to all overlapping genes is the presence of the initiation sequence for one gene embedded within the DNA sequence of another gene (Snustad and Simmons 2003). Thus, in overlapping genes, a given segment of DNA can contribute to the expression of two different genes. Similarly, nested genes are genes that are contained entirely within the noncoding, intron sequences of other genes (Portin 1993).

## Developmental Regulators: Transcription Factors and Paracrine Factors

In the early 1960s, Jacob and Monod introduced a distinction between structural genes and their regulatory elements. Structural genes code for the proteins generated during mRNA translation, but gene expression itself must be highly orchestrated and controlled. Jacob and Monod suggested that a second class of genes, that is, regulatory genes, may code for repressors whose function it is to control the activity of structural genes (Morange 2000).

Two classes of proteins that are particularly important in the regulation of development are special transcription factors and paracrine factors. As discussed earlier, transcription factors are expressed in the nucleus of cells and act to regulate the expression of other genes by binding enhancer sites. There are a number of different families of transcription factors that are related by their structural similarities and their functions (Gilbert 2006). Some of the major families of TFs that are expressed in the developing brain are HOX, PAX, EMX, LIM, and POU.

A second class of proteins that is important in brain development is paracrine factors. Paracrine factors are extracellular secreted proteins that can diffuse over short distances. When they are secreted into the intercellular space, they can establish signaling between cells. The four major families of paracrine factors are TGFB, WNT, SHH, and FGF. Extracellular secreted molecules transmit signals by binding to receptors on the extracellular membrane of target cells. Receptors are proteins whose structure spans the cell membrane. They have three components, or domains: the extracellular domain, the transmembrane domain, and the cytoplasmic domain (Figure 2.7). The extracellular domain can bind with specific signaling proteins (also called ligands), such as paracrine factors. The binding of the ligand induces a change in the shape of the receptor. That change in shape is transmitted through the transmembrane domain and in turn induces a change in the shape of the cytoplasmic domain of the receptor. The change in shape in the cytoplasmic domain induces enzymatic activity that can activate other proteins inside the cell. The activation of these proteins can set off a signaling cascade within the cell that eventually results in activation of transcription factors within the cell nucleus. It is the activation of transcription factors that modulates gene expression (Gilbert 2006).

## Pleiotropy and Conservation in Gene Expression

When one gene produces multiple effects or affects multiple aspects of developmental outcome, it is said to be pleiotropic (Snustad and

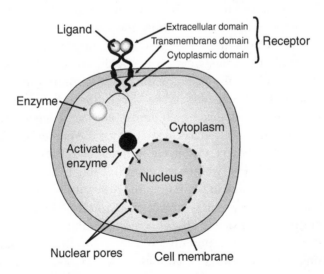

Figure 2.7. Structure of a receptor.

Simmons 2003). Such factors as differential transcriptional factor control of gene expression and alternative splicing contribute to pleiotropic variation in gene expression and function. It is estimated that 35 percent of human genes undergo alternative splicing (Croft et al. 2000; Gilbert 2006). Further, most genes require enhancers for expression, and many enhancers act in concert with multiple transcription factors. In development, the same genes play critical roles in the development of different body systems and/or play different roles within the same system at different times in development. Pleiotropy appears to be the rule among genes that regulate basic developmental processes. As Greenspan (2004) has noted, "The recognition of the ubiquity of pleiotropy in gene action means that . . . the summated action of the genes is not so much a jigsaw puzzle in which each piece fits together with its immediate neighbors . . . but is rather a flexible, multilayered network" (p. 98).

Genes are also highly conserved across species. Many of the critical developmental genes are common to a wide range of species, and in many but not all cases, they play homologous roles in development (Morange 2000). In the mid-1970s, Garcia-Bellido introduced the concept of "selector genes." Selector genes were described as a family of genes that controlled and regulated the early development of the body axis. By the early 1980s, Nusslein-Volhard and Wieschaus (1980) had identified a wide range of genes important to establishing the body pattern in *Drosophila*. The functions of one particularly important class of genes, homeotic genes, in establishing the segmental organization of the body were elaborated by a number of investigators, including Gehring (1976), Kaufman, Lewis, and Wakimoto (1980), and Lewis (1978). Their work set the stage for the investigation of the molecular structure of this family of genes and for the discovery that each member of the gene family contains a common molecular sequence. This sequence, which consists of 180 bases, was termed the homeobox. The discovery of the homeobox was made simultaneously by two groups. Matthew Scott and Amy Weiner working in Thomas Kaufman's lab at the University of Indiana in Bloomington (Scott and Weiner 1984) and a team of investigators working in Walter Gehring's lab in Basel, Switzerland (Gehring and Hiromi 1986), are credited with identifying the molecular structure of this important family of genes that are critical for - establishing the segmented organization of the body in *Drosophila*.

Critically, it has since been demonstrated that homeobox genes are highly conserved across species. Work from a number of different laboratories has identified a homologous set of genes in a wide range of species. Across mammalian species as varied as mouse and man, this family of genes is responsible for establishing the basic segmental organization of the nervous system (e.g., Kessel and Gruss 1990; Levine, Rubin, and Tjian 1984; McGinnis et al. 1984). Since the discovery of the homeotic gene family, a number of other highly conserved genes have been identified as critical for the regulation and control of development. Further, there is also evidence that multigene pathways, not single genes, are conserved (Gilbert 2000; Morange 2000).

The flexibility of function reflected in gene pleiotropy and the constancy of material inheritance observed in the interspecies conservation of genes evoke somewhat different notions of variation and constancy than we have considered thus far. Within the historical debate, questions about constancy and variation focused on transmission of specific characters or traits. From Mendel's peas to Morgan's white-eyed fly and Beadle and Tatum's single-enzyme effects, the goal was to identify the material unit of inheritance that could account for trait transmission. However, both pleiotropy and gene conservation focus on a very different set of issues that involve the inheritance of developmental processes rather than specific characters or traits. Pleiotropic genes participate in multiple functional networks; conserved gene functions are adapted to the demands of species. Both contribute in diverse ways to processes involved in development rather than to the instantiation of a specific character or trait. The processes may result in the emergence of a trait, but the relationship between the specific gene and the trait is indirect.

## Cellular Regulation and Epigenetic Inheritance

Over the past 10 years, it has become apparent that inheritance is not confined to nuclear DNA. Other factors also contribute to the process of transmission. First, what is inherited at conception is not only the genes but also the cellular machinery present in the dividing cell that allows for regulation and expression of genes (Keller 2000a; also see debates over the relative status of genetic versus cellular material, Jablonka 2002; Keller 2000b; Sarkar 2000). The nucleotide sequences that constitute DNA are, by themselves, inert; their expression requires the functioning of the complex cellular machinery that subserves gene transcription and translation. As Keller (2000a) has noted, "The gene can no longer be set above and apart from the processes that specify cellular and intercellular organization. That gene is itself part and parcel of processes defined and brought into existence by the action of a complex self-regulating dynamical system in which, and for which, the inherited DNA provides the crucial and absolutely indispensable raw material, but no more than that" (p. 71). It appears that Morgan's claim that development is controlled by factors in the cytoplasm was not entirely wrong after all. The cytoplasm does matter, and it matters because it is critical to the process of gene expression, which is, in turn, critical for the complex cascade of events that guides both biological and behavioral development.

Inheritance extends to other intra- and extracellular factors as well. Work on what has been termed epigenetic inheritance has shown that inheritance is not confined to the material substance of DNA. Epigenetic inheritance refers to heritable changes in gene expression that do not involve change in DNA sequences (Cheung and Lau 2005). One aspect of epigenetic inheritance that has received considerable attention concerns the role and functioning of cellular chromatin. Recall that chromatin contains the nucleotide sequences of DNA and histone protein complexes. The specific structure of chromatin can influence gene expression by controlling access to the nucleotide sequences of DNA. Highly compact regions of chromatin, called heterochromatin, limit access to DNA and contain few actively expressed genes, while less compact regions, called euchromatin, allow more open access to DNA and have many actively transcribing genes (Cheung and Lau 2005). Specific changes in chromatin composition (brought about, for example, by enzymatic modification associated with DNA methylation or histone acetylation) can alter local levels of compaction. DNA methylation can repress transcription and contribute to the stability of gene-expression states (Jaenisch and Bird 2003). Histone acetylation is prevalent within euchromatic regions and is closely associated with heightened levels of transcription activity. Importantly, during DNA replication, stable modifications in the chromatin of the parent can be transferred to the DNA of offspring.

Furthermore, change in chromatin markers can be induced by both cell-intrinsic and environmental factors (Jablonka 2001). It has been

shown that change in the proximity of euchromatic regions to heterochromatic regions by, for example, chromosomal rearrangement or
transposition can alter the transcriptional activity in euchromatic regions. Transcriptional silencing within a euchromatic region is observed when it is juxtaposed to a heterochromatic region. One example of environmental effects on chromatin marking comes from
studies of the expression of a gene that has been shown to modulate
coat color in mice, the agouti gene *(A)*. In normal or wild-type mice, *A*
is expressed in the hair follicles, and a dark coat color is typically observed (Jaenisch and Bird 2003). The effects of experimentally altering (mutating) the agouti gene depend on the state of chromatin
marking in the section of DNA that contains the altered *A* gene. When
the chromatin is "methylated" or marked, *A* expression is confined to
hair follicles, as it is in wild-type mice. The coats of these animals are
dark, and they are comparatively normal. If chromatin is unmarked, *A*
is expressed ubiquitously. The abnormally expressed agouti protein induces a complex gene signaling cascade that results in the expression
of a paracrine signaling factor that alters the synthesis of pigment-
producing factors (Morgan et al. 1999). This abnormal signaling cascade results in abnormalities in coat color, producing animals with
yellow or mottled fur. In addition, the widespread expression of agouti
is associated with obesity, increased levels of diabetes, and susceptibility to tumors. The distribution of coat patterns in the offspring of
these genetically altered animals is related to the maternal phenotype,
suggesting inheritance from the mother of epigenetic marking, as well
as the altered genes. Importantly, modification of the diet of the pregnant, genetically altered mothers by addition of methyl supplements
increases the number of offspring that show normal expression of *A*
(Cooney, Dave, and Wolff 2002; Wolff et al. 1998). The introduction of
a dietary factor presumably alters the marking of the segment of the
chromosome that contains the aberrant maternal gene. When that alteration is passed on to the offspring, it acts to mitigate the effects of
the abnormal gene.

Finally, a second example of the effects of chromatin marking
comes from a recent study of epigenetic profiles among monozygotic
human twins, which suggested that environmentally induced epigenetic
changes in chromatin marking may account for phenotypic difference
in genetically identical individuals (Fraga et al. 2005). Significant variation in chromatin marking was observed across a wide range of measures

in approximately one-third of the 40 pairs of twins (aged 3 to 74 years) who participated in the study. Importantly, the investigators found that the greatest variations occurred among twin pairs who were older, had different lifestyles, and had spent the least time living together.

## Changing Views of Genes and Inheritance

Early in the nineteenth century, the search for the identity of the material unit of inheritance had become a central theme of biological investigation. The work of Darwin and Mendel introduced two quite different but equally influential intellectual threads that would shape and guide the course of scientific inquiry for more than a century. By the beginning of the twentieth century, both the locus of the gene within the cell nucleus and its capacity for mutation and change were established. This emerging conception of the gene as a tangible, potentially measurable entity that could solve the problem of inheritance drove the focus of work in biology increasingly away from the study of embryological form and toward the search for the identity of the molecular substance that could support both intergenerational constancy and individual variation. In the 1940s, DNA was identified as the molecular substrate of the gene, and the functional association between individual genes and their products was defined in the form of the one-gene–one-enzyme hypothesis. In 1953, Watson and Crick's, double-helix model provided a means of conceptualizing a mechanism for gene expression in the form of a DNA template. Over the next decade, the basic model of DNA transcription and RNA translation was confirmed.

The gene of the 1950s and 1960s provided a tangible and straightforward mechanism for transmission of biological information. The structure of the gene specified in this model could also account for variability via the mechanism's allelic variation and mutation. The one-gene–one-protein account of biological inheritance resonated with earlier models in accounting for the transmission of specific characters or traits. In that sense, the early template model continued in the preformationist tradition in which genes are considered direct determiners of phenotypic outcome. However, subsequent work has shown that few genes fit this simple description in that few genes operate as unique and independent factors. Rather, genes are part of highly regulated and orchestrated cascades of expression and interaction. It has been argued by many scientists, historians, and philosophers of science that modern work in molecular biology has brought about the deconstruction or disintegration of the classical concept of the molecular, or nuclear, gene (Beurton 2000; Fogle 2000; Keller 2000a; Morange 2001; Moss 2003; Oyama, Griffiths, and Gray 2001; Rheinberger 2000). The concrete notion of the gene as originally defined when "the new molecular genetics had reached the heyday of its precocious simplicity" (Rheinberger 2000, p. 228) was quickly undermined by the wealth of data that challenged both the structural description of the unitary gene and its functional role in the development of the organism. Overlapping genes, nested genes, alternative splicing, and chromatin marking all serve to undermine any simple definition of the gene and to contribute to the deconstruction of the one-gene–one-polypeptide notion of the gene. The weight of evidence suggests that complex cascades of genetic expression both help direct the course of biological development and are influenced by it. Biological development is dynamic and interactive, and there is no simple mapping between the expression of nucleotide sequences and the development of specific phenotypes.

Yet in many ways, the familiar and accessible model of the unitary gene has remained a part of the popular conception of what genes are and how they function. The popular press and some scientific publications regularly refer to the "gene for $X$," where $X$ can be anything from language to eye color to depression. Although it is clear that current knowledge of gene structure and function renders this simple "one-gene/one-polypeptide/one-trait" model untenable, Moss has argued that this conception of the gene, which he calls Gene-P (for preformationist), may retain some utility, provided it is not confused or conflated with what he refers to as Gene-D (for development). Gene-D is defined by its molecular sequence and its precisely defined function in the genetic and developmental cascade. It does not bear an exact relationship to a specific phenotype, such as having blue eyes or suffering from depression (Moss 2003). According to Moss, the construct of the Gene-P retains "instrumental utility" within the specific context "where some deviation from a normal sequence results with some predictability in a phenotypic difference . . . [that is, it] serves as a kind of instrumental short hand with some predictive utility" (Moss 2003, p. 45). Using Moss's example, a "Gene-P for cystic fibrosis" can be defined on the basis of its predictive association between the disease and an abnormality at a particular gene locus. Furthermore, the predictive relationship is informative. It is medically useful for patients and doctors, and it provides a starting point for scientists seeking to understand the pathophysiology of the disease. However, it is inappropriate to conflate the associative information in the definition of Gene-P with the idea that it is a Gene-D, that is, a gene with a known specific function. Although the Gene-P concept usefully identifies an association between a genetic abnormality and a disease, it does not define a precise function for the gene.

In the case of cystic fibrosis, subsequent work has revealed the specific function of a gene that was initially identified by its Gene-P association. The gene (now identified as a Gene-D) has been identified as a "member of a 'family' of transmembrane ion-channel templates" (Moss 2001, p. 88). The disruption of expression of this gene leads to reduced chloride secretion that in turn interferes with hydration of the cell and results in abnormalities in the mucus within the airway, leading to some of the hallmark symptoms of the disease. Thus, although the Gene-P may be a useful construct in pointing to an association, it cannot be conflated with the Gene-D. The role Gene-D plays in understanding the problem of biological inheritance "is *not* one of preformationism but of epigenesis. Phenotypes are achieved through the complex interactions of many factors, the role of each being contingent upon the larger context to which it also contributes" (Moss 2003, p. 48). It is Gene-D, and not Gene-P, that best approximates the current knowledge of gene function and provides the most accurate current definition of the gene.

To return to the question that began this chapter: What, from a biological perspective, is inherited? Several centuries of work identified DNA as the carrier of what Johannsen called the gene and what Crick called genetic information. It is the absolutely essential particulate matter that carries the molecular code for the generation of proteins. However, DNA, by itself, is inert and cannot transmit the information encoded in its nucleotide sequences. Fortunately, DNA is not transmitted in isolation. It is transmitted within a cell that contains the biological machinery necessary for decoding the information in the genes. In that sense, biological inheritance includes not just the genes but also the first environment of the organism, that is, a cell that is capable of engaging in the biological processes that are necessary for the development and functioning of the organism.

As we will see in the chapters that follow, from the moment of conception—from the moment of biological inheritance—the dynamic processes that guide development begin to unfold. There is very little that is prescriptive or predetermined in the developmental processes that we will discuss. Rather, genes provide the template for making the proteins that enter into complex signaling cascades. It is these signaling cascades that serve to direct the development of cells, assemblies of cells, and connections among cells. The formation of these neural networks underpins and supports the behavior of the organism, and the behavior of the organism, in turn, influences the organization and functioning of the neural system. Early in development much of this signaling is intrinsic, originating from within the organism. But even very early, environmental factors in the form of nutrients or even toxins transmitted from the mother critically impact development. Furthermore, environment should be construed to encompass the multiple levels of the organism, as well as influences extrinsic to the organism. Cells signal and direct the fate of other cells. Connections between cells can alter signaling from cells originating from a third source. In short, the biological view of inheritance identifies and emphasizes the importance of the material factors that are transmitted from the parents, but it also recognizes that inheritance is only the first step of a much larger developmental process. Inherited resources and environmental input are essential to, but distinct from, the process of development. It is the complex, dynamic, and interactive signaling processes that are set in motion at the moment of conception that ultimately shape and direct the development of the mature organism.

## Chapter Summary

- Three central threads in the debate over the nature of biological inheritance are (1) the issue of accounting for both constancy and variability, (2) the question of defining the material nature of inheritance, and (3) differences in scientific focus arising from the specific level of inquiry: trait frequency and distribution versus individual trait variants versus developmental origins.

- Morgan identified the nuclear locus of genes and, with his student Mueller, demonstrated that gene structure can be affected by external agents.
- Avery and colleagues identified DNA as the material substance of genes. Beadle and Tatum demonstrated the specific association between genes and gene products, which was codified in their one-gene–one-enzyme hypothesis.
- Watson and Crick (1953) defined the structure of DNA and offered two important hypotheses about gene expression. The Sequence Hypothesis suggested that base sequences on the DNA molecules serve as a template for coding of the amino-acid sequences of proteins. The Central Dogma asserted that information can pass from DNA to RNA to protein, but transfer from protein to protein or from protein to DNA is not possible.
- Genes are contained within the chromatin of the cell nucleus. Chromatin is a complex of DNA and histone proteins. During transcription, the two strands of DNA separate, exposing a nucleotide template. A mirror copy of the DNA sequence, called a transcript, is transcribed by the nRNA. Once complete, the transcript is transported out of the cell nucleus as mRNA. The transcript is then translated into a protein that is produced at structures in the cell cytoplasm called ribosomes. Ribosomes are factories for assembling amino-acid sequences. The mRNA serves as the template for specifying the sequences of amino acids in proteins.
- Before being transported out of the cell nucleus, the nRNA transcript is edited to remove noncoding regions of DNA, called introns. The remaining regions of DNA, called exons, are reassembled into the edited transcript, which is then transported from the nucleus as mRNA. The resplicing of exon segments can vary, reflecting a process known as alternative splicing.
- Single genes can be expressed differently in different tissue systems or at different times in development and thus exhibit pleiotropy. Many genes are highly conserved across species.
- Recent studies suggest that there are nongenetic as well as genetic forms of inheritance. Studies of chromatin marking provide evidence of what is called epigenetic inheritance.

## References

Allen, G. E. 1975. *Life science in the twentieth century.* New York: Wiley.

———. 1986. "T. H. Morgan and the split between embryology and genetics, 1910–35." In *A history of embryology,* ed. T. J. Horder, J. A. Witkowski, and C. C. Wylie, 113–146. Cambridge: Cambridge University Press.

Avery, O. T., C. M. MacLeod, and M. McCarty. 1944. "Studies on the chemical nature of the substance inducing transformation of pneumococcal types: Induction of transformation by a deoxyribonucleic acid fraction isolated from pneumococcus type III." *Journal of Experimental Medicine,* 79: 137–158.

Beurton, P. J. 2000. "A unified view of the gene, or how to overcome reductionism." In *The concept of the gene in development and evolution: Historical and epistemological perspectives,* ed. P. J. Beurton, R. Falk, and H.-J. Rheinberger, 286–314. Cambridge: Cambridge University Press.

Brenner, S., F. Jacob, and M. Meselson. 1961. "An unstable intermediate carrying information from genes to ribosomes for protein synthesis." *Nature,* 190: 576–581.

Carlson, E. A. 1966. *The gene: A critical history.* Philadelphia: W. B. Saunders Company.

Cheung, P., and P. Lau. 2005. "Epigenetic regulation by histone methylation and histone variants." *Molecular Endocrinology,* 19: 563–573.

Cooney, C. A., A. A. Dave, and G. L. Wolff. 2002. "Maternal methyl supplements in mice affect epigenetic variation and DNA methylation of offspring." *Journal of Nutrition,* 132: 2393S–2400S.

Crick, F. H. 1958. "On protein synthesis." *Symposia of the Society for Experimental Biology,* 12: 138–163.

Croft, L., S. Schandorff, F. Clark, K. Burrage, P. Arctander, and J. S. Mattick. 2000. "ISIS, the intron information system, reveals the high frequency of alternative splicing in the human genome." *Nature Genetics,* 24: 340–341.

Falk, R. 2000. "The gene—A concept in tension." In *The concept of the gene in development and evolution: Historical and epistemological perspectives,* ed. P. J. Beurton, R. Falk, and H.-J. Rheinberger, 317–348. Cambridge: Cambridge University Press.

Fogle, T. 2000. "The dissolution of protein coding genes in molecular biology." In *The concept of the gene in development and evolution: Historical and epistemological perspectives,* ed. P. J. Beurton, R. Falk, and H.-J. Rheinberger, 3–25. Cambridge: Cambridge University Press.

Fraga, M. F., E. Ballestar, M. F. Paz, S. Ropero, F. Setien, M. L. Ballestar, D. Heine-Suner, J. C. Cigudosa, M. Urioste, J. Benitez, M. Boix-Chornet,

A. Sanchez-Aguilera, C. Ling, E. Carlsson, P. Poulsen, A. Vaag, Z. Stephan, T. D. Spector, Y. Z. Wu, C. Plass, and M. Esteller. 2005. "Epigenetic differences arise during the lifetime of monozygotic twins." *Proceedings of the National Academy of Sciences of the United States of America,* 102: 10604–10609.

Gamow, G., A. Rich, and M. Ycas. 1956. "The problem of information transfer from the nucleic acids to proteins." *Advances in Biological and Medical Physics,* 4: 23–68.

Gayon, J. 2000. "From measurement to organization: A philosophical scheme for the history of the concept of heredity." In *The concept of the gene in development and evolution: Historical and epistemological perspectives,* ed. P. J. Beurton, R. Falk, and H.-J. Rheinberger, 69–90. Cambridge: Cambridge University Press.

Gehring, W. J. 1976. "Developmental genetics of Drosophila." *Annual Review of Genetics,* 10: 209–252.

Gehring, W. J., and Y. Hiromi. 1986. "Homeotic genes and the homeobox." *Annual Review of Genetics,* 20: 147–173.

Gilbert, S. F. 1978. "The embryological origins of the gene theory." *Journal of the History of Biology,* 11: 307–351.

———. 2000. "Genes classical and genes developmental: The different use of genes in evolutionary syntheses." In *The concept of the gene in development and evolution: Historical and epistemological perspectives,* ed. P. J. Beurton, R. Falk, and H.-J. Rheinberger, 178–192. Cambridge: Cambridge University Press.

———. 2006. *Developmental biology.* 8th ed. Sunderland, MA: Sinauer Associates.

Greenspan, R. J. 2004. "E pluribus unum, ex uno plura: Quantitative and single-gene perspectives on the study of behavior." *Annual Review of Neuroscience,* 27: 79–105.

Griffith, F. 1928. "The significance of pneumococcal types." *Journal of Hygiene,* 27: 113–159.

Hershey, A. D., and M. Chase. 1952. "Independent functions of viral protein and nucleic acid in growth of bacteriophage." *Journal of General Physiology,* 36: 39–56.

Jablonka, E. 2001. "The systems of inheritance." In *Cycles of contingency: Developmental systems and evolution,* ed. S. Oyama, P. E. Griffiths, and R. D. Gray, 99–116. Cambridge, MA: MIT Press.

———. 2002. "Information: Its interpretation, its inheritance, and its sharing." *Philosophy of Science,* 69: 578–605.

Jacob, F., and J. Monod. 1961. "Genetic regulatory mechanisms in the synthesis of proteins." *Journal of Molecular Biology,* 3: 318–356.

Jaenisch, R., and A. Bird. 2003. "Epigenetic regulation of gene expression: How the genome integrates intrinsic and environmental signals." *Nature Genetics,* 33 (Suppl.): 245–254.

Johannsen, W. 1911. "The genotype conception of heredity." *American Naturalist,* 45: 129–159.

Kaufman, T. C., R. Lewis, and B. Wakimoto. 1980. "Cytogenetic analysis of chromosome 3 in *Drosophila melanogaster:* The homoeotic gene complex in polytene chromosome interval 84A–B." *Genetics,* 94: 115–133.

Keller, E. F. 1995. *Refiguring life: Metaphors of twentieth-century biology.* New York: Columbia University Press.

———. 2000a. *The century of the gene.* Cambridge, MA: Harvard University Press.

———. 2000b. "Decoding the genetic program; or, Some circular logic in the logic of circularity." In *The concept of the gene in development and evolution: Historical and epistemological perspectives,* ed. P. J. Beurton, R. Falk, and H.-J. Rheinberger, 159–177. Cambridge: Cambridge University Press.

Kessel, M., and P. Gruss. 1990. "Murine developmental control genes." *Science,* 249: 374–379.

Levine, M., G. M. Rubin, and R. Tjian. 1984. "Human DNA sequences homologous to a protein coding region conserved between homeotic genes of Drosophila." *Cell,* 38: 667–673.

Lewis, E. B. 1978. "A gene complex controlling segmentation in Drosophila." *Nature,* 276: 565–570.

Lewontin, R. C. 2000. *The triple helix: Gene, organism, and environment.* Cambridge, MA: Harvard University Press.

Maienschein, J. 1985. "History of biology." *Osiris, special volume on Historical Writing on American Science* (2nd series), 1: 147–162.

McClung, C. E. 1902. "The accessory chromosome-sex determinant?" *Biological Bulletin,* 3: 43–84.

McGinnis, W., C. P. Hart, W. J. Gehring, and F. H. Ruddle. 1984. "Molecular cloning and chromosome mapping of a mouse DNA sequence homologous to homeotic genes of Drosophila." *Cell,* 38: 675–680.

Morange, M. 2000. "The development gene concept: History and limits." In *The concept of the gene in development and evolution: Historical and epistemological perspectives,* ed. P. J. Beurton, R. Falk, and H.-J. Rheinberger, 193–215. Cambridge: Cambridge University Press.

———. 2001. *The misunderstood gene.* Cambridge, MA: Harvard University Press.

Morgan, H. D., H. G. Sutherland, D. I. Martin, and E. Whitelaw. 1999. "Epigenetic inheritance at the agouti locus in the mouse." *Nature Genetics,* 23: 314–318.

Morgan, T. H. 1909. "Recent experiments on the inheritance of coat colors in mice." *American Naturalist*, 43: 494–510.

———. 1910. "Sex limited inheritance in Drosophila." *Science*, 32: 120–122.

Moss, L. 1992. "A kernel of truth? On the reality of the genetic program." *Proceedings of the Biennial Meeting of the Philosophy of Science Association*, 1: 335–348.

———. 2001. "Deconstructing the gene and reconstructing molecular developmental systems." In *Cycles of contingency: Developmental systems and evolution*, ed. S. Oyama, P. E. Griffiths, and R. D. Gray, 85–97. Cambridge, MA: MIT Press.

———. 2003. *What genes can't do*. Cambridge, MA: MIT Press.

Nirenberg, M. W., and J. H. Matthaei. 1961. "The dependence of cell-free protein synthesis in E. coli upon naturally occurring or synthetic polyribonucleotides." *Proceedings of the National Academy of Sciences of the United States of America*, 47: 1588–1602.

Nusslein-Volhard, C., and E. Wieschaus. 1980. "Mutations affecting segment number and polarity in Drosophila." *Nature*, 287: 795–801.

Oyama, S., P. E. Griffiths, and R. D. Gray, eds. 2001. *Cycles of contingency: Developmental systems and evolution*. Cambridge, MA: MIT Press.

Portin, P. 1993. "The concept of the gene: Short history and present status." *Quarterly Review of Biology*, 68: 173–223.

Portugal, F. H., and J. S. Cohen. 1977. *A century of DNA*. Cambridge, MA: MIT Press.

Rheinberger, H.-J. 2000. "Gene concepts: Fragments from the perspective of molecular biology." In *The concept of the gene in development and evolution: Historical and epistemological perspectives*, ed. P. J. Beurton, R. Falk, and H.-J. Rheinberger, 219–239. Cambridge: Cambridge University Press.

Sarkar, S. 2000. "Information in genetics and developmental biology: Comments on Maynard Smith." *Philosophy of Science*, 67: 208–213.

Scott, M. P., and A. J. Weiner. 1984. "Structural relationships among genes that control development: Sequence homology between the Antennapedia, Ultrabithorax, and fushi tarazu loci of Drosophila." *Proceedings of the National Academy of Sciences of the United States of America*, 81: 4115–4119.

Snustad, D. P., and M. J. Simmons. 2003. *Principles of genetics*. 3rd ed. New York: J. Wiley.

Stamhuis, I. H., O. G. Meijer, and E. J. Zevenhuizen. 1999. "Hugo de Vries on heredity, 1889–1903: Statistics, Mendelian laws, pangenes, mutations." *Isis*, 90: 238–267.

Stevens, N. M. 1905. "A study on the germ cells of Aphis rosae and Aphis oenotherae." *Journal of Experimental Zoology*, 2: 313–333.

Van Speybroeck, L., D. De Waele, and G. Van de Vijver. 2002. "Theories in early embryology: Close connections between epigenesis, preformationism, and self-organization." *Annals of the New York Academy of Sciences*, 981: 7–49.

Volkin, E., and L. Astrachan. 1956. "Intracellular distribution of labeled ribonucleic acid after phage infection of Escherichia coli." *Virology*, 2: 433–437.

Watson, J. D., and F. H. Crick. 1953. "Genetical implications of the structure of deoxyribonucleic acid." *Nature*, 171: 964–967.

Wheeler, W. M. 1899. "Caspar Friedrich Wolff and the *theoria generationis*." *Biological Lectures delivered at the Marine Biological Laboratory, Wood's Hole, Mass.*: 265–284.

Wilson, E. B. 1895. *An atlas of the fertilization and karyokinesis of the ovum*. New York: Macmillan.

———. 1896. *The cell in development and inheritance*. New York: Macmillan.

———. 1905. "Studies on chromosomes II." *Journal of Experimental Zoology*, 2: 507–545.

Wolff, G. L., R. L. Kodell, S. R. Moore, and C. A. Cooney. 1998. "Maternal epigenetics and methyl supplements affect agouti gene expression in Avy/a mice." *FASEB Journal*, 12: 949–957.

# THREE

# Formation of the Neural Plate

BRAIN DEVELOPMENT IS a complex and protracted process that begins within days of conception and extends, arguably, throughout the
lifespan. This chapter and the next will consider the very first steps in
the cascade of biological events that eventually give rise to the mature
human brain. This series of events begins very early in development
with the processes that serve to differentiate the population of neural
progenitor cells that will later generate the cells of the central nervous
system (CNS). The interactions of the neural progenitor cells with
other cells will shape the basic organization of the developing neural
system. These early events are orchestrated by a complex interplay of
genetic signaling that is not fully understood. However, a number of
genes critical to regulating these important processes have been identified, and their main functions are well defined. The most basic and
best-understood of these genes and their roles in these important early
developmental events will be discussed.

The first steps in the story of brain development begin 14 days postconception (E14) and cover a period of approximately two weeks.
During this time, two major milestones in human embryonic development occur: gastrulation and neurulation. Gastrulation involves the
specialization and organization of relatively undifferentiated embryonic tissue into three distinct cell lines, each of which is capable of producing cells for different organ systems of the body. The process of
gastrulation in humans is complete at approximately E18. At that
point, a second, rather remarkable morphological change begins to

occur, marking the emergence of the first identifiable neural structure, the neural tube. The neural tube is the embryonic structure from which the CNS develops. The term *neurulation* is used to refer to the set of processes that give rise to the neural tube. Neurulation begins approximately 18 days after conception and is complete by E28. Together, these two very early events, gastrulation and neurulation, provide the foundation of all further milestones in brain development. They are so basic that the failure of either of these complex events can cause serious neural defects or in the most extreme cases can compromise the viability of the organism. This chapter will consider the events surrounding gastrulation, and Chapter 4 will discuss the processes involved in neurulation.

The processes that unfold during gastrulation affect all the tissues of the embryo, as well as the embryonic supporting tissue, or extraembryonic tissue. Thus gastrulation is an important stage in the development of all the organ systems of the embryo. Just before the onset of gastrulation, the cells of the embryo have not yet differentiated and are referred to as embryonic stem cells. Embryonic stem cells are pluripotent, that is, capable of generating all the cell lines in the body (note that it is the cells from this early period of embryonic development that are the focus of current scientific and political interest and debate). During gastrulation, the initially undifferentiated embryonic stem cells differentiate into three progenitor cell lines, the ectodermal, mesodermal, and endodermal progenitor cell lines. Progenitor cells are cells that are capable of dividing and can produce other cell types. They differ from embryonic stem cells in that the range of cell types that they can produce is more limited—their fate is more restricted. The three primary progenitor cell lines are organized into three distinct layers within the embryo, which are referred to as the primary germ layers. Each germ layer contains progenitor cells for different types of body tissue and are referred to as the ectodermal germ layer, the mesodermal germ layer, and the endodermal germ layer. The three-layered embryonic structure is called the trilaminar disc. The most dorsal layer (see Figure 1.1C) of the trilaminar disc is the ectodermal layer, which contains the cells that will become the neural progenitor cells. Neural progenitor cells are the subset of embryonic cells that will produce all the cells that form the CNS. Neural induction refers to the subset of processes that occur during gastrulation that specifically affect the development of the neural progenitor cells. This chapter will begin with a brief review of the basic processes of gastrulation that lead to the differentiation of the primary germ layers. It will then focus in greater depth on those processes that are specific to early brain development, the neural inductive processes.

## Gastrulation

In humans, gastrulation occurs during the third week of gestation (GW3). By the end of gastrulation, the three primary embryonic germ layers are specified and are organized into the three-layered trilaminar disc (Gilbert 2006; Sadler 2006). During the process of gastrulation, the major spatial axes of the developing embryo become specified such that by the end GW3 the embryo has clearly defined anterior-posterior, dorsal-ventral, and right-left axes (see Figure 1.1C). Both the germ layers and the major spatial axes can be identified by the differentiation and segregation of specific cell types into different locations within the embryo. Thus the rudimentary structural and functional plan for the embryo, defined in terms of both cell type and overall organization, is specified during gastrulation. During gastrulation, cells migrate to different regions of the embryo, using genetic signaling cues emanating from other cells to guide their movements. Other genetic cues provide signals that induce the cells to differentiate into a particular type. Thus for a given cell, both its target for migration and the determination of its cell type are specified by molecular signaling among cells.

## Setting the Stage for Gastrulation

Just before the onset of gastrulation, the fertilized egg undergoes a series of cell divisions via the process of cleavage. Cleavage of the egg serves to increase the number of cells that compose both the embryo and the emerging structures that will support its development, the extraembryonic structures. The process of cleavage produces two cell groups, an inner cell mass and an outer cell mass (called the trophoblast) that surrounds the inner cell mass. These two sets of cells together constitute the blastocyst. Cells in the inner cell mass will form the embryo and other extraembryonic structures, such as the amniotic cavity and the yolk sac. Cells of the trophoblast will form the chorion, which is the embryonic contribution to the placenta (Gilbert 2006). By E5, these two groups of cells separate, forming a large cavity in the center of the embryo called the blastocele, or blastocyst cavity (Sadler 2006).

By E13, the inner cell mass contains two distinct cell lines, epiblast cells and hypoblast cells. The epiblast cells will differentiate into the three principal germ layers from which the embryo will develop. The hypoblast cells will differentiate into extraembryonic structures. In humans, these two cell lines form a two-layered structure called the bilaminar disc (Figure 3.1A). By the onset of gastrulation, a subset of cells from the hypoblast layer has migrated to line the wall of the blastocyst cavity, thus transforming the blastocyst cavity into the primitive yolk sac. The yolk sac is an important structure in the early embryonic period. It is involved both in transport and metabolism of nutrients and in the production of embryonic blood cells (Palis and Yoder 2001). On the opposite side of the embryo adjacent to the epiblast layer, a small subset of epiblast cells, the extraembryonic epiblasts, has separated from the primary epiblast-cell layer to form a chamber that will become the amniotic cavity (Figure 3.1B).

## The Emergence of the Trilaminar Disc

During gastrulation, the two-layered embryo of the bilaminar-disc stage is transformed into a three-layered structure, called the trilaminar disc. As discussed at greater length in the following sections, each layer of the trilaminar disk contains a different progenitor cell line, each of which is capable of producing the cells for different parts of the developing embryo (see Table 3.1). The hypoblast layer of the bilaminar disc is replaced by the endodermal progenitor cells, thus forming the endodermal germ layer. Cells from this embryonic layer will generate the tissues of the gut. The cells of the epiblast layer are transformed into ectodermal cells and form the ectodermal germ layer. A subset of the ectodermal cells will further differentiate into the neural progenitor cell line, while the remaining ectodermal cells will become the progenitor cell line for the epidermal ectoderm and neural crest cells. A newly formed intermediate layer of cells, the mesodermal layer, is composed of mesodermal progenitor cells that will give rise to muscle and bone. The cells that will compose the mesodermal germ layer migrate from

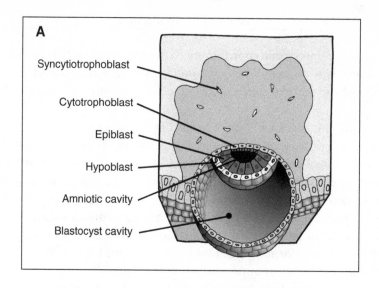

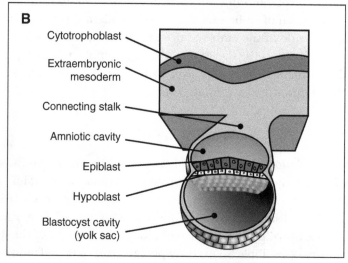

Figure 3.1. A. Human blastocyst at E7.5. The two layers of the bilaminar disc, the hypoblast and the epiblast, are well defined. The amniotic cavity is beginning to emerge. The extraembryonic tissues of the trophoblast have invaded the uterine wall and are establishing a connection with the maternal vascular system. B. Human blastocyst at E13. The connecting stalk and the extraembryonic mesoderm form from hypoblast-layer cells. The connecting stalk anchors the embryo to the uterine wall. The extraembryonic mesoderm combines with the trophoblast layers to form the chorion, the embryonic portion of the placenta. The definitive yolk sac and the amniotic cavities are well defined.

Table 3.1 Major derivatives of the primary germ layers

Endoderm:
- The epithelial lining of the gastrointestinal tract, respiratory tract, and urinary bladder
- Parenchyma of thyroid, parathyroids, liver, and pancreas
- Tympanic cavity and auditory tube

Mesoderm:
- Paraxial mesoderm forms somites
- Somites give rise to muscle, cartilage, bone, and subcutaneous tissue of the skin
- Vascular system
- Urogenital system—kidneys, gonads, and their ducts
- Spleen

Ectoderm consists of two broad subcategories:
Neural tissue:
- Central nervous system
- Peripheral nervous system (Ectodermal Neural Crest)

Epidermal tissue:
- Sensory epithelium of the ear, nose, and eye
- Epidermis, nails, and hair
- Pituitary, mammary, and sweat glands
- Enamel of teeth

Source: T. W. Sadler, *Langman's medical embryology,* 10th ed. (Philadelphia: Lippincott Williams & Wilkins, 2006).

the epiblast layer, moving down and forming a new layer of cells between the epiblast and hypoblast layers of the bilaminar disc. As these cells migrate, they send out molecular messages that instruct the cells that remain in the epiblast layer to differentiate into either neurectodermal or epidermal precursor cells. The details of this complex signaling process, which are discussed in the following sections, illustrate the kinds of dynamic interactions that characterize this earliest stage of neural development.

### Formation of the Primitive Streak and Node

The onset of gastrulation is signaled by the formation of the primitive streak on the surface of the epiblast layer (Figure 3.2). The primitive streak begins as a midline thickening at the posterior end of the embryo that gradually extends anteriorly. A depression forms in the streak that is referred to as the primitive groove. Once elongation of the primitive streak is complete, the anterior end thickens and forms a structure referred to as the node. At the center of the node, a depression called the primitive pit emerges by about E16. The primitive pit provides an opening through which migrating cells can leave the epiblast layer. The primitive streak provides the initial definition of the spatial coordinates of the embryo. Its position on the surface of the bilaminar disc defines both the anterior-posterior and the right-left axes. The surface opening at the node provides the dorsal landmark that marks the dorsal-ventral dimension (see Figure 1.1C).

*Cell Migration and the Formation of the Third Cell Layer*
On E14, the first epiblast cells begin to migrate toward the primitive streak (Gilbert 2006). These cells move from the dorsal surface of the epiblast layer—and thus the dorsal surface of the embryo—to more ventral regions (Figure 3.2B). The first cells to leave the epiblast layer initially move ventrally (down) and then migrate anteriorly between

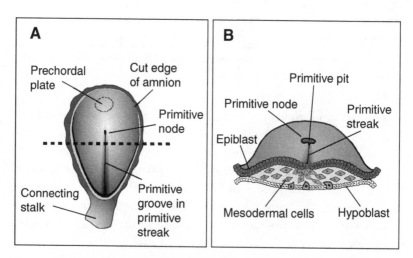

Figure 3.2. Two views of the embryo on E15–16. A. Dorsal view of the embryo looking down on the epiblast layer (the amnion has been cut away). The primitive streak and the primitive node are evident. B. A cross section of the embryo just posterior to the node (the dotted line in A indicates the level of the cross-sectional view).

the epiblast and hypoblast layers of the embryo (Figures 1.1C and 3.2B). When they reach the anterior region of the embryo, these earliest migrating cells displace cells within the lower hypoblast layer. The migration of these cells initiates the formation of the anterior region of the endodermal germ layer, which is called the pharyngeal endoderm. The next wave of migrating cells will form part of a newly emerging intermediate layer, the mesodermal germ layer (Figure 3.2B). These cells migrate ventrally and then anteriorly between the epiblast and hypoblast layers and along the midline of the embryonic disc. They will form two embryonic structures important for early neural development, the prechordal plate mesoderm and the chordamesoderm (together, they constitute the dorsal mesoderm. As discussed later, the prechordal plate cells play an important role in specifying cell types in anterior regions of the nervous system (brain). The chordamesoderm, which is located immediately behind the prechordal plate, plays a crucial role in specifying a posterior neural fate (hindbrain and spinal cord) for cells in the overlying ectodermal layer.

The next waves of epiblast cells arrive in two layers. A deeper layer of migrating endodermal progenitors displaces the remaining hypoblast cells to complete the formation of the endodermal germ layer, while a more superior layer of migrating mesodermal progenitor cells completes the intermediate, mesodermal germ layer. Cells that remain in the epiblast layer form the third of the three primary germ layers, the ectodermal germ layer.[1] Together, these three primitive germ layers constitute the embryonic trilaminar disc. The three germ layers will later give rise to different subsets of structures in the embryo. Major derivatives of each layer are shown in Table 3.1.

### Formation of the Notochord

Near the end of the period of cell migration, the primitive streak begins to regress toward the posterior end of the embryo (Sadler 2006). As the primitive streak regresses, the cells in the region of the underlying

---

1. The genetics of primary germ layer induction is complex and may vary across species. Although the topic is well beyond the scope of this book, the reader is referred to several excellent reviews of the genetics of germ layer induction and other inductive processes that occur during gastrulation: Gilbert 2006; McLaren 2003; Tiedemann et al. 2001.

chordamesoderm begin to proliferate and then detach from the underlying endoderm. The cells then condense and form a solid cord of cells called the notochord (Figure 3.3). This process of notochord formation begins at the anterior end of the chordamesoderm and progresses posteriorly. The notochord is an important embryonic structure that will be critical later in development during the formation of the hindbrain and the spinal column.

The major product of gastrulation is the generation of the primary germ layers and their organization in coordinate space. The organism now has the three progenitor cell lines necessary for generating all the major organ systems of the body. However, by the end of gastrulation, the degree of specification within the primitive neural progenitor tissue is more detailed than this simple description suggests. For the developing nervous system, neural progenitor cells have emerged, and there is considerable evidence of region-specific constraints on the types of cells that they can produce. By the end of gastrulation, different subpopulations of neural progenitor cells will selectively produce cells appropriate for particular regions of the CNS. Progenitors

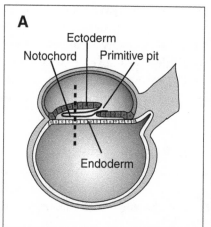
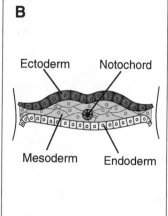

Figure 3.3. Two views of the formation of the notochord. A. A sagittal view (anterior-posterior at the midline of the embryo), E17. The chordamesoderm is the precursor to the notochord, which develops in caudal regions of the embryo. B. A cross-section of the embryo showing the fully formed notochord. (The dotted line in A indicates the level of the cross-section.)

located in posterior regions of the embryo will produce cells for the hindbrain and the spinal column, while those in more anterior regions will produce cells for the brain and the neocortex. The differentiation of neural progenitor subtypes emerges through the processes of neural induction.

## Neural Induction and Initial Patterning of the Central Nervous System

The most significant changes observed in the embryonic nervous system during gastrulation are those associated with the cells that form the ectodermal germ layer, the most dorsal layer of the trilaminar disc. As indicated in Table 3.1, all the cells that will give rise to the CNS are derived from this embryonic layer. Although the prospective ectodermal cells appear to be the least active subset of epiblast cells during gastrulation, they are critically affected by the activities of the cells that migrate to the more ventral embryonic layers and thus pass immediately beneath them. Most important, during gastrulation, cells in the epiblast layer receive signals from the cells migrating beneath them that will determine their fate as either neural or epidermal progenitor cells, that is, as cells that can produce either mature neural or epidermal cells. The epiblast cells that are located along the midline of the epiblast layer become neural progenitors, while cells in more lateral regions become epidermal progenitors. The processes that are involved in determining the fate of the emerging ectodermal layer cells are referred to collectively as neural induction.

In addition to the establishment of the neural progenitor cell line, the processes of neural induction also serve to further establish the basic organization of the primitive nervous system along the major spatial axes: dorsal-ventral, right-left, and anterior-posterior. Although spatial patterning of the embryo can arguably be said to begin at the moment of fertilization, the first patterning in the embryonic nervous system emerges during gastrulation and is closely related to the neural inductive processes. Specifically, by the end of gastrulation, not only have the neurectodermal cells differentiated and become spatially separated from underlying mesodermal and endodermal tissue along the dorsal-ventral axis, but also the initial specification of primitive right-left and anterior-posterior axes of the embryonic nervous system is complete.

## Specifying the Neural Progenitor Cells

The question of how undifferentiated epiblast tissue is transformed into the two primary ectodermal progenitor cell lines, neural progenitor cells and epidermal progenitor cells, was the subject of investigation for nearly a century. For many years, the key question concerned the problem of neural induction, or how neural progenitors differentiate and become specified. The focus of research was the search for the molecular cues that could signal, or "induce," undifferentiated epiblast cells to become neural progenitor cells. In the 1920s, an important series of experiments by the German biologist Hans Spemann and his colleague, Hilde Mangold, initiated a quest for the "neural organizer" that would continue for more than 60 years.

## Hans Spemann and the Discovery of the Organizer

The phenomenon of neural induction was first identified by Hans Spemann and Hilde Mangold (1924) in a series of studies with amphibian (newt) embryos that involved transplanting tissue from a donor embryo to a host embryo during the period of gastrulation. In a seminal study, they took a section of tissue from the node (which is called the blastula lip in newts) of the donor embryo and transplanted it to a position on the epiblast surface of the host embryo that would normally become epidermis (Figure 3.4). Recall that the node is the structure on the epiblast surface of the bilaminar disc that is the point where migrating cells move out of the epiblast layer to form the more ventral endodermal and mesodermal germ layers of the trilaminar disc. It had long been thought that the node provided signals to migrating cells that in some way altered their identity and their capacity to signal other cells. Thus the effect of Spemann and Mangold's transplantation experiment was to artificially provide the host embryo with two copies of the structure that is integrally involved in establishing the primary germ layers during gastrulation. Specifically, after the transplant procedure, the host embryo had two nodes, one located in the normal position and one grafted abnormally in a region of the developing ectodermal layer that would normally have given rise to epidermal structures. The results of these experiments were remarkable and somewhat surprising. Spemann and Mangold's host embryo developed two complete nervous systems, one at the normal site and one at the site of the transplanted nodal tissue. Further, Spemann confirmed that the tissue of the second nervous system was composed of cells derived from the host animal rather than the donor. This was important because it confirmed that it was not the case that the transplanted tissue simply generated a second neural system on its own. Rather, something in the transplanted tissue signaled a change in the surrounding tissue that resulted in the formation of the second nervous system.

Subsequent studies demonstrated that the timing of the transplant affects the pattern of induction and suggested that the function of the node may change somewhat across the period of gastrulation. Tissue transplantation completed during early gastrulation resulted in organisms with a second complete head and nervous system, while transplants during late gastrulation produced only the more posterior

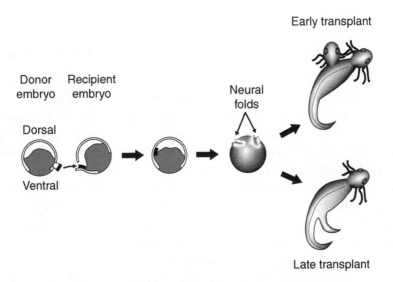

Figure 3.4. Spemann and Mangold's 1924 transplantation study. Nodal tissue taken from a donor embryo at the onset of gastrulation was transplanted to a host embryo (also during gastrulation). The host embryo developed two separate nervous systems, one signaled by its original nodal tissue and one signaled by the transplanted nodal tissue. The timing of the transplant affected the parts of the neuraxis that developed. (Note: The shape of the amphibian blastocyst-stage embryo is cylindrical, while that of human embryos is disk shaped. Beddington and Robertson 1998 have demonstrated, however, the topological equivalence of the basic structures in the embryos from four species: mouse, chick, xenopus (newt), and zebrafish.)

"tail" regions of the CNS (Figure 3.4). On the basis of his transplant studies, Spemann proposed that the transplanted tissue served as the "organizer" for neural induction (in mammals the equivalent structure is referred to as the "organizer node"). He suggested that the organizer creates an "organization field" in otherwise neutral tissue (Stern 2001). He proposed that something in the organizer signals the transformation of the ectodermal tissue to a neural, as opposed to an epidermal, fate. This series of studies precipitated a search for the "neural inducer" that would define the course of investigation for the next 60 years. Many different candidate "inducer" substances were systematically tested. The difficulty with the growing body of work was a failure to identify a reasonable single candidate substance as the organizer. Rather, many of the substances tried, including a number of unlikely candidates, appeared to induce a neural fate in ectodermal tissue (Brown, Keynes, and Lumsden 2001). Thus the puzzle of the organizer remained.

## An Unexpected Answer to the Question of Neural Induction

The search for the key to the problem of neural induction continued for more than half a century. In the mid-1990s, Hemmati-Brivanlou and Melton conducted a series of studies examining the role of a particular family of secreted molecules in signaling the fate of ectodermal cells in vertebrates (Hemmati-Brivanlou and Melton 1997a, 1997b; Hemmati-Brivanlou and Thomsen 1995). The molecules they studied were collectively called transforming growth factor beta (Tgfb). Although their original studies were intended to examine the effects of *Tgfb* expression on mesodermal tissue, over the course of their experiments, Hemmati-Brivanlou and colleagues discovered a surprising solution to the decades-old question of neural induction. Specifically, they found that the role of Tgfb proteins was not to instruct ectodermal cells to become neural progenitor cells; rather, the Tgfb proteins signaled the specification of epidermal progenitor cells. Thus in the absence of a signal provided by the Tgfb proteins, the default fate for ectodermal cells is to become neural, while the induction of an epidermal fate requires the intervention of the Tgfb signal. This work demonstrated that neural induction is the default pathway for ectodermal cells, and the 60-year-old puzzle had been solved by the identification of the "epidermal inducer."

After screening a variety of candidate members of the Tgfb superfamily, Hemmati-Brivanlou and colleagues determined that a specific protein, bone morphogenic protein 4 (Bmp4) was a particularly effective inducer of epidermal fate. Bone morphogenic proteins were originally discovered when they were found to play a critical role in bone formation (Urist 1965). However, they are now known to be a ubiquitous and highly conserved family of proteins that is found in different organ systems and in species as divergent as coral and man (Yamamoto and Oelgeschlager 2004). Bmp4, like proteins produced by other members of the Tgfb superfamily, is a secreted molecule that initiates a signaling cascade by binding to receptors in the wall of a target cell. The signal is then transmitted through the receptor to other proteins, called Smads, which are located in the cytoplasm of the cell. This signal triggers the conversion of the Smad proteins to transcription factors. Smad transcription factors then enter the cell nucleus, where they activate particular genes. The proteins produced by those genes in turn induce epidermal differentiation of the cell, and they suppress genes that would induce a neural differentiation.

### Protecting Neurectodermal Cells from the Effects of Bmp4

The discovery that Bmp4 acts to induce ectodermal cells to become epidermal rather than neural led to the question of how the emerging neurectodermal cells are protected from the Bmp4 signaling. Hemmati-Brivanlou and colleagues and many other groups began to focus on both the further elucidation of the role of Bmp4 and the search for other protein signals that might alter Bmp4 activity. At the onset of gastrulation, the Bmp4 protein is widely distributed throughout the regions of the embryo that will become the ectodermal and mesodermal germ layers of the trilaminar disc. However, as gastrulation progresses, the distribution of Bmp4 activity becomes restricted to the ventrolateral regions of the trilaminar disc, that is, to areas notably distant from dorsomedial regions of the embryo that express neural characteristics (Gilbert 2006; Yamamoto and Oelgeschlager 2004). This sequestering of Bmp4 away from emerging neural tissue suggested that logical candidates in the search for neural organizers were Bmp4 antagonists, that is, gene products that block the activity of other gene products, in this case gene products that block the activity of Bmp4. Within a few years, three different secreted molecules had been identified, noggin (Nog), chordin (Chrd), and follistatin (Fst). All are Bmp antagonists that bind directly and with high affinity and thus prevent Bmp4 from binding with its target receptors. Ectodermal cells exposed to Bmp4 antagonists are thus protected from Bmp4 signaling and differentiate into neurectodermal cells.

### Where Do the Bmp4 Antagonists Come From?

All three Bmp4 antagonists are expressed in the cells of the organizer, that is, in the ventrally migrating cells that form the endodermal and mesodermal germ layers of the embryo (Brown, Keynes, and Lumsden 2001; Yamamoto and Oelgeschlager 2004). The earliest cells to migrate include both endodermal precursors that form the pharyngeal endoderm and mesodermal progenitors that form the dorsal mesoderm, and thus have been referred to collectively as mesendodermal cells (Brown, Keynes, and Lumsden 2001). These cells derive from nodal tissue (Gilbert 2006; see Robb and Tam 2004 for discussion of the changes in the murine organizer across gastrulation), and together the cells of the node and the mesendoderm constitute the neural organizer. Mesendodermal cells migrate along the midline toward the anterior regions of the embryo. They form the pharyngeal endoderm and the dorsal mesoderm structures (including the prechordal plate mesoderm and the chordamesoderm, Figure 3.5). As the cells migrate, they express Bmp4 antagonists that block the epidermal differentiation of the cells in the ectodermal tissue overlying their path of migration. By blocking Bmp4 activity, these migrating cells indirectly support the production of neural progenitors. Ectodermal cells in the region above the mesendoderm become neural progenitors, and that region of the ectodermal layer is transformed into the presumptive neural plate. Thus the migrating cells of the organizer node provide the molecular signals that

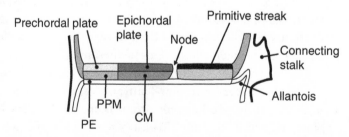

Figure 3.5. BMP4 antagonist signaling eminates from the pharyngeal endoderm (PE) and the dorsal mesoderm (which includes the prechordal plate mesoderm [PPM] and chordamesoderm [CM]).

protect the emerging neural progenitor cells from effects of Bmp4 signaling.

The role of Bmp4 antagonists in establishing the embryonic nervous system has been further demonstrated in studies that experimentally manipulate the levels of Bmp4 and Bmp4 antagonists in the developing organism. Animals with gene mutations that interfere with *Bmp4* expression display "dorsalized" phenotypes; that is, the mutation reduces the amount of available Bmp4 and results in animals with disproportionately large CNS and dorsal mesodermal structures. By contrast, interference with production of the Bmp4 antagonist Chrd results in animals with enlarged ventral mesoderm and reduced CNS structures (Oelgeschlager et al. 2003). These kinds of studies suggest that dorsal-ventral patterning in the developing embryo may be orchestrated by an interactive balance, a kind of competition, between a number of different factors that control the fate of different classes of cells in different ways. Bmp4 is a modulator of dorsal cell fate in that it signals epidermal fate and represses neural fate. When production of this dorsal modulator is suppressed, dorsal features are overexpressed. Similarly, Bmp4 antagonists are ventral modulators in that they block the effects of Bmp4. When production of the ventral modulators is suppressed, dorsal features are underexpressed. Studies examining the roles of dorsal and ventral modulators have also shown that interaction of Bmp4 and Bmp4 antagonists may affect more than just the establishment of the CNS. Bmp4 signaling plays an essential role in establishing the dorsal-ventral organization of all the tissues in the embryo.

## Organization of the Embryo along the Major Spatial Axes

The process of gastrulation establishes the principal spatial axes of the embryo. As discussed earlier, Bmp4 signaling is important for establishing an epidermal fate in ectodermal cells. However, as discussed in the next section, the graded expression of Bmp4 throughout the dorsal-ventral extent of the embryo also signals the differentiation of multiple cell lines that will give rise to different organ systems within the embryo. Primitive left-right patterning also emerges during gastrulation. Differential signaling cascades on the two sides of the presumptive neural plate serve to establish left-sided and right-sided characteristics. Finally, patterning along the anterior-posterior dimension sets up the basic organization of the CNS. As will be discussed below, the migrating cells of the organizer not only signal the neural fate of cells along the axial midline of the ectodermal layer, but differential signaling by these same cells also establishes the fate of cells at different locations along the presumptive neural plate to give rise to brain, midbrain, or spinal cord.

## Dorsal-Ventral Patterning of the Embryo

The effects of Bmp4 and Bmp4 antagonist signaling extend beyond the emerging CNS. These interactions are essential for establishing the fundamental dorsal-ventral organization of all of the organ systems of the embryo. The three Bmp4 antagonists are all secreted molecules that diffuse in a gradient that extends from the production source in the mesendoderm through more ventral regions of the embryo. The effect of this expression pattern of Bmp4 antagonists is to induce a countergradient of effective Bmp4 signaling. That is, as the concentration of antagonists diminishes in a graded fashion as it extends out from the source of expression, the concentration of Bmp4 increases. The effect of this counterposed gradient is critical for the normal development of the ventral structures of the embryo. In addition to its role in epidermal induction, Bmp4 activates the expression of genes that induce differentiation in the ventral mesoderm structures. At different concentrations, the Bmp4 protein induces different types of tissue; that is, it acts as a local morphogen. Specifically, at low dosage Bmp4 induces muscle, at medium dosage kidney is induced, and at high dosage blood cells are formed (Gilbert 2006; Yamamoto and Oelgeschlager 2004). Within the developing embryo, the dosage level of Bmp4 is modulated by the activity of Bmp4 antagonists derived from the "neural" organizer. However, the effects of that modulation extend beyond nervous system formation and include many of the major organ systems. Thus the interaction of the secreted Bmp4 protein and its antagonists affects dorsal-ventral specification of the embryo beyond the level of the neurectoderm. The counterposed gradients serve to establish the dorsal-ventral pattern of organization throughout the entire embryonic axis.

## Right-Left Patterning of the Embryo

Vertebrate bodies exhibit left-right asymmetries. In humans, for example, the liver is typically on the right, while the spleen and pancreas are on the left. Left-right asymmetries begin to emerge very early in development, and the principal genes associated with left- or right-sidedness are consistent across species. The transcription factor snail (Snai) is characteristically present on the right lateral plate mesendoderm of gastrulating embryos and is believed to be critical for establishing right-sided characteristics. The transcription factor Pitx2 and three secreted molecules, Nodal, Lefty1, and Lefty2, are associated with left lateralization (Figure 3.6). Across species, the gene activity that establishes the left-right axis of organization is the product of a complex cascade of activity in which complementary sets of genes on

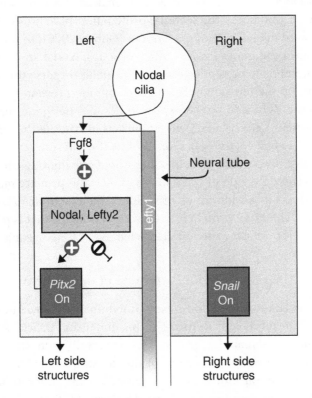

Figure 3.6. Cascades of gene expression regulate right-left patterning in the embryo. Snail proteins are largely responsible for specifying right-sided characteristics. A signaling cascade emanating from the node specifies left-sided characteristics. Left-sided expression of *Lefty1* prevents the signaling cascade on the left from influencing cells on the right. (From Gilbert 2006. Adapted with the permission of Sinauer Associates, Inc.)

the right or left side of the body are upregulated or downregulated in an orderly sequence. This process has been best described in avian species. However, although the final determiners of left- or right-sided characteristics appear to be common across vertebrate species, the precise pattern of gene activity that ultimately results in the expression of these left- and right-sided determiner molecules is known to vary across species. Although less fully delineated, the basic processes involved in left-right differentiation have been described in mammals.

In mammals, the mechanical activity of the cilia (hairlike structures) within the node appears to be an important determiner of left-right patterning. The activity of the cilia produces a right-to-left flow of fluids (Robb and Tam 2004). It is thought that this directional flow may create a gradient of the secreted protein fibroblast growth factor 8 (Fgf8) toward the left side of the embryo (Gilbert 2006). In the mouse, Fgf8 activates the genes for two other proteins, Nodal and Lefty2, in the left lateral plate mesendoderm. The proteins disperse through the mesoderm on the left side of the embryo but are prevented from diffusing to the right side by the expression of another gene that codes for the protein Lefty1. Lefty1 effectively acts to confine the activity of Nodal and Lefty2 to the left side. Within the left-side lateral mesoderm, Lefty2 blocks Snai proteins, thus effectively limiting the activity of Snai to the right side of the embryo. *Snai* is the primary marker of right-sidedness in a wide range of species. Nodal activates *Pitx2* gene expression. The Pitx2 protein is a transcription factor that is primarily responsible for defining the left-sided character of the organism.

## Anterior-Posterior Patterning of the Embryo

The third axial dimension to be established during gastrulation is the anterior-posterior axis. Patterning in this dimension provides the initial organizational plan that gives rise to the very different structures of the anterior and posterior regions of the neural system. Thus far, the discussion of neural induction has focused on the differentiation of the epiblast layer into the well-defined subregions that compose the emerging ectodermal germ layer, specifically, the neurectoderm and the epidermal ectoderm. As discussed earlier, migrating mesendodermal cells of the organizer express Bmp4 antagonists. The antagonists prevent Bmp4 from inducing an epidermal fate in the overlying ectoderm and thus promote the emergence of a midline band of neurectodermal cells that will later give rise to the neural plate. However, the cellular differentiation of neurectodermal cells is more specific. During gastrulation, distinct cell lines emerge within spatially discrete subregions of the neurectoderm. Cells within anterior regions will give rise to such structures as the forebrain and the midbrain, while cells in posterior regions will produce such structures as the hindbrain and the spinal column. The signaling pathway for anterior-posterior specification involves both temporally and spatially varying cues that induce the differentiation of the neural progenitor cells arranged along the developing neural axis.

The first suggestion that there might be different signaling systems for neurectodermal cells in anterior and posterior regions of the embryo came very early in the search for the neural organizer. Indeed, some of Hans Spemann's own studies pointed to this possibility. As discussed earlier, after the initial transplantation studies that produced duplicate head and central-axis structures in the developing newt embryo, Spemann conducted a series of studies in which he varied the timing of the organizer node tissue transplantation (Figure 3.4). This experimental manipulation led to a somewhat surprising result. The early transplants produced embryos very much like the original studies, specifically, embryos with duplicate head and central-column structures. However, the late transplants produced embryos in which only the posterior structures were duplicated, that is, animals with duplicate tails but not heads. At the time, Spemann speculated about whether these effects reflected the action of two separate organizers, one functioning as a "head organizer" and the other as a "tail organizer." Alternatively, the findings could indicate a change in the organization and functioning of a single organizer over time.

A large body of work has pointed to the possibility of separate pathways, but not necessarily separate organizers, for anterior-posterior specification. Work by Nieuwkoop and colleagues (1952) defined a two-step model in which tissue along the entire neurectodermal axis is initially neuralized and anteriorized, and then, in a second step, the posterior regions are exposed to agents expressed in a later gradient that serve to establish posterior identity (Brown, Keynes, and Lumsden 2001; Gilbert 2006; Kiecker and Niehrs 2001). As discussed next, more recent work has suggested that a related but somewhat different and more complex model of neurectodermal differentiation may account for the observed changes in the organization of the anterior-posterior axis during gastrulation.

### Specific Signals for Anterior or Posterior Specification

A critical step in the process of understanding and defining anterior-posterior specification was the identification of candidate molecules that might function as either posteriorizing or anteriorizing signals. Table 3.2 provides a summary of the major classes of molecules that have been implicated in establishing the anterior-posterior axis. The table indicates the major function of each molecule and its sites of expression. There is a larger number of anteriorizing than of posteriorizing agents, and their expression sites are less restricted.

Wnts are a class of secreted molecules that have been shown to suppress head induction in a variety of species and are thus candidates for posteriorizing agents. Overexpression of Wnts leads to repression of anterior structures, while overexpression of Wnt antagonists leads to repression of posterior structures. Other factors important for posterior specification include a specific fibroblast growth factor protein (Fgf8) and retinoic acid (RA). Fgf8 appears to modulate the Wnt signaling pathway by inducing other cells to respond to Wnt signals, while RA, a derivative of vitamin A, is present in posterior regions and influences hindbrain organization.

As discussed earlier, Nog and Chrd are expressed by the organizer and are critical for neural induction, but they also play an important role in anterior specification. However, neither alone is a potent head inducer in that mutations of either the *Nog* or *Chrd* gene have little effect on anterior specification. However, in organisms with mutation of both genes, there is failure of forebrain induction (Bachiller et al. 2000). It has been suggested that Nog and Chrd may play a role in maintaining rather than inducing early anterior patterning. A number of other molecules crucial for normal anterior specification are indicated in Table 3.2. Mutation of these genes results in failure of head induction. They are expressed in a variety of anterior sites at differing points during gastrulation.

### Expression Gradients Affect Anterior-Posterior Specification

In the model of neural induction discussed earlier, neurectodermal tissue is specified by deactivation of a potent and widely distributed epi-

**Table 3.2** Major classes of posterior and anterior signaling molecules

| Posterior Signaling Molecules | | |
| --- | --- | --- |
| Molecule | Function and Expression Pattern | Region |
| Wnt (secreted molecule) | Posteriorizing agent<br>Expressed in an anterior < posterior gradient in the embryo | CM<br>LVM |
| Fgf8 (secreted molecule) | Posteriorizing agent<br>May be mediated through Wnt | CM |
| Retinoic acid | Posteriorizing agent<br>Derived from maternal vitamin A<br>Signaling observed in posterior regions only | CM |
| Anterior Signaling Molecules | | |
| Nog (secreted molecule) | Neuralizing (Bmp antagonist)<br>Anteriorizing but produces only primitive forebrain characteristics<br>Nog gene mutation does not affect development, but in combination with Chrd mutation causes failure of forebrain development | CM<br>ON |
| Chrd (secreted molecule) | Neuralizing (Bmp antagonist)<br>Anteriorizing but produces only primitive forebrain characteristics<br>Chrd gene mutation does not affect development, but in combination with Nog mutation causes failure of forebrain development | PPM<br>CM<br>ON |
| Cer (secreted molecule) | Anteriorizing agent (Wnt, Bmp, Nod antagonist)<br>Overexpression produces multiple heads, but abnormal (single eye); cannot fully induce head characteristics | PE<br>AVE |
| Dkk1 (secreted molecule) | Anteriorizing agent (Wnt antagonist)<br>Overexpression produces large heads<br>Suppression leads to microcephaly; knockout causes failure of head expression | AVE<br>PE<br>PPM<br>ON |

Table 3.2 *(continued)*

| Anterior Signaling Molecules | | |
|---|---|---|
| Molecule | Function and Expression Pattern | Region |
| Oxt2 | Anteriorizing agent | |
| (transcription factor) | Gene mutation causes failure of head | AVE |
| | expression | EPI |
| Lhx1 | Anteriorizing agent | AVE |
| (transcription factor) | Gene mutation causes failure of head | PPM |
| | expression | EPI |
| Hesx1 | Anteriorizing agent, important for | AVE |
| (transcription factor) | forebrain development | |
| | Important in establishing AVE | EPI |
| Lefty1 | Anteriorizing agent (encodes Nod | AVE |
| (secreted molecule) | antagonists) | |
| | | PPM |

Structures expressing anterior and posterior signaling molecules.
Organizer structures—from most anterior to most posterior: PE = pharyngeal
endoderm; PPM = prechordal plate mesoderm; CM = chordamesoderm;
ON = organizer node.
Structures outside organizer: LVM = lateral ventral mesoderm; AVE = anterior
visceral endoderm (develops before the primitive streak and is important in
establishing initial anterior characteristics); EPI = epiblast layer.

dermalizing agent, Bmp4. Bmp4 antagonists, which are expressed along the dorsal midline by mesendodermal organizer tissues, create a gradient of Bmp4 signaling that serves both to define the dorsal-ventral axis of the organism and, because of variation in Bmp4 concentration, to induce cell types for different body structures. An analogous counterposed gradient model has been proposed for anterior-posterior neuraxis specification. *Wnts* are expressed along the length of the anterior-posterior axis in the embryo during early gastrulation. However, the concentration of Wnt varies in a graded fashion, with the highest concentration in the posterior regions (Kiecker and Niehrs 2001). *Wnt* expression induces posterior characteristics in neurectodermal tissue, but like *Bmp4*, the specific outcomes are affected by concentration. At different dosage levels, the expression of anterior versus posterior neural cell markers is altered. High concentrations of Wnt induce hindbrain and spinal-column progenitors, at midlevel dosage midbrain progenitors are induced, and at low levels forebrain progenitors are generated. Thus, the morphogenic effect of *Wnt* gradient expression contributes to the differentiation of cell types along the anterior-posterior axis of the embryo. However, the modulation of *Wnt* expression is somewhat more complex than that of *Bmp4* expression. As was the case for dorsal-ventral specification, the organizer tissues are directly involved, but different parts of the organizer participate differentially in modulating *Wnt* expression. Further, a second structure that develops prior to the onset of gastrulation, the anterior visceral endoderm (AVE), appears to play a significant role in establishing anterior identity.

As discussed earlier, gastrulation involves the migration of mesendodermal cells from the region of the primitive streak to form an intermediate embryonic germ layer. The first waves of cells to migrate are derived from nodal tissue and are considered part of the organizer. There is a spatiotemporal association between the time of migration of these cells and their eventual location in the embryo. The cells that migrate earliest move to the most anterior position in the embryo, and successively later groups of cells form more posterior parts of the structure. This spatiotemporal arrangement of cells also has functional consequences because different groups of migrating cells receive different signals from the node. As a result, the successive substructures that compose the mesendoderm set up somewhat different signaling pathways. Organizer cells that migrate early form the pharyngeal endoderm and the prechordal plate mesoderm, while cells that migrate later form the chordamesendoderm (Figure 3.5). As discussed earlier, along their full extent, the mesendodermal organizers have the capacity for neural induction; that is, they send signals to block Bmp4 activity and thus specify a neural fate for the cells in the overlying ectodermal cell layer. However, different portions of the organizer also regulate the expression of posteriorizing signals.

The most anterior portions of the mesendoderm are considered head-induction centers because they express the highest numbers and concentrations of proteins that block posterior-fate-inducing factors such as Wnt. Cells within the most anterior region of the mesendoderm, the pharyngeal endoderm, express the *Cerberus (Cer)* gene. Cer is a secreted protein that binds Wnt. When the mRNA of *Cer* is injected into the ventral side of a newt embryo, multiple heads without tail structures are formed. However, the heads are incomplete, with only one eye, suggesting that Cer cannot fully induce head structures. The Dickkopf (Dkk1) protein ("big head" in German) is expressed in the prechordal plate mesoderm. It blocks the Wnt receptor. Blocking the activity of Dkk1 results in animals with microcephaly (small heads). The posterior-fate-blocking capacity of the anterior organizer structures is consistent with the gradient model of anterior-posterior induction proposed earlier. The presence of secreted molecules with the capacity to bind Wnts provides a means for establishing the observed posterior-anterior gradient of *Wnt* expression. The gradient model suggests that the default path for neural progenitor cells may be an anterior fate. When Wnt activity is blocked completely, neural progenitor cells express an anterior fate. However, as the concentration of Wnt antagonists diminishes, concentrations of Wnt rise and cells expressing a progressively more posterior fate emerge. These findings suggest that the default pathway for neural progenitor cells is to become anteriorized, and only when they are exposed to Wnts do they express a posterior fate.

## The Anterior Visceral Endoderm

Although the mesendoderm organizers appear to have the capacity to regulate the expression of factors that induce posterior fate, thus specifying the basic anterior-posterior pattern of the embryo, there is evidence that a second structure may also be important in specifying the fate of anterior structures in mammals. This structure is referred to as the anterior visceral endoderm (AVE). The AVE develops in the most anterior region of the visceral endoderm very early in embryonic development, before the emergence of the primitive streak. The AVE is derived from extraembryonic tissues and thus is not part of the embryo, but it expresses an important set of genes that contribute to the patterning in anterior regions of the embryo, particularly in regions that contribute to the development of the neurectoderm (Yamaguchi 2001). After the onset of gastrulation, the AVE is displaced outside the embryo by the ingressing endodermal cells (Yamaguchi 2001). Recent work suggests that the AVE may act as an early channel for suppressing posterior differentiation in anterior regions of the primitive epiblast layer and thus may be an important early factor in promoting anteriorization. *Cer* and *Lefty1* are expressed in the AVE. Both encode antagonists for *Tgfb* superfamily members (which include Nodal). *Nodal* is expressed in the epiblast early in gastrulation. Nodal is necessary for mesoderm formation, but it is also a potent posteriorizing agent. Thus one function of the AVE may be to suppress posterior differentiation of anterior epiblast cells before the formation of the primitive streak. The AVE expresses a number of transcription factors that are critical for head development, including Otx2, Hesx1, and Lhx1. *Otx2* and *Lhx1* are also expressed in the anterior mesendoderm; *Otx2* and *Hesx1* are expressed in the anterior epiblast layer. *Otx2* expression in the AVE is required for initiating the specification of anterior patterning in the neural plate (Simeone and Acampora 2001). In mice, failure to express *Otx2* results in failure of development of the rostral neurectoderm.

Although the AVE appears to be important in early anterior specification, a question remains whether it constitutes a second organizer structure. One requirement of the organizer is the ability to express factors that induce neural fate. Transplantation studies have failed to confirm that the AVE by itself has the capacity for neuraxis induction (Tam and Steiner 1999). Surgical removal of the AVE results in the loss of forebrain markers but does not result in major abnormalities (Beddington and Robertson 1998). Thus, although the AVE is important in the early specification of anterior structures, it does not appear to function as a second organizer. Rather, it provides early protection from posteriorizing signals and later appears to act in concert with the anterior portions of the mesendoderm to specify anterior regions of the developing neurectoderm.

## Clinical Correlation: Holoprosencephaly

Holoprosencephaly is a serious brain malformation characterized by failure of the cerebral hemispheres to separate. As will be discussed in Chapter 4, the separation of the hemispheres begins soon after closure of the anterior end of the neural tube and is complete by the end of the fifth week of gestation. Abnormalities or injury to cells of the anterior midline of the neural plate during gastrulation (Sadler 2006) or defects associated with formation of the anterior end of the neural tube somewhat later in the embryonic period (Menkes, Sarnat, and Maria 2006) can result in holoprosencephaly. Holoprosencephaly is

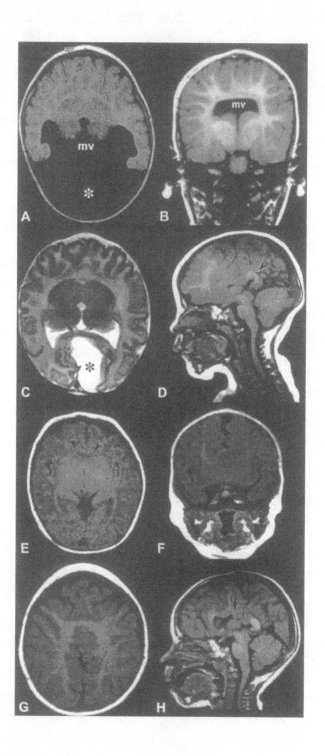

the most common defect of forebrain and facial structures. It is estimated that it occurs in 1 out of 250 pregnancies (Hahn and Plawner 2004). However, only 3 percent of cases survive to delivery. Thus the frequency among live births is approximately 1 in 10,000. Of those, two-thirds have the most severe form of the malformation.

## Types of Holoprosencephaly

Holoprosencephaly manifests with differing degrees of severity. The classical designation includes three levels of disorder: from most to least severe, alobar, semilobar, and lobar holoprosencephaly. Alobar holoprosencephaly is characterized by complete lack of separation between the hemispheres, a single undivided midline ventrical, undifferentiated ventral forebrain structures (e.g., basal ganglia), and absent central fissure and corpus callosum. In severe cases, a large dorsal cyst is common (Figures 3.7A, 3.7B). In semilobar holoprosencephaly, the anterior hemispheres fail to separate, but there is some separation in posterior regions. The corpus callosum is missing in the front but evident in the back of the brain (Figures 3.7C, 3.7D). In the mildest of the classical forms, lobar holoprosencephaly, most of the hemispheres are separated except in the most rostral and ventral regions. Most of

---

Figure 3.7. *(Opposite Page)* MRI images of the brains of children with holoprosencephaly, ordered by level of severity. A, B. Images of two children with alobar holoprosencephaly, illustrating the failure of the hemispheres to separate and the presence of a large single ventricle (monoventricle, mv). C, D. Images of two children with semilobar holoprosencephaly. The axial image in C shows the failure of hemispheric separation in anterior, but not posterior, regions. The saggital image in D shows the absence of all of the corpus callosum except the most caudal region of the splenium indicated by the arrow. E, F. Images of a child with lobar holoprosencephaly in which the interhemispheric fissure is present but underdeveloped. G, H. Images of two children with middle interhemispheric variant holoprosencephaly, where separation of the hemispheres is present in anterior frontal, and occipital regions, but not in posterior frontal, or parietal regions. The saggital image in H shows only the genu and splenium of the corpus callosum have formed. (From Kinsman, Plawner, and Hahn 2000. Reprinted with permission of Lippincott Williams & Wilkins.)

the corpus callosum is present, though the most posterior segment may be missing (Figures 3.7E, 3.7F). A fairly recently defined holoprosencephaly variant is referred to as the middle interhemispheric variant (MIH). In these cases, the anterior frontal and most posterior (occipital) cerebral lobes separate, but the posterior frontal and parietal lobes fail to do so (Figures 3.7G, 3.7H).

## Causes of Holoprosencephaly

Both genetic and environmental causes have been suggested for holoprosencephaly. The data appear to be more consistent with genetic than environmental factors. One consistent and well-documented environmental factor is maternal diabetes. Diabetic mothers have a 1 percent risk of having a child with holoprosencephaly, a hundredfold increase in risk over the typical population. A number of toxins have been associated with increased risk for holoprosencephaly, including maternal ingestion of alcohol, some anticonvulsant medications, and ingestion of cyclopamine (a cancer drug). It has been suggested that these toxins may interfere with the synthesis of SHH. Toxins disrupt cholesterol synthesis, and cholesterol is necessary for SHH synthesis. (The role of SHH in embryonic patterning will be discussed in greater detail in Chapter 4.)

Chromosomal abnormalities are frequent in holoprosencephaly; approximately 40 percent of children have documented anomalies, of which half are trisomy 13 (Hahn and Plawner 2004). In addition, at present, seven gene mutations have been identified in humans. Many of them are associated with SHH signaling, suggesting that the holoprosencephalic disorder may be associated with a failure of the ventral specification pathway. In *Shh* mutant mice, ventral specification along the whole neuraxis is disrupted. Within the spinal cord, expression of dorsal markers is normal. However, within the forebrain, both ventral and dorsal expression are disrupted. This is likely related to differences in the dorsal-ventral specification pathway in these two regions. In typical development, the separation of the hemispheres is achieved as dorsal midline cells migrate ventrally and divide the brain into the right and left hemispheres (Hayhurst and McConnell 2003). Accompanying this division, midline structures such as the choriod plexus, a structure necessary for production of cerebrospinal fluid (CSF), and the hippocampus, an important memory structure, form independently within the two hemispheres. In *Shh* mutants, the hemispheres fail to separate and midline structures fail to form. Loss of *Shh* also leads to a failure of anterior neural cells to express *Fgf8* (Ohkubo, Chiang, and Rubenstein 2002). Gunhaga (2003) showed that *Wnt* expression is critical for the specification of telencephalic fate, but that the expression initially of *Fgf8* from the anterior medial telencephalon and later of *Bmps* from the medial telencephalon is necessary to specify dorsal midline cells. Thus failure of the Shh pathway could account for the separation failures associated with the development of midline structures and the cerebral hemispheres. Other gene mutations associated with holoprosencephaly include several *Nodal* pathway-related genes, likely reflecting an important role for *Nodal* in the *Shh* pathway (Hayhurst and McConnell 2003).

## Developmental Outcomes

Children with holoprosencephaly have a range of medical, neurological, and cognitive problems, but the severity of deficit in each of these areas varies with the form of the disorder. A recent prospective study of a large cohort of children with holoprosencephaly studied at the Carter Centers for Brain Research in Holoprosencephaly and Related Malformations (Plawner et al. 2002) provided a cohesive overview of the impact of different types of the disorder on subsequent development. Children with holoprosencephaly have a variety of medical problems, including craniofacial malformations, motor system abnormalities, feeding and swallowing problems, and endocrine system problems, such as diabetes and growth-hormone deficiency (Hahn and Plawner 2004). The risk and severity of the disorder are associated with the type of holoprosencephaly. Craniofacial abnormalities are common in children with holoprosencephaly, and these manifestations reflect the failure of separation of the two halves of the brain and cranial region. The most severe cases include cyclopia, or the formation of a single central eye, formation of a single nostril, or cleft lip and palate. The severity of craniofacial disorders varies with the form of holoprosencephaly. Children with the most severe disorders typically do not survive infancy.

Virtually all children with alobar forms of the disorder in the Carter Centers sample had serious motor impairment, and all had oral motor problems that created difficulties in feeding. None of the children in the alobar group were able to sit unsupported, and they could do little more than bat at objects with their hands. Children in the semilobar group also had difficulty sitting unassisted, but their upper-body motor abilities were comparatively better. Motor problems were also common, but much less severe, among children with lobar and MIH forms. About half the children with lobar holoprosencephaly could walk independently or with assistance, and half had normal or only mildly impaired upper-body motor functioning. Feeding problems were comparatively rare in both these groups.

Endocrine disorders in children with holoprosencephaly are associated with defects in midline structures, such as the hypothalamus and the pituitary gland. Disorders of the posterior pituitary place children at risk of diabetes, while anterior pituitary dysfunction can lead to growth-hormone deficiency and hypothyroidism. Endocrine disorders were found in three-quarters of children with classic forms of holoprosencephaly in the Carter Centers sample, though frequency increased with severity of type. Children with MIH did not have endocrine disorders.

Neurological problems included seizures and epilepsy, microcephaly, and hydroencephaly associated with the presence of large dorsal cysts. Again, the type and severity of the disorder were associated with the form of holoprosencephaly. Microcephaly was present in 80 percent of children with semilobar or lobar forms but significantly less common among children with alobar holoprosencephaly. This is likely because of the high incidence of dorsal cysts and associated hydrocephalus among the alobar group. Nearly two-thirds of that group required CSF shunting, compared with under 10 percent in the other classic forms of the disorder. About half the children with holoprosencephaly had at least one seizure, and approximately one-quarter had chronic epilepsy.

Cognitive and linguistic outcomes are also associated with the degree of severity. Children with alobar holoprosencephaly had severe to profound developmental delay and mental retardation (Hahn and Plawner 2004). Deficits were much less pronounced in milder forms of the disorder. In the Carter Centers sample, there was an inverse relationship between the grade of holoprosencephaly and the level of cognitive function. Children with alobar forms made little or no advance in spoken language beyond production of vowel sounds; language was also severely impaired among children in the semilobar group. About half the children in the lobar group and three-quarters of the children in the MIH group were able to produce words or even multiword utterances. There is some suggestion that among the less compromised groups there is relative sparing of receptive language and social communicative skills, but compromise of visual reasoning and nonverbal problem solving (Hahn and Plawner 2004).

In summary, holoprosencephaly is a serious developmental disorder that involves compromise of forebrain areas very early in gestation. The two cerebral hemispheres fail to separate, creating a single band of neural tissue within cortical and, in several cases, subcortical areas. The frequency of the disorder among children surviving to birth is comparatively low. However, it has been estimated to affect as many as 1 in 250 pregnancies, making it a fairly common cause of early miscarriage. The disorder appears to reflect a failure of dorsal-ventral patterning and has been associated with mutation or disruption of the SHH signaling pathway. Both genetic and environmental factors have been implicated. Different levels of severity of the disorder have been defined. Medical, neurological, and behavioral outcomes are all directly related to the severity of the disorder.

## Chapter Summary

- The third prenatal week marks the beginning of CNS development. The two major events occurring that week are the induction of the neural progenitor cell lines, located along the midline axis of the embryonic ectodermal germ layer, and the emergence of initial organization along the three primary spatial axes. Both of these events are precipitated by signals derived from an important embryonic structure, the organizer. The organizer emerges on the posterior end of the embryonic disc at the beginning of the third week of development. It generates a set of structures, the pharyngeal endoderm and the dorsal mesoderm (including the prechordal plate and chordamesoderm), referred to collectively as the mesendoderm. The cells that form these structures migrate under the epiblast layer of the embryo and together with

epiblast cells that migrates later form a three-layered structure
known as the trilaminar disc.

- The induction of neurectodermal tissue requires genetic signaling that originates from the organizer tissues in the mesendoderm. For many years, it was thought that the default fate of epiblast cells was to become epidermal, and that a specific signal was
required to change the fate of epiblast cells from epidermal to
neural. It is now clear that the default fate of epiblast cells is to
become neural, but expression of a widely distributed transforming growth factor, Bmp4, signals the change to an epidermal
fate. The role of the organizer is to block the Bmp4 signal. The
organizer cells lie along the axial midline of the embryo. They
express a number of genes, such as *Nog*, *Fst*, and *Chrd*, that have
the capacity to block Bmp4 activity. The genes produce secreted
molecules that signal cells in the axial epiblast layer. This signaling process establishes the primitive neurectoderm, the progenitor cells of the CNS.

- The activity of Bmp4 antagonists creates a dorsal-to-ventral gradient of Bmp4 within the embryo. Bmp4 signaling is weakest in
dorsal regions and strongest in ventral regions. This patterning is
important for brain development, but it is also critical for the development of other organ systems. Organ systems that are derived from mesodermal germ tissue are sensitive to concentrations of Bmp4. Thus the establishment of the Bmp4 gradient
allows for differentiation of mesodermal tissue into different
organ types. The migration of cells to form the deeper embryonic layers and the vertical signaling between the mesendoderm
and epiblast layer establish the early dorsal-ventral organization
of the embryo. During this time, asymmetrical patterns of gene
expression also establish the initial right-left axis of organization.

- The early anterior-posterior patterning of the gastrula embryo is
also critical for the establishment of the CNS. Members of the
Wnt family of secreted molecules play a central role in establishing the anterior-posterior axis of the embryo. *Wnts* are expressed in the chordamesoderm and are widely dispersed
throughout the anterior-posterior extent of the embryo. As was
the case with Bmp4, Wnt antagonists expressed in the organizer
create a gradient of Wnts along the anterior-posterior axis of the

embryo that gives rise to different neural cell lines. However, the expression patterns are somewhat more complex for the *Wnt* antagonists. Just before the onset of gastrulation, a structure derived from extraembryonic tissue, the AVE, is present in the anterior endoderm of the embryo. The AVE appears to establish the early anterior fate of the epiblast cells by expressing genes that block posteriorizing signals. This structure is displaced outside the embryo with the migration of cells from the organizer. Later in development, cells in the pharyngeal endoderm and prechordal plate mesoderm express the Wnt antagonists, thus preserving the anterior fate of the anterior neurectodermal cells.

- Thus both the initial specification of neurectodermal cells and their subspecification into cell types appropriate for different levels of the neuraxis derive from the establishment of two orthogonal gradients of secreted proteins. The gradients are the product of a complex set of gene interactions that have been greatly simplified here for clarity. The organization that emerges at the end of the third embryonic week sets the stage for the next major event in brain development, the emergence of the neural tube.

- Formation of the three-layered neural plate is the primary outcome of the process of gastrulation. Along the axial midline of the ectodermal layer of the trilaminar disc are the neurectodermal cells, the neural progenitor cells. With the closure of the neural tube, these cells will form a single layer at the center of the tube that will become the neural proliferative zone. Most of the cells of the CNS will be produced in this region.

## References

Bachiller, D., J. Klingensmith, C. Kemp, J. A. Belo, R. M. Anderson, S. R. May, J. A. McMahon, A. P. McMahon, R. M. Harland, J. Rossant, and E. M. De Robertis. 2000. "The organizer factors Chordin and Noggin are required for mouse forebrain development." *Nature*, 403: 658–661.

Beddington, R. S., and E. J. Robertson. 1998. "Anterior patterning in mouse." *Trends in Genetics*, 14: 277–284.

Brown, M., R. Keynes, and A. Lumsden. 2001. *The developing brain*. Oxford: Oxford University Press.

Gilbert, S. F. 2006. *Developmental biology.* 8th ed. Sunderland, MA: Sinauer Associates.

Gunhaga, L., M. Marklund, M. Sjodal, J. C. Hsieh, T. M. Jessell, and T. Edlund. 2003. "Specification of dorsal telencephalic character by sequential Wnt and FGF signaling." *Nature Neuroscience,* 6: 701–707.

Hahn, J. S., and L. L. Plawner. 2004. "Evaluation and management of children with holoprosencephaly." *Pediatric Neurology,* 31: 79–88.

Hayhurst, M., and S. K. McConnell. 2003. "Mouse models of holoprosencephaly." *Current Opinion in Neurology,* 16: 135–141.

Hemmati-Brivanlou, A., and D. Melton. 1997a. "Vertebrate embryonic cells will become nerve cells unless told otherwise." *Cell,* 88: 13–17.

———. 1997b. "Vertebrate neural induction." *Annual Review of Neuroscience,* 20: 43–60.

Hemmati-Brivanlou, A., and G. H. Thomsen. 1995. "Ventral mesodermal patterning in Xenopus embryos: Expression patterns and activities of BMP-2 and BMP-4." *Developmental Genetics,* 17: 78–89.

Kiecker, C., and C. Niehrs. 2001. "A morphogen gradient of Wnt/beta-catenin signalling regulates anteroposterior neural patterning in Xenopus." *Development,* 128: 4189–4201.

Kinsman, S. L., L. L. Plawner, and J. S. Hahn. 2000. "Holoprosencephaly: Recent advances and new insights." *Current Opinion in Neurology,* 13: 127–132.

McLaren, A. 2003. "Primordial germ cells in the mouse." *Developmental Biology,* 262: 1–15.

Menkes, J. H., H. B. Sarnat, and B. L. Maria, eds. 2006. *Child neurology.* 7th ed. Philadelphia: Lippincott Williams & Wilkins.

Nieuwkoop, P. D., E. C. Boterenbrood, A. Kremer, F. F. S. N. Bloemsma, E. L. M. J. Hoessels, G. Meyer, and F. J. Verheyen. 1952. "Activation and organization of the central nervous system in amphibians. Part III. Synthesis of a new working hypothesis." *Journal of Experimental Zoology,* 120: 83–108.

Oelgeschlager, M., H. Kuroda, B. Reversade, and E. M. De Robertis. 2003. "Chordin is required for the Spemann organizer transplantation phenomenon in Xenopus embryos." *Developmental Cell,* 4: 219–230.

Ohkubo, Y., C. Chiang, and J. L. Rubenstein. 2002. "Coordinate regulation and synergistic actions of BMP4, SHH and FGF8 in the rostral prosencephalon regulate morphogenesis of the telencephalic and optic vesicles." *Neuroscience,* 111: 1–17.

Palis, J., and M. C. Yoder. 2001. "Yolk-sac hematopoiesis: The first blood cells of mouse and man." *Experimental Hematology,* 29: 927–936.

Plawner, L. L., M. R. Delgado, V. S. Miller, E. B. Levey, S. L. Kinsman, A. J. Barkovich, E. M. Simon, N. J. Clegg, V. T. Sweet, E. E. Stashinko, and

J. S. Hahn. 2002. "Neuroanatomy of holoprosencephaly as predictor of function: Beyond the face predicting the brain." *Neurology*, 59: 1058–1066.

Robb, L., and P. P. Tam. 2004. "Gastrula organiser and embryonic patterning in the mouse." *Seminars in Cell and Developmental Biology*, 15: 543–554.

Sadler, T. W. 2006. *Langman's medical embryology*. 10th ed. Philadelphia: Lippincott Williams & Wilkins.

Simeone, A., and D. Acampora. 2001. "The role of Otx2 in organizing the anterior patterning in mouse." *International Journal of Developmental Biology*, 45: 337–345.

Spemann, H., and H. Mangold. 1924. "Über Induktion von Embryonalanlagen durch Implantation artfremder Organisatoren." *Roux' Archiv für Entwicklungsmechanik*, 100: 599–638.

Stern, C. D. 2001. "Initial patterning of the central nervous system: How many organizers?" *Nature Reviews Neuroscience*, 2: 92–98.

Tam, P. P., and K. A. Steiner. 1999. "Anterior patterning by synergistic activity of the early gastrula organizer and the anterior germ layer tissues of the mouse embryo." *Development*, 126: 5171–5179.

Tiedemann, H., M. Asashima, H. Grunz, and W. Knochel. 2001. "Pluripotent cells (stem cells) and their determination and differentiation in early vertebrate embryogenesis." *Development, Growth and Differentiation*, 43: 469–502.

Urist, M. R. 1965. "Bone: Formation by autoinduction." *Science*, 150: 893–899.

Yamaguchi, T. P. 2001. "Heads or tails: Wnts and anterior-posterior patterning." *Current Biology*, 11: R713–R724.

Yamamoto, Y., and M. Oelgeschlager. 2004. "Regulation of bone morphogenetic proteins in early embryonic development." *Naturwissenschaften*, 91: 519–534.

# FOUR

# Formation of the Neural Tube

THE NEURAL TUBE is the embryonic structure from which the central nervous system (CNS) develops. The formation of the neural tube involves a process called neurulation. Neurulation actually begins with the induction of the neural progenitor cells during gastrulation, but the major morphological changes involved in tube formation begin approximately 18 days after conception and are complete by E28. The onset of neurulation is marked by the formation of two longitudinal ridges that run along the anterior-posterior midline of the flat, three-layered embryonic disc. The ridges are formed from the neurecto-dermal cells on the surface of the disc. Over the course of several days, the ridges fold over and fuse to form a hollow tube. The neural progenitor cells, the cells that will give rise to the CNS, line the center of the tube. With the closure of the neural tube, the basic, three-dimensional shape of the embryo has become well defined. Neurulation, in concert with the earlier processes surrounding gastrulation, provides the foundation of all further milestones in brain development. Gastrulation and neurulation are so basic that the failure of either of these complex events can cause serious neural defects or in the most extreme cases can compromise the viability of the organism.

Although the basic organization of the embryo is evident by the end of neurulation, over the next month, the embryo undergoes rapid growth. At the end of neurulation, the average embryonic length is 3 to 5 mm, and by the end of the eighth week of development it grows to 27 to 31 mm, nearly a tenfold increase. Accompanying this growth are significant changes in the shape and organization of the fetus and specifically of the developing brain. The second part of this chapter will examine change in the overall morphology of the embryo, providing a kind of macroanalytic look at the major changes that take place during this period. It will begin with an examination of the changing shape of the developing nervous system, focusing on the differentiation of the primary brain vesicles, or neural subdivisions. The emergence of the primary vesicles is accompanied by a very dramatic expansion of the brain region of the embryo. The processes that underlie that rapid expansion will also be considered. The final macroanalytic topic will be the changing morphology of the whole embryo and the relationship of the developing neural system to the other body systems. This very brief discussion will not cover the emergence of specific nonneural systems in any depth; rather, it is intended to place the brain in its developmental context.

## Neurulation: The Emergence of the Embryonic Nervous System

Neurulation is the set of events that begins in late gastrulation with the formation of the neural plate and culminates with the generation of the primitive nervous system structure called the neural tube. Neurulation is typically divided into two sets of processes described as primary neurulation and secondary neurulation. During primary neurulation, neurectodermal cells give rise to the portions of the embryonic neural tube from which the brain and most of the spinal column (to the level of the sacrum in the very low back) will develop. Because the development of most of the CNS depends on primary neurulation, this chapter will focus on those processes. Secondary neurulation involves formation of the remainder of the neural tube that will give rise to the most caudal segment of the spinal column, including most of the sacral and all of the coccygeal regions (Copp, Greene, and Murdoch 2003). The structures that arise during secondary neurulation are derived from a type of mesodermal tissue, the mesenchyme, rather than ectodermal cells, and the process of tube formation is quite different from that of primary neurulation. The cells that will form the caudal portion of the tube first coalesce into a solid core that then hollows out to form a central lumen, or canal. In humans, primary neurulation begins on approximately E18 and is complete by E28. Secondary neurulation begins as primary neurulation ends and extends until the seventh week of gestation (Gos and Szpecht-Potocka 2002), at which point the two parts of the tube fuse to form a single structure.

There are four basic processes involved in primary neurulation: (1) formation of the neural plate, (2) shaping of the neural plate, (3) bending of the neural plate, and (4) closure of the neural tube (Colas and Schoenwolf 2001; Copp, Greene, and Murdoch 2003; Gilbert 2006; O'Rahilly and Müller 2002). The formation of the neural plate involves the neural inductive processes that occur during gastrulation. These processes were discussed at length in the last chapter. The remaining three processes reshape the flat, three-layered embryonic plate into a closed cylinder with a hollow center that is referred to as the lumen. After tube closure, the neurectodermal cells line the center of the tube and form a region called the ventricular zone. The layer of neurecto-dermal cells is initially surrounded by concentric layers of mesodermal and then epidermal ectodermal cells. Cells in the neurectodermal layer are the neural progenitors that, over the next few months, will produce all the cells that make up the CNS.

## Shaping of the Neural Plate

The neural plate is made up of cells called neuroblasts that are collec-tively referred to as the neuroepithelium. The first step in the shaping of the neural plate involves the elongation of the neuroblast cells. This happens at the end of gastrulation and results in a thickening of the plate (Colas and Schoenwolf 2001). When the plate is initially formed, it has a "spadelike" shape of roughly equal length and breadth when viewed dorsally (Figure 4.1A). Just before the tube begins to form, the embryo begins to elongate through a process called convergent exten-sion. During convergent extension, neuroblast cells move toward the midline of the neural plate and become interleaved, or intercalated, with one another (Figure 4.1C). A similar process occurs at the same time in the underlying mesoderm. The result is the elongation and nar-rowing of the neural plate (Figures 4.1A, 4.1B). The narrowing of the neural plate is a necessary part of neural tube formation. Mice with gene mutations that interfere with the genetic pathway that controls convergent extension have abnormally wide neural plates that disrupt neural tube closure (Wallingford 2004).

## Bending of the Neural Plate

Bending of the neural plate begins while shaping is still ongoing. Bending begins in humans on approximately E19 with the elevation of two neural folds of tissue (Figure 4.2A). The two neural folds rise up on either side of the midline of the neural plate, extending along the anterior-posterior axis. The elevation of the folds creates a central neural groove that will eventually form the center of the closed tube (Figure 4.2B). Recent studies suggest that the specific mechanism that brings about the bending differs at different levels of the CNS (Copp, Greene, and Murdoch 2003). Within regions of the neural plate that will become the spinal column, three inflection points located at the base and sides of the neural groove control bending. Within regions that will form the brain, expansion of the underlying mesodermal tissue induces bending.

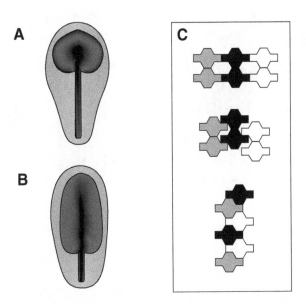

Figure 4.1. The changing shape of the embryo during neural tube formation. A. The plate begins as a "spadelike" structure of equal length and breadth (dorsal view). B. As the tube begins to form, the embryo elongates. C. During convergent extension, neuroblast cells intercalate to form a more compact layer.

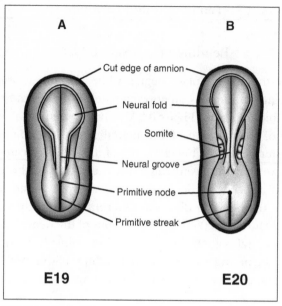

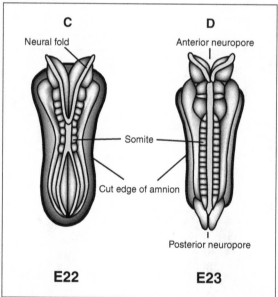

Figure 4.2. Closure of the neural tube. A. Closure of the neural tube begins with the elevation of the neural folds that run along the anterior-posterior midline axis of the embryo. B. By E20, the central portion of the fold begins to come together, and the first somites appear. C. Fusion of the neural tube begins in central regions and extends toward both anterior and posterior regions. D. The last regions of the neural tube to fuse are the anterior neuropore (E25) and the posterior neuropore (E28).

At the middle level of the spinal column, bending is initiated with the formation of the median hinge point. The median hinge point overlies the notochord and the prechordal plate and runs for most of the extent of the spinal column (Colas and Schoenwolf 2001). The notochord induces the median hinge point cells to become wedge shaped, thus forming an anchor point for the base of the neural groove (Figure 4.3A).

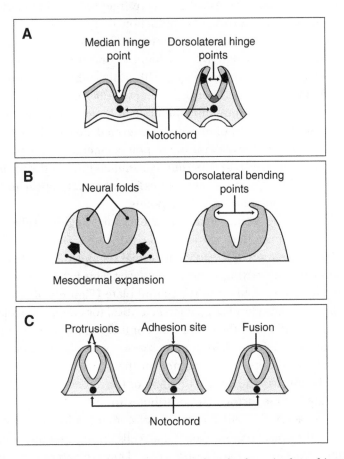

Figure 4.3. Bending the neural tube. A. Bending in the spinal cord involves the median hinge points at the base of the neural tube. Bending of the elevated portion occurs at the two dorsolateral hinge points. B. Bending in the cranial regions involves expansion of the underlying mesodermal layer, which results in folding and bulging of the neural plate. C. The neural tube fuses at the tips of the folds. (From Copp, Greene, and Murdoch 2003. Adapted with the permission of Nature Publishing Group.)

Bending of the elevated portion of each neural fold is accomplished by formation of a dorsolateral hinge point. Within each fold, the dorsolateral hinge point forms near the point of contact between the neural plate and the rest of the ectoderm. Each is anchored to the ectoderm, and like the median hinge point cells, the cells of the dorsol lateral hinge points change their shape and become wedgelike. At the upper levels of the spinal cord, where the spinal cord converges with the brain, only the median hinge point forms. The induction of the dorsolateral hinge points is controlled by the concentration of Shh. *Shh* is expressed from the notochord in a gradient, with the highest concentration at the upper spinal levels. In high concentrations, Shh inhibits the formation of the dorsolateral hinge points (Ybot-Gonzalez et al. 2002). Thus in the upper levels of the spinal column, only the median hinge point is evident. As the concentration of Shh diminishes at intermediate spinal levels of the spinal column, the dorsolateral hinge points emerge. Local release of Shh in lower spine levels in experimental animals inhibits the formation of dorsolateral hinge points. *Shh* expression does not appear to be involved in induction of median hinge points.

Bending of the neural plate in the cranial regions relies on a different mechanism than in the spinal cord (Copp, Greene, and Murdoch 2003). Elevation of the folds in cranial regions is preceded by expansion of the underlying mesodermal layer. This expansion causes a bulging and then a folding of the neural plate (Figure 4.3B). This expansion of the mesoderm appears to be critical for cranial neurulation. Mice with mutations of the genes that control expansion of the mesodermal tissue (*Twist* or *Cart1*) have serious cranial, but not spinal, neural tube disorders. The next step in the formation of the cranial neural tube involves the inward bending of the upper edges of the fold (Figure 4.3C). One factor that contributes to the bending is the contraction of actin microfilaments in cells. Actin microfilaments are present in the apical regions (top) of all cells throughout the neuroepithelium (Ybot-Gonzalez and Copp 1999). They are part of the cell's cytoskeleton, and, therefore, one of their functions is to support the cell's shape. The contraction of actin microfilaments in the apex of a cell changes the cell's shape from a cube to a wedge. When contraction occurs in a sheet of cells, the shape of the whole structure can change. Actin microfilament contraction has long been associated with bending within the neural tube and particularly within cranial regions, but the gene that controls actin contraction has only recently been identified (Haigo et al. 2003). Mice with a mutation of the *Shroom* gene exhibit anencephaly, a catastrophic loss of forebrain structures that results from failure of the rostral end of the neural tube to close. Injection of Shroom antagonists on one side of the embryo causes unilateral failure of bending. *Shroom* is expressed in the neural plate just before tube closure. The concentration is low throughout most of the plate, except in cranial regions undergoing bending. The mechanism for selective up-regulation of expression at these sites is not understood, but may be related to either *Shh* or *Lim2* expression (Martin 2004).

A second factor that contributes to cranial bending is naturally occurring cell death, or apoptosis. Apoptosis is distinct from necrotic, or pathological, cell death and is an important factor in later brain development, where it serves to regulate the size and organization of cell populations (Oppenheim 1991). Apoptosis is observed in dorsolateral regions of the cranial plate at the time of cranial bending (Copp, Greene, and Murdoch 2003) and is thought to facilitate the secondary bending at the top of the tube. In mice with mutations that either increase or decrease cell death, tube closure is disrupted. Finally, proliferation of the neuroblast cells themselves may contribute to cranial bending. Throughout the period of neural tube formation, the neuroblast cells proliferate, steadily increasing the number of neural progenitor cells. Genetic mutations that either result in excessive proliferation or reduce the number of dividing cells disturb the process of neural tube closure.

## Closure of the Neural Tube

The last step in the formation of the neural tube is the fusion of the tissues at the tips of the neural folds. At the tips of the folds, a neurectodermal cell layer lies immediately adjacent to and below the surface ectodermal layer. Fingerlike cellular protrusions on the tips of the two opposing folds, called lamellipodia, contact each other and become interleaved, fusing the folds on the two sides of the emerging tube (Figure 4.3C). The cells of the surface ectoderm fuse first, followed by the neurectodermal cells (Finnell et al. 2002). The two layers remain adjacent for a period of time and then are separated by an intervening mesodermal cell layer. Some of the observed cell death in the dorsal region of the newly closed tube may serve to separate the layers and allow for the establishment of continuous and independent sheets of the ectodermal and neurectodermal cells, along with the eventual intervening layer of mesodermal cells.

## Fusion of the Neural Tube

The sequence of neural tube fusion has been described in a number of species. For many years, data from avian species served as the model. Fusion of the avian neural tube begins at the level of the future midbrain and proceeds both rostrally (toward the head) and caudally (toward the tail) in a process that has been described as "zipping up" the neural tube in two directions. Tube closure in rostral regions precedes closure in caudal regions. In avians, the openings at the two ends of the tube, referred to as the anterior and posterior neuropores, are the last sites to fuse. Fusion of the neuropores completes the closure of the neural tube.

Recent work with mammalian species, especially the mouse, suggests a more complex pattern of neural tube fusion. The neural tube in mice forms between E8 and E10 (Finnell et al. 2002). A number of studies have identified at least four closure sites in mouse models (Finnell et al. 2002): a cervical site, which is consistent with the principal cervical site described in the avian model, a second cervical closure point just rostral to the first, a site at the junction of the midbrain and the hindbrain, and one at the most rostral end near the anterior neuropore. Evidence for this multisite-closure model in a mammalian species suggested that the pattern of closure for humans may also be more complex than previously thought (Golden and Chernoff 1995; Juriloff and Harris 2000; Van Allen et al. 1993). This was of considerable clinical interest because it was thought that the multisite model might better explain patterns of neural tube defects (NTDs) in human populations. NTDs are a common human birth defect, but the cause of the disorders is not well understood. NTDs occur at different levels within the nervous system and result in different specific disorders. Failure of anterior neuropore closure results in very serious cranial NTDs such as anencephaly; NTDs associated with more posterior failures of closure include spina bifida (Nakatsu, Uwabe, and Shiota 2000; also see the section "Clinical Correlation" in this chapter).

Two recent studies, though not completely consistent with each other, have provided further insight into the process of human neural tube closure. The first study identified two fusion points (O'Rahilly and Müller 1987). The first (termed α) was found near the somite pairs that develop earliest, somites 2–3, and the second site (β) was at the rostralmost tip of the embryo. Fusion from site α proceeds caudally toward the posterior neuropore and rostrally toward the anterior neuropore, while fusion from site β proceeds caudally, approaching the wave of fusion from site α (Figure 4.4). A second study by Nakatsu and colleagues (2000) identified fusion sites in positions roughly comparable with sites α and β (in this model these sites are called A and C), but also reported an additional site, B, between A and C (Figure 4.4). A and C had fusion patterns similar to those of the other study. Fusion from site B extended both rostrally and caudally, and the fusion of tissue between sites A and B occurred very early, well in advance of the

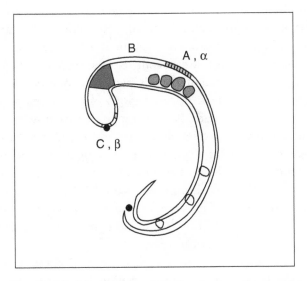

Figure 4.4. Two models of human neural tube closure. One model posits two fusion sites, α and β. The other includes two points that correspond to the first model, here called A and C, but also includes a third, intermediate point, B. In both models the anterior neuropore closes (E25) before the caudal neuropore (E28). (From O'Rahilly and Müller 2002. Adapted with the permission of John Wiley & Sons.)

closure of either the anterior or the posterior neuropore. Although
these studies are not entirely consistent, they suggest that a modified
version of the zipper model may best describe the progress of neural
tube closure in humans. A bidirectional wave of fusion extends from
either one or two sites just rostral to the cervical region of the neural
plate. The wave of fusion proceeds rostrally and meets a caudally proceeding wave of fusion emanating from the fusion site at the rostral tip
of the embryo. Fusion of the caudal extent of the tube proceeds from
the original fusion site ($\alpha$ or A) to the posterior neuropore. Finally,
closure of the anterior and posterior neuropores completes the process of tube closure. The anterior neuropore closes on approximately
E25, and the posterior neuropore on E28 (see Figure 4.2D for the sites
of the neuropores just before closure).

## New Structures and Cell Lines
## That Emerge during Neurulation

In addition to the actual creation of the neural tube, two other important embryonic features emerge during neurulation. They are the establishment of a new class of cells, the neural crest cells, and the formation of an important but transient set of structures that guide the
development of the segmented body plan, the somites. Neural crest
cells originate in the most dorsal regions of the developing neural
tube along its entire length. A wide range of structures are derived
from neural crest cells, including the peripheral nervous system,
endocrine system structures, pigment producing cells, facial bone and
cartilage, smooth muscle, fatty tissue of the head and neck, and connective tissue of the eye, mouth, and skin. The cranial neural crest
cells migrate away from their point of origin to targeted regions of the
head before closure of the tube, while those in the spinal cord migrate
to targets in the trunk after tube closure.

Somites form out of mesodermal tissue located lateral to the notochord. At the beginning of tube formation, the notochord extends
from the base of the head region to the most caudal extent of the
neural plate. As the neural folds begin to appear, the mesodermal
tissue adjacent to the notochord begins to segregate into blocks of cells
called somites (Gilbert 2006). In humans, the first somites appear near
the rostral end of the notochord on approximately E20. They develop

as paired structures flanking the notochord on both sides (Figures 4.2B, 4.2C, 4.2D). New pairs of somites develop at the rate of approximately 3 per day through E30, yielding a total of 42–44 somite pairs (Larsen 2001). The most caudal somites disappear quickly, leaving a total of approximately 37 somite pairs in humans. Somites are transient embryonic structures that help define the segmented portion of the nervous system (the hindbrain and spinal column). They serve to guide migrating neural crest cells and the spinal nerve axons. In addition, they give rise to cells that form vertebrae and ribs, as well as skin and skeletal muscles of the back and muscles of the body trunk and limbs.

## Rapid Growth and Morphologic Change after Neural Tube Closure

This section examines large-scale changes in the size and shape of the developing embryo as the second month of gestation begins. Two kinds of change will be considered. The first is the emerging differentiation of the neural tube into the classically defined embryonic subdivisions. The neural tube first divides into three subdivisions called the primary vesicles. Then the primary vesicles further subdivide into the five secondary vesicles. This process of partitioning is accompanied by the rapid expansion of the anterior regions of the brain, which presages the rapid growth of the brain that will occur in the upcoming months. As this major partitioning of the embryo proceeds, other changes are also occurring that alter the shape and organization of both the embryo and the extraembryonic structures that support the embryo. These changes are quite dramatic but in some ways not intuitive, making it hard to visualize the rapidly changing morphology of the embryo. The human embryo begins as a flat disc and morphs into a complex three-dimensional structure that contains all the organ systems of the body. Attempting to track these changes within the context of a single system, such as the CNS, can be difficult. Placing the CNS changes within the context of changes in other body systems makes the CNS changes easier to follow. The second part of this section will attempt to place the changes in the CNS within the context of changes in other embryonic systems and in extraembryonic structures. The intent is not to discuss the development of nonneural systems in any depth, but to provide a guide for understanding and contextualizing anatomical changes in the CNS.

## Differentiation of the Neural Tube

Early in neurulation, the shape of the developing neural tube along the anterior-posterior axis is comparatively uniform. However, before the closure of the anterior neuropore (E25), the anterior end of the tube begins to change in shape, expanding rapidly to form the three primary vesicles. Vesicle is a general anatomical term describing a structure that forms a pouch. In the case of the primary vesicles, it refers to the three anatomical subdivisions that emerge along the anterior-posterior axis within the anterior region of the neural tube (Figure 4.5A). The most anterior of these embryonic vesicles is called the prosencephalon and is the embryonic precursor of future forebrain structures. The middle vesicle is the mesencephalon and is the precursor of midbrain structures. The most posterior is the rhombencephalon and will become the hindbrain.

The rapid expansion of the anterior neural tube is not the product of a sudden increase in the amount of neural tissue being generated in those regions. Rather, it comes about by the stretching or inflation of the central cavity of the anterior tube. At approximately the time of anterior neuropore closure, a portion of the lumen, or central opening of the tube, becomes completely occluded for a brief period of time. A section of the tube extending from approximately the third to the ninth somite, or approximately 60 percent of the length of the tube, collapses on itself, completely blocking the movement of fluid within the tube (Desmond 1982; Desmond and Levitan 2002). Fluid rapidly builds up in the anterior portion of the tube, and the pressure causes it to balloon out. The occlusion is temporary, and by approximately E30 it is no longer evident. The temporary blockage and accumulation of fluids account for the rapid expansion of anterior brain regions during the formation of the primary and secondary vesicles.

The three primary vesicles further subdivide into the five secondary brain vesicles. This comes about by the partitioning of two of the primary vesicles (Figure 4.5B). The prosencephalon divides into the telencephalon and the diencephalon, and the rhombencephalon divides into the metencephalon and the myelencephalon. The mesencephalon does not further divide. These five subdivisions are aligned along the anterior-posterior axis of the embryo and establish the primary organization of the CNS. Table 4.1 provides a summary of the major derivatives of each of the secondary vesicles. The major derivatives of the telencephalon are the cerebral hemispheres and the basal ganglia. Important diencepalic structures include the thalamus and the hypothalamus. The mesencephalon contains the fiber tracts as they extend between the brain and the spinal column. The metencephalon will give rise to the pons and the cerebellum, and the myelencephalon will produce the medulla. At the center of each of these vesicles, the hollow opening of the neural tube will be transformed to become a part of the interconnected network of ventricles. The ventricles are filled with cerebrospinal fluid. The ventricles associated with each of the secondary vesicles are indicated in Table 4.1.

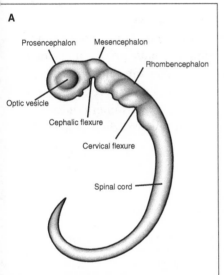

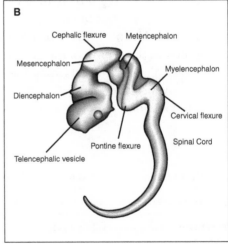

Figure 4.5. A. The primary vesicles are the three initial anatomical subdivisions. They are aligned along the anterior-posterior axis of the embryo. The most anterior is the prosencephalon, which is the embryonic precursor of the forebrain. The middle is the mesencephalon, which is the precursor of midbrain structures, and the most posterior is the rhombencephalon, which will become the hindbrain. B. Secondary vesicles emerge from the primary vesicles. The prosencephalon divides into the telencephalon and the diencephalon, and the rhombencephalon divides into the metencephalon and myelencephalon.

With the formation of the primary and secondary vesicles, the developing neuraxis also begins to bend quite dramatically in three regions (Figure 4.5B). The first bend, or flexure, occurs at the time of primary vesicle differentiation in the region of the midbrain. This flexure, which is called the cephalic flexure, results in a pronounced downward bending of the most rostral regions of the embryo. The second flexure arises somewhat later, after the secondary vesicles have differentiated in anterior regions but before the rhombencephalic differentiation emerges. This flexure again entails a downward bending of the tube, but here it is in the more posterior regions and is thus referred to as the cervical flexure. The final flexure bends the embryo in the opposite direction to the first two flexures, folds the rhombencephalon in the region of what will become the junction of the pons and the medulla, and is called the pontine flexure.

The rapid anterior expansion of the CNS observed during the formation of the primary and secondary vesicles presages the later expansion of those regions. Between the second month of gestation and birth, the anterior brain regions undergo dramatic growth and development. Much of this expansion occurs within the telencephalic region with the growth of the cerebral hemispheres. However, unlike the earlier phase of neural expansion during the establishment of the primary vesicles, growth of the cerebral hemispheres does reflect the rapid addition of neural tissue.

Table 4.1  Primary and secondary subdivisions of the neural tube

| Primary Vesicle | Secondary Vesicle | Mature Derivatives | Central Cavity |
| --- | --- | --- | --- |
| Prosencephalon | Telencephalon | Cerebral cortex Basal ganglia Basal forebrain | Lateral ventricles |
| | Diencephalon | Thalamus Hypothalamus | Third ventricle |
| Mesencephalon | Mesencephalon | Midbrain-Tectum | Cerebral aqueduc |
| Rhombencephalon | Metencephalon | Hindbrain pons, cerebellum | Fourth ventricle |
| | Myelencephalon | Medulla | Fourth ventricle |
| Spinal cord | Spinal cord | Spinal cord | Central canal |

## Changing Shape of the Embryo

Changes in the shape and organization of the CNS happen in the context of other changes occurring throughout the embryo and in the extraembryonic tissue. When the nervous system is considered in isolation, it can be difficult to appreciate how the changing neural morphology fits with changes in other body systems. This section will consider both changes in the organization of the surrounding extraembryonic tissues and changes in the nonneural embryonic tissues (see also Kostovic and Rakic 1990 for review).

During the first month postconception, all the cell lines that will give rise to the embryo are generated. In addition, the progenitor cells for a number of important extraembryonic structures also differentiate. The epiblast cells of the bilaminar disc give rise to the amnion. The amniotic cavity initially sits dorsal to the embryonic disc (Figure 4.6, E13), but by the beginning of the second month postconception the amniotic cavity surrounds and insulates the developing embryo (Figure 4.7A). Hypoblast cells give rise to the connecting stalk and the yolk sac. Early in development, the connecting stalk is the embryo's anchor to the tissues that line the wall of the uterus; later it will lengthen and form part of the umbilical cord. The yolk sac is an important structure during the early embryonic period. It transports and metabolizes serum proteins and macromolecules derived from the mother. It is also the source of red blood cells in the early embryonic period, and it provides the mechanism for blood circulation. The chorion develops from two cell types, hypoblast cells and trophoblast cells (cells that surrounded the inner cell mass just before the onset of gastrulation). The chorion attaches to the wall of the uterus and forms the embryonic component of the placenta; the maternal component is formed of endometrial cells of the uterine wall.

At the onset of gastrulation (E13), primitive versions of extraembryonic structures can be seen (Figure 4.6). The amniotic cavity has formed dorsal to the embryonic bilaminar disc, and the yolk sac has formed ventral to it. The embryo is attached to the uterine wall tissue by the connecting stalk. In addition, the primitive trophoblast (two layers) and hypoblast cells have begun to line the uterine wall, and they will later form the chorion. This developing chorion encircles the structure comprising the embryonic amniotic cavity, the embryonic disc, and the yolk sac. The space between the outer emerging chorion and the inner embryonic structure is called the chorionic cavity (Figure 4.7A shows the chorionic cavity at E30).

By E25, much of neurulation is complete (Figure 4.6), and the embryo has begun to acquire its characteristic pattern of flexure. As the embryo bends, the surrounding amniotic cavity also begins to surround the embryo, and the top of the yolk sac begins to contract. The connecting stalk has moved toward the gut regions of the embryo. The major vessels of the future umbilical cord, two arteries and one vein, form within the stalk. By E30, the primary and secondary vesicles are visible, and flexure of the neural tube has advanced (Figure 4.6). The amniotic cavity surrounds most of the embryo except for the region of the connecting stalk and the mouth of the yolk sac.

Looking at the development of the embryo relative to the immediately adjacent embryonic and extraembryonic tissue gives a sense of how the initially layered and disc-shaped structure can change and fold into a complex, nested three-dimensional organism. To get a

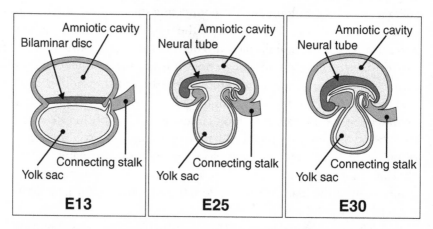

Figure 4.6. The changing shape of the embryo between E13 and E30. The embryo begins as a disc and gradually becomes elaborated and folded to the characteristic shape of the human fetus. The neural tube structures form the dorsal surface of the embryo, and the head and brain form from the most anterior structures of the neural tube. Ventral to the neural tube structures are the tissues that will give rise to the gut and organ systems. During the embryonic period, the yolk sac forms ventral to the embryonic structures.

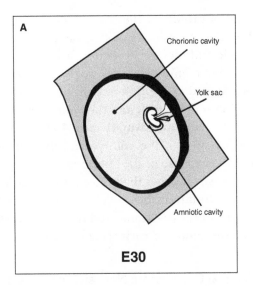

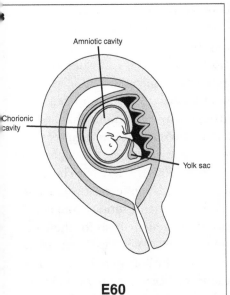

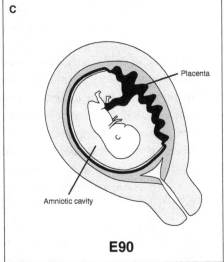

Figure 4.7. The changing shape and size of the embryo between E30 and E90. A. By E30, the embryo is 3–5 mm in length, and the chorionic cavity is larger than the amniotic cavity. B. By E60, the amniotic cavity is larger than the chorionic cavity, and the embryo has grown to 25–30 mm. C. By E90, the fetus is 70–80 mm long, and the amniotic cavity has displaced the chorionic cavity.

sense of the rate of growth of the embryo during this time, and to make clear the relative positions of the embryo/fetus and the supporting embryonic and uterine structures, it is necessary to consider more distal extraembryonic structures, such as the chorion and the uterine wall. At the end of the first month, the embryo is quite small (approximately 5 mm in length), and the chorionic cavity is considerably larger than the amniotic cavity (Figure 4.7A). Over the next several weeks, the size of both the embryo and the amniotic cavity expands rapidly at the expense of the chorionic cavity (Figure 4.7B). By E60 the amniotic cavity is larger than the chorionic cavity, and the embryo has grown to 25 mm. By the end of the third month of gestation (E90), the fetus measures 70–80 mm, and the amniotic cavity has completely displaced the chorionic cavity (Figure 4.7C).

## Clinical Correlation: Neural Tube Defects

NTDs are caused by the failure of neural tube closure. They are among the most common human birth defects, second only to congenital cardiac defects. Serious NTDs affecting neural tissues are estimated to occur in 1 of 1,000 pregnancies worldwide. NTDs can cause several malformations and in the most severe cases can compromise viability. The risk of NTDs varies by ethnic and socioeconomic group, but they are frequent in all population subgroups. The rate is somewhat higher in females than in males, and the risk of recurrence in families with one affected pregnancy is heightened to approximately 3 to 8 percent for subsequent pregnancies (Mitchell et al. 2004). There have been reports of increased risk for second- and third-degree relatives. These findings point to a complex genetic basis for this serious congenital malformation, but little is known about the genetic basis for these defects in humans. In the mouse, more than 100 genes have been associated with failure of neural tube closure (Juriloff and Harris 2000; Mitchell et al. 2004). Specific mutations in mice appear to result in disorders specific to different levels of the neuraxis. Although this work is promising, very few human homologues of these genes have been studied, and no clear pattern of association between gene mutation and specific NTDs has been identified (Mitchell et al. 2004).

Although the epidemiological data from human studies suggest that family history is one of the stronger risk factors for NTDs, other factors

have been implicated as well. There is substantial evidence that inadequate levels of maternal folate during early pregnancy are strongly associated with the occurrence of NTDs. A wide range of studies have
shown that folic acid supplements (synthetic folate) can reduce the
risk of NTDs by as much as 70 percent if they are taken daily beginning
two months before conception and continuing throughout pregnancy
(Sadler 2006). These findings have led to widespread changes in government guidelines concerning recommended daily levels of dietary
folate that, when implemented effectively, have reduced the frequency
of NTDs significantly (Castilla et al. 2003; Ray and Blom 2003; Rosano
et al. 1999). They have also led to a focus on the role of folate metabolism pathway genes in NTDs. A large number of genes have been identified; some are associated with maternal and others with embryonic
factors. However, as yet no clear pattern of association between gene
defect and NTDs has been established (Mitchell et al. 2004).

Two other major factors that have been associated with increased risk
for NTDs are maternal diabetes and certain types of anticonvulsant
medications. Diabetic mothers have a twofold increase in the risk of
having a child with an NTD. This effect appears to be related to heightened blood glucose concentrations early in pregnancy, but it is not
clear how this affects neural tube closure. The metabolic pathway for
valproic acid, an anticonvulsant medication, is also not clear. However,
there is some evidence that it may interfere with folate metabolism. A
range of other factors have been implicated in NTDs, including obesity,
exposure to mycotoxins (toxic agents produced by some types of mold),
and elevated temperature from fever or external sources such as hot
tubs or saunas (Mitchell et al. 2004). The wide range of factors that
have been implicated in NTDs suggest a complex underlying developmental pathway that is not yet well defined.

## Types of Neural Tube Defects

Neural tube defects can occur at any level of the developing nervous
system. The resulting disorder varies in both type and severity depending on the level of the NTD. When the tube fails to close in the
most caudal regions, the resulting disorder is termed spina bifida.
Failure of closure in more rostral regions of the hindbrain and the
spinal column results in a disorder termed rachischisis. NTDs in the

region of the brain lead to anencephaly. Mouse models indicate that specific genetic mutations result in failure of tube closure at specific levels along the rostral-caudal axis of the developing nervous system, resulting in NTDs characteristic of one of these classes of disorder (Juriloff and Harris 2000).

## Spina Bifida

The term *spina bifida* is used to indicate a range of NTDs that affect spinal regions. The hallmark of spina bifida is failure of the vertebral arch to close (Sadler 2006). The vertebral arch is a bony structure that normally encloses the spinal cord on the dorsal side. The separation of the peaks of the arch exposes the underlying cord. In some cases, the neural tissue is further involved; in others, it is not (Figure 4.8). Spina bifida occulta is the least debilitating of the spinal NTDs. In spina bifida occulta, although the vertebral arch is open, the neural tissue is not directly involved (Figure 4.8A), and the NTD is covered with skin. The frequency of this defect is surprising, with estimates as high as 10 to 20 percent of the population (because they do not involve neural tissue, occurrences of spina bifida occulta are not usually included in the prevalence estimates for NTDs). Though there have been few systematic studies in this patient group, outcomes are generally considered to be good. However, there is some recent evidence of persistent difficulties with pain and incontinence (Verhoef et al. 2004). There may also be some problems with malformation of the spinal cord and nerve roots or localized doubling of the cord. Spina bifida cystica is a more serious NTD that does involve either neural tissue or the membranes that surround and protect the spinal cord, the meninges. When only the meninges protrude through the open vertebral arch, the defect is referred to as spina bifida with meningocele (Figure 4.8B). When both neural tissue and meninges protrude, it is called spina bifida with meningomyelocele (Figure 4.8C). Finally, in rare cases the effects on neural tissue are more significant. Spina bifida with rachischisis refers to cases where the neural tissue underlying the vertebral arch fails to fold and form that section of the neural tube (Figure 4.8D).

The great majority of spina bifida cystica cases, an estimated 95 percent, involve meningomyelocele; 5 percent involve meningocele (Menkes, Sarnat, and Maria 2006). The appearance of meningomyelocele is most often a saclike protrusion located at any point along the spinal column. The sac is usually covered by a thick membrane that is prone to tearing, which can result in both infection and leakage of cerebrospinal fluid. Most children with meningomyelocele have the Arnold-Chiari II malformation, in which the cerebellum extends through the foramen magnum, the opening in the base of the skull through which the spinal column extends. Because the cerebellum is

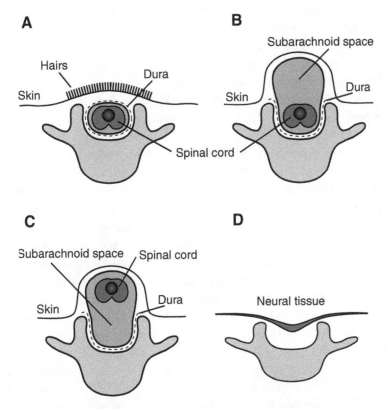

Figure 4.8. Types of neural tube disorders. A. In spina bifida occulta, the vertebral arch is open, but the neural tissue is not directly involved and the neural tube defect is covered with skin. B. In spina bifida cystica with meningocele, the meninges protrude outside the vertebral arch. C. In spina bifida cystica with meningomyelocele, both the meninges and neural tissue protrude. D. In spina bifida with rachischisis, the neural tissue fails to fold and the tube in that region does not form. (From Sadler 2006. Adapted with the permission of Lippincott Williams & Wilkins.)

drawn through the foramen magnum, the flow of cerebrospinal fluid (CSF) is blocked. CSF is a watery substance present in the ventricles, the open cavities in the center of the brain and spinal column. It is continuously produced in the ventricles and then reabsorbed, providing a continuous supply of fresh CSF. Blockage of CSF circulation can lead to a condition called hydrocephaly in which CSF builds up in the ventricles and is not reabsorbed. The accumulation of fluids can cause pressure to build in the brain, and that pressure can damage neural tissue. Hydrocephaly is a common complication of meningomyelocele. Finally, approximately 65 percent of children with meningomyelocele have dysgenesis of the corpus callosum. The corpus callosum is the large neural fiber bundle that connects the two cerebral hemispheres and allows for communication between the two sides of the brain. In children with meningomyelocele, the most anterior and posterior portions of the corpus callosum are typically missing (Fletcher, Barnes, and Dennis 2002).

Functional outcomes in children with meningomyelocele are associated with level of spinal lesion. Approximately 66 percent have severe motor handicaps such that by adolescence they depend upon wheelchairs. On measures of cognitive and linguistic functioning, children with meningomyelocele present a mixed profile with relative strengths and weaknesses, but there is also considerable individual variability. Level of function is highly associated with the anatomical position of the NTD. On standardized IQ measures, children typically perform better on verbal than performance subtests. They have difficulty with tasks that require focused attention and reconstructive memory. In areas of academic achievement, they have relative strengths in phonological decoding in reading, and fact retrieval in math but have difficulty with reading comprehension and execution of mathematical procedures. Their basic language skills are good. Their grammatical and lexical mastery is high, but they have difficulty with discourse-level pragmatics (Fletcher, Barnes, and Dennis 2002).

## Exencephaly and Anencephaly

A failure of neural tube closure in cerebral regions is referred to as exencephaly. In this condition, fetal forebrain development ceases to progress. The mesodermal tissues do not differentiate, and thus the skull fails to form, exposing the neural tissue to amniotic fluid (Copp, Greene, and Murdoch 2003; Gilbert 2006; Menkes and Sarnat 2000; Sadler 2006). The exposed neural tissue gradually degenerates, leading to a devastating condition known as anencephaly. The brainstem structures in these children can remain intact, and thus children are born alive, though they do not typically survive beyond early infancy. This condition is far more frequent in females than in males. There is no effective medical treatment.

## Diagnosis and Treatment

Serious NTDs involving an open malformation, such as meningomyelocele or anencephaly, can be diagnosed before birth by measuring levels of a substance called α-fetoprotein in both maternal blood and the amniotic fluid. α-fetoprotein is the major blood-serum protein produced in early embryonic life. It normally passes from fetal serum into fetal urine and then into the amniotic fluid, but concentrations outside the infant's body should remain relatively low. Elevated levels in either maternal blood or the amniotic fluid suggest the presence of an open neural-tube malformation. When high levels of α-fetoprotein are detected, confirmation of the NTD can be achieved through the use of ultrasonography (Mitchell et al. 2004).

It is common practice to surgically close spinal defects within 48 hours of birth. Closing of the defect does not reverse the neurological damage already present, but it appears to prevent further loss of function. With surgery, 87 percent of children with meningomyelocele survive one year and 78 percent survive into the teen years (Wong and Paulozzi 2001). However, approximately 80 percent of children operated on to close NTDs require subsequent ventricular shunt placement for hydrocephaly (Rintoul et al. 2002), thus underscoring the continuing neurological risk for the population. Recently, procedures have been developed to repair NTDs before birth. These involve opening the uterus and surgically closing the NTD lesion. Although the number of cases studied to date is not large, the results are promising. Rates of shunting in the prenatally operated group were approximately 43 to 54 percent, as compared to 80 percent in postnatally operated cases. However, larger and more systematic samples of children need to be studied before full evaluation of the procedure is possible (Mitchell et al. 2004).

In summary, NTDs are one of the most common human birth defects and constitute a major health risk worldwide. The origin of these disorders is not well understood, but progress is being made in a number of different areas. The most important prevention tool to date has been the introduction of dietary folic acid. Where this policy has been implemented by adding it to staple food products, the frequency of NTDs has been significantly reduced. Treatment of NTDs has also advanced. The introduction of new surgical procedures has improved the prognosis substantially. A number of large studies of cognitive development in this population are also under way. Work on the genetics of NTDs is complicated, but the number of animal models has increased dramatically in the past 10 years, and these promise to be an important tool in deciphering the complex genetic interactions that contribute to this devastating neurodevelopmental disorder.

## Chapter Summary

- As discussed in the last chapter, formation of the three-layered neural plate is the primary outcome of the process of gastrulation. Along the axial midline of the ectodermal layer of the trilaminar neural plate are the neurectodermal cells, the neural progenitor cells. With the closure of the neural tube, these cells will form a single layer at the center of the tube that will become the neural proliferative zone. Most of the cells of the CNS will be produced in this region.
- The process of neurulation refers to the formation of an early embryonic structure known as the neural tube. The process of neurulation begins during gastrulation with the specification of the neural progenitor cell lines. Neurulation involves two sets of processes, primary and secondary neurulation. Primary neurulation consists of those processes that give rise to the brain and most of the spinal column. Secondary neurulation consists of a somewhat different and distinct set of processes that give rise to the most caudal regions of the spinal column. Primary neurulation involves four basic processes that emerge in sequence: the formation of the neural plate, the shaping of the neural plate, the bending of the neural plate, and closure of the neural tube.

- Just before the tube begins to form, the embryo begins to elongate as the cells in both the neurectoderm and the underlying mesoderm become interleaved. This elongation is necessary for the subsequent formation of the neural tube. Bending of the plate begins on approximately E19 in humans with the formation of neural folds. The neural folds are elevated ridges that form on either side of the axial midline of the neural plate. The mechanisms that underlie the bending of the plate are different at different levels of the nervous system. Within the spinal column, *SHH*, which is expressed by the notochord, directs the formation of the lateral hinge points that allow for the smooth inward bending of the neural folds into a single tube. Within cranial regions, expansion of the underlying mesoderm brings about the initial folding. The production and contraction of actin microfilaments serve to redefine the shape of cells, and in turn direct the inward folding of the sides of the emerging tube. Both rapid neural proliferation and naturally occurring cell death also contribute to neural-tube formation in the cranial regions.

- Fusion of the tube occurs along the central midline as the folds from each side extend cellular structures that serve to guide their convergence. The cells of the surface ectoderm fuse first, followed by the neurectodermal cells. After initial fusion, these two cell lines are separated by an intervening layer of mesodermal tissue.

- For many years, avian species were the model for neural tube closure. In avians, closure begins centrally and "zips" up and down the neuraxis, with closure first in rostral regions and later in caudal regions. The pattern of closure in humans is somewhat controversial, but it appears that there is at least one and possibly two additional initial points of fusion in rostral regions. Fusion extends bidirectionally from all sites except the most rostral.

- The second embryonic month is a time of rapid change in both the size and shape of the embryo. Soon after the neural tube closes, the anterior regions of the developing nervous system undergo rapid expansion. The primary vesicles emerge and subdivide the embryo along the anterior-posterior axis. The three primary vesicles, ordered from anterior to posterior, are the

prosencephalon, the mesencephalon, and the rhombencephalon.

- By E35, further subdivision of the embryo is complete as the secondary vesicles emerge. The prosencephalon divides into the telencephalon and the diencephalon, and the rhombencephalon
divides into the metencephalon and myelencephalon. The resulting five subdivisions define the basic organization for the developing nervous system. A series of flexure points along the
neural tube contribute to the characteristic shape of the embryo.
- Extraembryonic tissues play essential roles in the development of
the embryo. The amniotic sac, yolk sac, and chorion all serve as
support systems that provide nutrients and essential blood elements to the embryo.

## References

Castilla, E. E., I. M. Orioli, J. S. Lopez-Camelo, G. Dutra Mda, and J. Nazer-
Herrera. 2003. "Preliminary data on changes in neural tube defect
prevalence rates after folic acid fortification in South America." *American Journal of Medical Genetics A,* 123: 123–128.

Colas, J. F., and G. C. Schoenwolf. 2001. "Towards a cellular and molecular understanding of neurulation." *Developmental Dynamics,* 221:
117–145.

Copp, A. J., N. D. Greene, and J. N. Murdoch. 2003. "The genetic basis of
mammalian neurulation." *Nature Reviews Genetics,* 4: 784–793.

Desmond, M. E. 1982. "Description of the occlusion of the spinal cord
lumen in early human embryos." *Anatomical Record,* 204: 89–93.

Desmond, M. E., and M. L. Levitan. 2002. "Brain expansion in the chick
embryo initiated by experimentally produced occlusion of the spinal
neurocoel." *Anatomical Record,* 268: 147–159.

Finnell, R. H., W. M. Junker, L. K. Wadman, and R. M. Cabrera. 2002.
"Gene expression profiling within the developing neural tube." *Neurochemical Research,* 27: 1165–1180.

Fletcher, J. M., M. Barnes, and M. Dennis. 2002. "Language development in
children with spina bifida." *Seminars in Pediatric Neurology,* 9: 201–208.

Gilbert, S. F. 2006. *Developmental biology.* 8th ed. Sunderland, MA: Sinauer
Associates.

Golden, J. A., and G. F. Chernoff. 1995. "Multiple sites of anterior neural
tube closure in humans: Evidence from anterior neural tube defects
(anencephaly)." *Pediatrics,* 95: 506–510.

Gos, M., and A. Szpecht-Potocka. 2002. "Genetic basis of neural tube defects. I. Regulatory genes for the neurulation process." *Journal of Applied Genetics*, 43: 343–350.

Haigo, S. L., J. D. Hildebrand, R. M. Harland, and J. B. Wallingford. 2003. "Shroom induces apical constriction and is required for hingepoint formation during neural tube closure." *Current Biology*, 13: 2125–2137.

Juriloff, D. M., and M. J. Harris. 2000. "Mouse models for neural tube closure defects." *Human Molecular Genetics*, 9: 993–1000.

Kostovic, I., and P. Rakic. 1990. "Developmental history of the transient subplate zone in the visual and somatosensory cortex of the macaque monkey and human brain." *Journal of Comparative Neurology*, 297: 441–470.

Larsen, W. J. 2001. *Human embryology*. 3rd ed. New York: Churchill Livingstone.

Martin, P. 2004. "Morphogenesis: Shroom in to close the neural tube." *Current Biology*, 14: R150–R151.

Menkes, J. H., and H. B. Sarnat. 2000. *Child neurology*. 6th ed. Philadelphia: Lippincott Williams & Wilkins.

Menkes, J. H., H. B. Sarnat, and B. L. Maria. 2006. *Child neurology*. 7th ed. Philadelphia: Lippincott Williams & Wilkins.

Mitchell, L. E., N. S. Adzick, J. Melchionne, P. S. Pasquariello, L. N. Sutton, and A. S. Whitehead. 2004. "Spina bifida." *Lancet*, 364: 1885–1895.

Nakatsu, T., C. Uwabe, and K. Shiota. 2000. "Neural tube closure in humans initiates at multiple sites: Evidence from human embryos and implications for the pathogenesis of neural tube defects." *Anatomy and Embryology*, 201: 455–466.

Oppenheim, R. W. 1991. "Cell death during development of the nervous system." *Annual Review of Neuroscience*, 14, 453–501.

O'Rahilly, R., and F. Müller. 1987. *Developmental stages in human embryos, including a revision of Streeter's Horizons and a survey of the Carnegie Collection*. Washington, DC: Carnegie Institution of Washington.

———. 2002. "The two sites of fusion of the neural folds and the two neuropores in the human embryo." *Teratology*, 65: 162–170.

Ray, J. G., and H. J. Blom. 2003. "Vitamin B12 insufficiency and the risk of fetal neural tube defects." *QJM*, 96: 289–295.

Rintoul, N. E., L. N. Sutton, A. M. Hubbard, B. Cohen, J. Melchionni, P. S. Pasquariello, and N. S. Adzick. 2002. "A new look at myelomeningoceles: Functional level, vertebral level, shunting, and the implications for fetal intervention." *Pediatrics*, 109: 409–413.

Rosano, A., D. Smithells, L. Cacciani, B. Botting, E. Castilla, M. Cornel, D. Erickson, J. Goujard, L. Irgens, P. Merlob, E. Robert, C. Siffel, C. Stoll, and Y. Sumiyoshi. 1999. "Time trends in neural tube defects prevalence in relation to preventive strategies: An international study." *Journal of Epidemiology and Community Health*, 53: 630–635.

Sadler, T. W. 2006. *Langman's medical embryology*. 10th ed. Philadelphia: Lippincott Williams & Wilkins.

Van Allen, M. I., D. K. Kalousek, G. F. Chernoff, D. Juriloff, M. Harris, B. C. McGillivray, S. L. Yong, S. Langlois, P. M. MacLeod, D. Chitayat, J. M. Friedman, R. D. Wilson, D. McFadden, J. Pantzar, S. Ritchie, and J. G. Hall. 1993. "Evidence for multi-site closure of the neural tube in humans." *American Journal of Medical Genetics*, 47: 723–743.

Verhoef, M., H. A. Barf, M. W. Post, F. W. van Asbeck, R. H. Gooskens, and A. J. Prevo. 2004. "Secondary impairments in young adults with spina bifida." *Developmental Medicine and Child Neurology*, 46: 420–427.

Wallingford, J. B. 2004. "Closing in on vertebrate planar polarity." *Nature Cell Biology*, 6: 687–689.

Wong, L. Y., and L. J. Paulozzi. 2001. "Survival of infants with spina bifida: A population study, 1979–94." *Paediatric and Perinatal Epidemiology*, 15: 374–378.

Ybot-Gonzalez, P., P. Cogram, D. Gerrelli, and A. J. Copp. 2002. "Sonic hedgehog and the molecular regulation of mouse neural tube closure." *Development*, 129: 2507–2517.

Ybot-Gonzalez, P., and A. J. Copp. 1999. "Bending of the neural plate during mouse spinal neurulation is independent of actin microfilaments." *Developmental Dynamics*, 215: 273–283.

# FIVE

# Molecular Patterning of the
# Primary Spatial Dimensions
# of the Embryo

BY THE END of neurulation, the basic organization of the developing embryo has been established. The primary germ layers have formed and become segregated, providing the three types of progenitor cells that, along with the newly differentiated neural crest cells, will produce the cells for all the organs in the body. The major dimensional axes have been specified in the initial dorsal-ventral, right-left, and anterior-posterior patterning of the embryonic disc. The neural tube has closed, and the basic shape of the embryo is becoming defined. Rostral portions of the neural tube are undergoing rapid expansion as the neocortex begins to emerge within the dorsal telencephalon.

Although the basic patterning of the embryo was initiated during embryonic plate formation, those initial definitions were very crude. During the late embryonic period and the early fetal period, specification of the major axes becomes much more refined. The emergence of both dorsal-ventral and anterior-posterior specification has been studied most extensively in the spinal cord, but along each spatial axis, similar changes are happening within more anterior regions as well. Specification along the dorsal-ventral axis establishes the primary sensory and motor organization of the hindbrain and the spinal column. It also sets up the initial differentiation of important anterior structures such as the basal ganglia, which are located in ventral regions of the brain and are crucial for movement and coordination. Specification along the anterior-posterior axis serves to establish the segmented organization of the hindbrain and the spinal column. It also establishes the anterior-posterior polarity of the midbrain regions and sets up the initial pattern of regionalization within the developing neocortex.

All these changes add to the growing complexity of the developing nervous system. As was the case for the study of earlier embryonic periods, knowledge of the genetic underpinnings of the changes that will be discussed in this chapter is growing rapidly and indeed extends far beyond the scope of this book, but some of the best-understood and most important genes will be discussed. Interestingly, a number of the genes involved in development during this next period will be familiar. Many of the genes that were crucial for setting up the embryonic nervous system again play important roles in the refinement of the early system. Further, as was observed during the patterning of the neural plate, signaling often involves gradients of signaling molecules, and in some cases countervailing gradients of different molecules work jointly to establish the organization of the neural tube.

## Dorsal-Ventral Specification

In caudal regions of the neural tube, differentiation of cells in dorsal and ventral regions gives rise to the characteristic patterns of sensory and motor segregation. Within dorsal regions of the caudal neural tube, the neurons of the sensory tracts will aggregate in the alar plate. In ventral regions, neurons of the motor system will establish the major motor pathways within the basal plate (Figure 5.1). The border of the two regions is marked by a structure called the sulcus limitans. This region will contain interneurons that serve as a conduit to relay information between the sensory and motor systems. Dorsal-ventral specification also occurs in more rostral regions of the neural tube. It has been studied less extensively than dorsal-ventral specification in more caudal regions. However, some of the same signaling pathways that are expressed in caudal regions have been implicated in specification of ventral-anterior structures, such as the basal ganglia.

## Dorsal-Ventral Specification of the Spinal Cord

When the neural tube closes, the circular layer of neuroepithelial cells is flanked by two structures that are important for the process of dorsal-ventral specification (Figure 5.2). The first is the notochord, which lies ventral to the neural tube and runs along the anterior-posterior midline of the caudal tube. The second structure, which is composed of epidermal cells, is positioned dorsally above the neural tube. Each of these structures secretes signaling molecules that will specify the fate of cells within different regions of the tube.

The notochord expresses the secreted protein sonic hedgehog (Shh). Initially, *Shh* expression induces cells in the medial hinge point (MHP; see Chapter 4) to form a new structure, the floor plate (Figure 5.2A). Floor-plate cells then establish a second Shh signaling center in the most ventral regions of the neural tube. Shh is secreted in a gradient from the ventral signaling centers. The highest concentration of Shh is in the most ventral regions of the neural tube, and the concentration diminishes as Shh diffuses toward more dorsal regions. A countergradient of a different class of secreted molecules is established in dorsal regions. The epidermis overlying the dorsal region of the neural tube expresses the secreted molecules Bmp4 and Bmp7. These molecules, Bmp4 in particular, played a central role in initial specification of the primary germ layers in the neural plate. During this later period of development, the expression of *Bmp4* and *Bmp7* induces the formation of a new dorsal midline structure, the roof plate (Figure 5.2A). The roof-plate cells establish a second dorsal signaling center

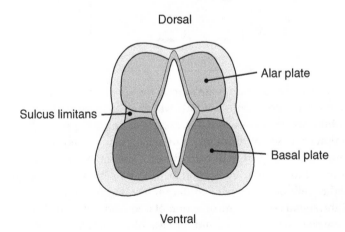

Figure 5.1. Organization of the spinal cord. The sensory tracts form in the dorsal alar plate and the major motor pathways will form within the ventral basal plate. The sulcus limitans marks the border between the two regions.

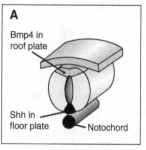

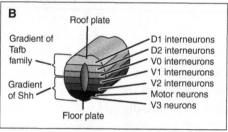

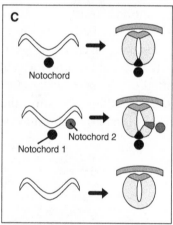

Figure 5.2. Dorsal and ventral signaling in the spinal cord. A. In the ventral region, the notochord expresses Shh, which induces formation of the floor plate, which also expresses Shh. The dorsal roof plate expresses Tgfs. B. The interaction of these two diffusing gradients of secreted molecules creates a morphogenic effect. Different concentrations of the two molecules induce expression of different transcription factors and consequently the production of different neuron types at different levels within the dorsal-ventral axis of the spinal cord. C. Introduction of a second notochord creates an extra ventral signaling center, and removal of the notochord blocks ventral specification. (A, B from Gilbert 2006. Adapted with the permission of Sinauer Associates, Inc. C from Kintner and Lumsden 1999. Adapted with the permission of Elsevier.)

that begins to express Bmp4. This, in turn, induces the expression of related Tgfb family proteins (recall that Bmp4 is a member of the Tgfb family of signaling molecules) in adjacent tissues. The Tgfb proteins are all secreted molecules that diffuse in a gradient, with highest concentration in the most dorsal regions.

The interaction of these two diffusing gradients, Shh ventrally and Tgfbs dorsally, induces the expression of different transcription factors in cells at different levels of the neural tube. The specific transcription factor expressed at a given level, in turn, activates intrinsic programs within the cells that cause them to adopt specific cell fates. For example, expression of the transcription factor Pax6 signals the cell's progression to a dorsal fate, while the expression of Nkx6.1 signals a ventral fate (Rallu, Corbin, and Fishell 2002). Cells in the immediate vicinity of the floor plate are exposed to high concentrations of Shh and very little Tgfb. That induces them to express the transcription factors Nkx6.1 and Nkx2.2 and blocks the expression of other transcription factors, including Pax6, Pax7, Dbx1, and Dbx2. That combination of signals causes those cells to differentiate into a particular type of ventral neuron, V3 neurons (Gilbert 2006; Zigmond et al. 1999). The concentrations of Shh and Tgfb are slightly different in the region just above the V3 neurons, and thus a different transcription factor is expressed and those cells become motor neurons. In the most dorsal region, the low concentrations of Shh produce a reversed pattern of expression. Ventral transcription factors are not signaled and dorsal transcription factors are not repressed, resulting in the induction of dorsal cell types. In all, the interaction of the Shh and Tgfb gradients at different levels of the neural tube induces seven different cell types (Figure 5.2B), and the arrangement of those cell types gives rise to the dorsal-ventral organization of the caudal neural tube.

The roles of both the notochord in specifying the ventral fate of cells and the roof plate in specifying dorsal fates have been confirmed experimentally (Figure 5.2C). Early removal of the notochord represses ventral fate expression in neural tube cells, with the result that all cells within the neural tube express a dorsal fate. Further, experimental implantation of a second notochord adjacent to the first induces the formation of an additional column of ventral neurons. The grafted notochord first induces a second floor plate, and then cells begin differentiating in a graded fashion above the floor-plate signaling center. Together, these studies suggest that *Shh* works in concert with dorsal organizers to induce different cell types along the dorsal-ventral axis.

The role of the roof plate in specifying dorsal fates has also been examined. Early removal of the roof plate results in the elimination of the dorsal cell types and their replacement by cells usually found in the midline of the neural tube (Brown, Keynes, and Lumsden 2001, p. 83; Lee, Dietrich, and Jessell 2000). As was the case in the early formation of the neural plate, Bmp4 appears to be an important organizing factor. However, Bmp4's role earlier in development during neural plate formation was to direct a nonneural fate within the ectodermal layer. Induction of neurectodermal cells required blocking of Bmp4 activity. In contrast, Bmp4's contribution to establishing the dorsal-ventral axis of organization within the neural tube appears to involve the induction of specific types of interneurons. Thus at different points in development, the same signaling molecules can play very different roles.

## Dorsal-Ventral Patterning in Anterior Regions

Dorsal-ventral patterning within the telencephalon begins soon after the closure of the anterior neuropore with the appearance of three primitive ventral telencephalic structures (Figure 5.3). The first to appear is the medial ganglionic eminence (MGE). The MGE is located along the midline of the ventral telencephalon just above the prechordal plate. Soon after the appearance of the MGE, the lateral ganglionic eminence (LGE) and the caudal ganglionic eminence (CGE) emerge immediately above and behind the MGE, respectively (Kohtz et al. 1998; Rallu et al. 2002). In the developing embryo and fetus, these three structures will become the source of important interneurons and oligodendrocytes. Later in development, interneurons produce inhibitory neurotransmitter substances and thus are critical components of both cortical and subcortical circuits. Oligodendrocytes compose the myelin sheaths that engulf the axons of cranial neurons and improve the speed and efficiency of neural signaling. The MGE, LGE, and CGE will later give rise to important structures in the mature brain, the basal ganglia. The basal ganglia are ventral telencephalic structures that are important for movement and coordination. They are composed of two main substructures, the globus pallidus and the striatum. The globus pallidus arises from the embryonic MGE, and the striatum arises from the embryonic LGE and CGE. The dorsal regions of the embryonic telencephalon will give rise to the cerebral cortex.

Throughout the rostral-caudal extent of the neuraxis, *Shh* expression is required for induction of ventral structures. Within forebrain regions, mutant mice that lack the *Shh* gene fail to express ventral telencephalic brain structures, and the experimental introduction of abnormally high levels of Shh to dorsal telencephalic regions induces the expression of ventral markers (Rallu et al. 2002). However, until recently, little was known about either the timing or the source of *Shh* expression in forebrain regions. As discussed earlier, in caudal regions of the neural tube, ventral patterning derives from the expression of *Shh* in the notochord and the floor plate. However, the notochord ends at the rostral midbrain border and does not extend into the forebrain. Thus it cannot serve as the source of Shh signaling in forebrain

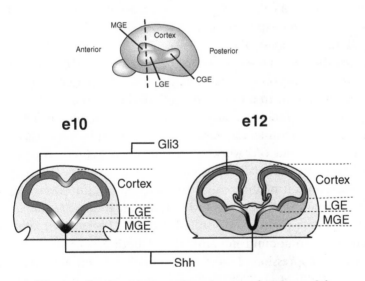

Figure 5.3. The ganglionic eminences form in ventral regions of the telencephalon. During development, these structures will be important proliferative regions, generating interneurons and oligodendrocytes. In the mature organism, these structures will become the basal ganglia. (From Rallu, Corbin, and Fishell 2002. Adapted with the permission of Nature Publishing Group.)

regions. The question then becomes, how is the differentiation of ventral structures in the forebrain accomplished? Because the mechanism for dorsal-ventral specification in the spinal cord is well understood, it had been a model for the study of dorsal-ventral patterning in the forebrain. However, recent work suggests that patterning within the telencephalon may be somewhat different.

*Shh* is first expressed during gastrulation in the midline mesoderm, and it is thought that early signaling serves to provide initial ventral fate signaling throughout the telencephalon (Gunhaga et al. 2003). However, that early signaling may not be sufficient to fix cell fate in all regions of the telencephalon. As neurulation proceeds, the prechordal plate mesoderm expresses *Shh* (Rally, Corbin, and Fishell 2002). Near the end of the embryonic period, *Shh* is expressed in the cells of the ventral telencephalon. There is evidence that unlike the profile observed in the spinal column, specification of cell fate within the telencephalon may be determined by the timing of Shh exposure rather than its concentration (Kohtz et al. 1998). Specifically, the levels of susceptibility of cells to exposure to Shh seem to change with development, and later exposure appears to be associated with specification of LGE rather than MGE progenitors.

As was the case in the spinal cord, modulation of *Shh* appears to involve the interaction of genetic factors, but the patterns of interaction are different. In a wide range of species, members of the transcription factor family Gli are required for Shh signaling. Three Gli family transcription factors have been identified in mice, *Gli1*, *Gli2*, and *Gli3*. *Gli1* and *Gli2* work as activators, while *Gli3* is a repressor. Only mutation of *Gli3* disrupts telencephalic development, resulting in the expansion of the ventral telencephalon into dorsal regions. That pattern is the opposite of what is obtained with *Shh* mutants, in which ventral signaling is disrupted and dorsal regions expand. Surprisingly, in compound mutants, where both *Shh* and *Gli3* are disrupted, the expression of most aspects of dorsal-ventral patterning is restored (Rallu et al. 2002). This finding suggests that the relationship between Shh and Gli3 cannot be one of simple reciprocal competition to set up dorsal or ventral fates. Rather, this reciprocal signaling pathway must work in conjunction with some other factor or factors that must also work to establish dorsal-ventral patterning within the telencephalon. Recent studies have suggested that another secreted factor, Fgf8, may act in conjuction with Shh to specify the ventral fate of progenitors in the telencephalon (Gutin et al. 2006). Fgf8 is produced downstream of Shh, and its expression may account for the rescue of ventral telencephalic progenitors in *Shh* and *Gli3* null mutants.

Furthermore, recent work suggests that another somewhat surprising factor may be involved in dorsal telencephalic specification, Wnt signaling (Gunhaga et al. 2003). Recall that earlier in development, during the gastrula stage, Wnts expressed in the epiblast layer specify a posterior fate for developing neurectoderm cells. Expression of an anterior fate requires blockage of *Wnt* expression by antagonists expressed in the underlying mesendoderm. During this same period, Shh signaling specifies a ventral fate for all prospective telencephalic cells (Gunhaga, Jessell, and Edlund 2000). During the neural fold stage, the prospective dorsal telencephalic cells are exposed to Wnt signaling that emanates from cells in the overlying epidermal ectoderm. However, the function of Wnt signaling in specifying the dorsal telencephalon appears to be very different than it was during gastrulation. Wnt signaling emanating from the epidermal ectoderm blocks the expression of ventral characteristics in the prospective dorsal telencephalic cells. Further, during the neural tube stage, *Wnt* is expressed in the dorsal telencephalic cells themselves. Finally, midline dorsal telencephalic cells are exposed to Fgf signaling from a signaling center in the anterior dorsal midline. The combined Wnt and Fgf signaling appears to fix the dorsal fate of cells in the dorsal telencephalon (Figure 5.4).

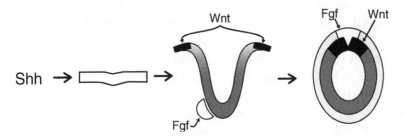

Figure 5.4. Complex signaling involving Shh, Gli3, Fgf, and Wnts results in differentiation of the dorsal telencephalon. (From Gunhaga et al. 2003. Adapted with the permission of Nature Publishing Group.)

## Anterior-Posterior Specification

Earlier in development, during neural plate formation, rudimentary specification of the anterior-posterior axis was established. The expression of posteriorizing agents such as Wnt was blocked in anterior regions of the embryo by antagonists such as Nog, Chrd, and Fst, thus restricting Wnt activity to posterior regions. Expression of factors such as Otx2 served to specify an anterior fate of neurectodermal cells. However, this initial specification is very global and does not correspond with any precision to the regional differentiation that emerges with the formation of the primary and secondary vesicles. As the neural tube forms, differentiation along the anterior-posterior extent of the neuraxis becomes more specific. Differentiation is observed within the prosencephalon at the junction of the telencephalon and the diencephalon, at the midbrain-hindbrain junction, and within the rhombencephalon with the differentiation of both hindbrain and spinal-cord segments. As was the case for the study of dorsal-ventral specification, the process of anterior-posterior specification is best understood in hindbrain and spinal-cord regions, but there is also considerable information on specification in more anterior regions.

## Anterior-Posterior Specification in the Hindbrain and the Spinal Cord

Within the posterior regions of the developing nervous system, progressive segmentation and compartmentalization of the neural tube begin to become apparent immediately after tube closure (Brown, Keynes, and Lumsden 2001). This compartmentalization is most clearly observed in the hindbrain, where a series of eight divisions, called rhombomeres, emerges. Rhombomeres are transient embryonic structures that serve an important organizational function early in development (Kiecker and Lumsden 2005). The three rostral rhombomeres will give rise to the metencephalon including the pons and cerebellum, and the five caudal rhombomeres will form the myelencephalon. Each rhombomere is a parcellated group of cells that constitutes a separate functional unit. Cells within a rhombomere make contact and communicate with each other, but they are segregated from cells in adjacent rhombomeres. Cells within a rhombomere have a specific and common functional fate that differs from the fate of cells in other rhombomeres. For example, different rhombomeres give rise to functionally distinct cranial nerves (Gilbert 2006).

Rhombomeres begin to emerge as the tube closes, and the full set of eight is fully established by the end of the sixth week of gestation (Figure 5.5). By convention, rhombomeres are numbered from 1 to 8 in order from anterior to posterior (r1–r8). The formation of each rhombomere begins with an initial wave of neuron proliferation, but the onset of neuron proliferation differs across rhombomeres. Proliferation occurs in two waves, beginning first in r2, r4, r6, and r8 and then in r1, r3, r5, and r7. Cells within a rhombomere do not intermingle with cells in neighboring rhombomeres. This segregation begins when the rhombomere boundaries first appear and continues through the end of neurogenesis. Initial segmentation begins with an increase in the space between cells at the rhombomeres' borders that reflects what has been

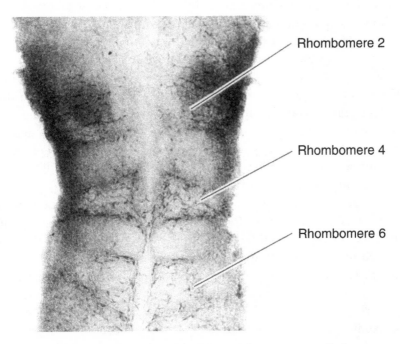

Rhombomere 2

Rhombomere 4

Rhombomere 6

Figure 5.5. The hindbrain is parcellated into eight segments called rhombomeres. (From Lumsden and Keynes 1989. Reprinted with the permission of Nature Publishing Group.)

described as an adhesion differential, that is, the tendency for some cells to adhere and others to be repelled. The segregation of cells is further amplified by differential expression of Eph receptor tyrosine kinases (enzymes that act as receptors in transmembrane signaling pathways) and their ligands (factors that can either permit or block specific enzyme activity). Three Eph receptors are expressed in odd-numbered rhombomeres, while their ligands are expressed in even-numbered rhombomeres. The receptor-ligand interaction at the borders enhances the repulsive interactions between cells in adjacent rhombomeres.

## The Role of HOX Genes

The specification of cell function (also referred to as the "positional value" of the cell) within each rhombomere is brought about by the expression of an important and evolutionarily highly conserved set of genes, *Hox* (for the mouse, *HOX* for humans) genes. *Hox* genes are a particular family of homeobox genes. Homeobox genes are so named because they all contain a specific 180-nucleotide-pair sequence called a homeobox, and they encode transcription factors that all contain a specific 60-amino-acid sequence called the homeodomain (recall that during mRNA translation each amino acid that is incorporated into the growing protein chain is initially associated with a nucleotide triplet of tRNA, called an anticodon, that pairs with a nucleotide triplet in the mRNA called a codon). *Hox* genes are a highly conserved set of genes that were originally identified as critical for patterning of the anterior-posterior body axis in *Drosophila*, the fruit fly. In the fly, the set of genes was termed homeotic selector genes, *Homc* genes, because of their role in changing the shape or structure of the organism.

*Hox* genes are closely related both structurally and functionally to *Homc* genes. In mammals, they serve a similar role in setting up the anterior-posterior organization of the central nervous system (McGinnis and Krumlauf 1992). In the fly, eight genes constitute the set of *Homc* genes. They are distributed in an ordered sequence along the chromosome that reflects the position of their expression along the anterior-posterior axis (Figure 5.6A, first set). The major evolutionary change observed in mammals with regard to the set of homeotic selector genes is the number of copies of the genes that act to establish the anterior-posterior patterning. While one copy of each *homc* gene is found in the fly, up to four copies of the homologous genes are found in mice *(Hox)* and in humans *(HOX)* (Figure 5.6A; compare the single fly set with the four sets for the mouse). The four sets of mammalian *Hox* genes are termed *Hoxa, Hoxb, Hoxc,* and *Hoxd.* Figure 5.6A is organized to indicate the genes in the fly and the multiple equivalent genes in the mouse. Thus the gene that is called *lab* in the fly and *Hoxa1, Hoxb1,* and *Hoxd1* in the mouse are all equivalent genes, and they have similar, although not identical, expression patterns along the anterior-posterior axis. Further, the equivalent genes from the mouse sets (e.g., *Hoxa1, Hoxb1,* and *Hoxd1*) together form what is called a paralogous group. Thus *a1, b1,* and *d1* form a paralogue group, as do *a4, b4, c4,* and *d4,* and so forth. In mammals, there are 13 paralogue groups, each containing from two to four genes and most corresponding to a particular *Homc* gene.

*Hox* genes encode TFs that are expressed along the neuraxis beginning at the midbrain-hindbrain border (MHB) and extending through the spinal cord. *Hox* genes are expressed in the notochord, the prechordal plate, and the neural tissue. Critically for anterior-posterior patterning, there are very specific differences in the extent of anterior expression for each of the genes. The expression patterns for the set of genes form a nested sequence in which expression of different constellations of genes is confined to specific rhombomeres or spinal-cord segments. The patterns of expression are consistent across the fly and the mouse in that mouse and fly equivalents are expressed in similar anterior-posterior regions. Figure 5.6B shows the gene expression patterns for fly *Homc* genes and for one of the mouse *Hox* sets, *Hoxb.* The patterns of *Hox* gene expression give rise to the differentiation of cells within each of the rhombomeres and spinal-cord segments and thus serve both to determine the positional value of the cells and to specify their derivatives (Schilling and Knight 2001). Mutations of specific *Hox* genes lead to failure of rhombomere differentiation and the subsequent failure of structures that would have derived from the rhombomere to emerge. For example, a mutation of *Hoxb1,* which is normally expressed in r4, leads to a loss of specification of r4. Alternatively, the introduction of Hoxb1 transcripts into r2 leads to the anomalous expression of r4 characteristics within r2 (Brown, Keynes, and Lumsden 2001).

The means by which *Hox* genes are activated have not been fully described. However, a number of transcription factors have been identified that modulate *Hox* gene activity. First, there is evidence of cross-regulation among *Hox* genes (Schilling and Knight 2001) in that the

**A**

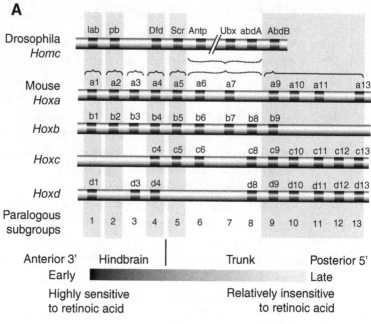

**B**

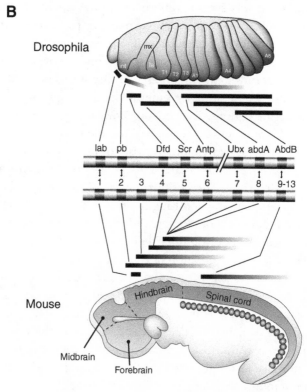

combined activity of different sets of *Hox* genes at different levels of the neuraxis serves to determine the positional value of cells (Gavalas et al. 2003; Lumsden and Krumlauf 1996). In addition, two transcription factors, Krox20 and Kreisler, have been found to have very localized effects on hindbrain patterning and appear to work by regulation of specific *Hox* gene expression. Krox20 has been shown to regulate the activity of Hoxa2, Hoxb2, and Hoxb3 within r3 and r5. Inactivation of *Krox20* leads to failure of r3 and r5 formation. Further, Krox20 has been shown to activate transcription of one Eph tyrosine kinase receptor gene in r3 and r5. Recall that the enzyme products of the Eph tyrosine kinase receptor gene act to establish rhombomere boundaries by promoting repulsive interactions between cells. Krox20 thus acts to regulate expression of the receptors that promote boundary formation. Introduction of Krox20 to even-numbered rhombomeres converts them to odd-number identity (Giudicelli et al. 2001). Kreisler modifies the expression of the three paralogous group 3 genes within r5. *Kreisler* mouse mutants show marked abnormalities of hindbrain development that involve failure of rhombomere formation posterior to the r3-r4 boundary (McKay et al. 1994).

*Retinoic Acid Modulates* Hox *Gene Expression*
One other important regulator of *Hox* gene expression is retinoic acid (RA). RA is a powerful posteriorizing agent that is present in a gradient along the neuraxis from the anterior hindbrain border through the extent of the spinal cord (Glover, Renaud, and Rijli 2006). RA is derived from vitamin A, and cannot be produced in animal cells (Sakai et al.

---

Figure 5.6. *(Opposite Page)* Comparison of *Drosophila Homc* and mouse *Hox* gene expression patterns. A. *Drosophila* have eight *Homc* genes aligned along one chromosome. Mammals have up to four copies of the eight genes found in *Drosophila*. In mammals, equivalent genes located on different chromosomes constitute a paralogous group. B. The anterior-posterior expression patterns for the *Homc* family of genes in *Drosophila* and the *Hoxb* family in the mouse are similar. (A from Krumlauf 1993. Adapted with the permission of Elsevier; and from Gilbert 2006. Adapted with the permission of Sinauer Associates, Inc. B from McGinnis and Krumlauf 1992. Adapted with the permission of Elsevier; and from Gilbert 2006. Adapted with the permission of Sinauer Associates, Inc.)

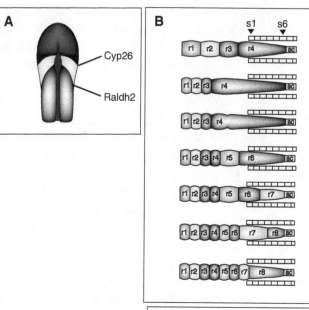

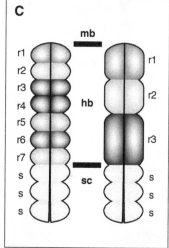

Figure 5.7. RA regulates *Hox* gene expression and rhombomere formation.
A. Raldh2 is present at the spinal cord-hindbrain border and promotes synthesis of RA. Cyp26 degrades RA in more rostral regions. B. Rhombomeres
emerge in a sequence at the spinal cord-hindbrain border, with each new
rhombomere moving the earlier rhombomere farther away from the source
of RA. Earlier rhombomeres are exposed to RA for shorter durations than
those produced later. C. Depletion of vitamin A from the maternal diet

2001). Rather, it is ingested in the form of vitamin A, which must then be metabolized through a series of steps to form RA. The level of RA in the body is regulated by two enzymes. The first is Raldh2, which completes the final step in RA synthesis and thus is associated with increases in the level of RA. The second is Cyp26, which acts to degrade RA and thus reduces levels of RA. These two enzymes are expressed in complementary regions of the neuraxis. *Raldh2* is expressed in caudal regions and provides the RA needed for posterior specification. The anterior border of Raldh2 expression is the spinal-cord–hindbrain border. *Cyp26* is expressed in the rostral forebrain, where it actively degrades RA, thus blocking its posteriorizing effects (McCaffery et al. 2003; Sakai et al. 2001). Between these two expression areas is a gap region where neither of the two enzymes is expressed. The gap corresponds precisely to the position where the hindbrain will form (Figure 5.7A).

Two possible explanations of RA's role in the anterior-posterior patterning of the hindbrain have been suggested (Glover, Renaud, and Rijli 2006). The first is that the expression patterns of these two competing enzymes act together to create a gradient of RA within the gap region and that variation in the concentration of RA results in expression of different *Hox* genes within different rhombomeres. However, the RA gradient has been hard to document, and various studies of mutant mice have produced results that are inconsistent with a simple gradient model (Gavalas 2002; Maden 2002). Alternatively, it has been suggested that rhombomere differences in *Hox* gene expression may be linked to the duration of cell exposure to RA. It has been shown that rhombomeres emerge in a region adjacent to the spinal cord–hindbrain border in a strict anterior-posterior sequence. As each rhombomere emerges, it moves away from the source of RA at the level of the spinal cord (Figure 5.7B). Thus the cells that form the more posterior rhombomeres may be exposed longer to RA than are the earlier-produced cells of the anterior rhombomeres. This model suggests that it is the duration of exposure to RA that induces the enhanced posterior characteristic in later-developing rhombomeres (Gavalas 2002).

---

Figure 5.7. *(Opposite Page)* depletes RA and leads to failure of posterior rhombomere formation. Mb=midbrain; hb=hindbrain; sc=spinal cord. (A, C from McCaffery et al. 2003. Adapted with the permission of Blackwell Publishing. B from Gavalas 2002. Adapted with the permission of Elsevier.)

RA appears to regulate the overall expression of *Hox* genes in a dose-dependent fashion such that different *Hox* genes are expressed depending on the concentration of RA. RA thus regulates the *Hox* gene modulation of positional information for cells at different levels of the neuraxis. RA can diffuse across cell membranes to regulate transcription activity in the cell (Brown, Keynes, and Lumsden 2001). Experimental manipulation of vitamin A availability dramatically alters patterning in the hindbrain. Depletion of dietary vitamin A during the period of hindbrain formation results in the loss of rhombomeres posterior to the r3-r4 border and expansion of the anterior rhombomeres to fill the open space (Figure 5.7C; McCaffery et al. 2003). An excess of RA can be equally devastating. Exposure to high levels of RA produces malformations in all hindbrain structures, most commonly dysgenesis of the cerebellum (McCaffery et al. 2003). Thus RA plays a critical role in patterning of the posterior nervous system via its graded regulation of *Hox* gene expression.

## Establishing the Midbrain-Hindbrain Border

Induction and organization of structures at the border between hindbrain and midbrain regions are not under the control of *Hox* genes. Rather, a number of other genes play central roles in establishing the border between these two brain regions and in the induction of the major structures that arise from them (Brown 1975; Nakamura et al. 2004). The cerebellum will arise from the most anterior portion of the hindbrain in r1. The tectum will arise from the midbrain structures of the mesencephalon. The border between the two regions (see Figure 5.8A), which is referred to as the isthmus, is defined by the opposition of two homeobox transcription factors, Otx2 and Gbx2 (these are unrelated to the *Hox* homeobox genes). As discussed previously, *Otx2* is expressed in the AVE and in the anterior mesendoderm and plays an important role in the very early specification of anterior characteristics. At this later point in development, within anterior regions of the neural plate, *Otx2* expression extends throughout the midbrain up to the border with the hindbrain. By contrast, *Gbx2* is expressed posterior to the region of *Otx2* expression. The two molecules act to block each other's expression, thus establishing the border between the two brain regions.

Two other transcription factors, En1 and En2, are critical for establishing regional identity within the midbrain and the anterior hindbrain (see Figure 5.8B). They are expressed in a gradient that extends through both regions; *En1* is expressed earlier in development than *En2*. Mutation of *En1* results in agenesis of both the tectum and the cerebellum, while mutation of *En2* results in loss of only the cerebellum. The graded expression of *En1* and *En2* is controlled by two other secreted molecules expressed at the border, Fgf8 and Wnt1. Fgf8 proteins are essential for initiation of *En* expression, while Wnt1 is necessary for maintenance of *En* expression in the region. *Wnt1* is expressed in the anterior, *Otx2*-positive region, while *Fgf8* is expressed in the posterior, *Gbx2*-positive region (Wurst and Bally-Cuif 2001). They are initially broadly expressed through each region, but each becomes restricted to a narrow band at the immediate border between the midbrain and

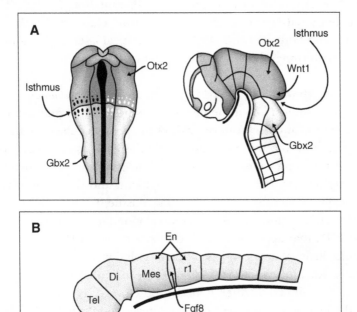

Figure 5.8. A. The isthmus is the border between the midbrain and the hindbrain. Opposing concentrations of Otx2 and Gbx2 define the isthmus. The cerebellum will arise from r1, immediately caudal to the isthmus, and the tectum will arise from the region of the mesencephalon immediately rostral to the isthmus. B. Gradients of En1 and En2 contribute to defining the midbrain-hindbrain border. (From Brown, Keynes, and Lumsden 2001. Adapted with the permission of Oxford University Press.)

hindbrain. Finally, the protein products of three *Pax* genes, *Pax2*, *Pax5*, and *Pax8* participate in both the establishment of the border and in its maintenance.

## Anterior-Posterior Specification of Forebrain Structures

During the development of the neural plate, a number of factors were found to be critical in specifying rudimentary anterior-posterior patterning. Repression of the activity of the posteriorizing agent Wnt by Wnt antagonists expressed in the underlying mesoderm was critical for blocking posterior fates in anterior regions. Further, expression of *Otx2* in the anterior visceral endoderm (AVE), the mesendoderm, and the neurectoderm was critical for expression of anterior fate, as evidenced by failure of head expression with mutation of *Otx2*. These rudimentary patterns of organization become elaborated with development, and both *Wnt* and *Otx2* are also critical later in development in early patterning of the forebrain structures.

### Differentiation of the Telencephalon and the Diencephalon

Very little is known about the mechanisms by which segmentation occurs along the anterior-posterior axis of the prosencephalon (Braun et al. 2003). However, there is evidence that as early as the neural plate stage, gene expression patterns begin to presage the much-later-emerging division between the telencephalon and the diencephalon. Specifically, during the neural plate stage, tissue that will later give rise to the telencephalon expresses a transcription factor, Foxg1 (formerly called Bf1), that appears to mark the boundaries of the future telencephalic tissue. When *Foxg1* is blocked, deletion of the ventral telencephalon and substantial reduction in the size of the cerebral hemispheres are observed. After neural tube closure, *Fgf*s are expressed from the most anterior extent of the telencephalon, a region called the anterior neural ridge. *Fgf* expression appears to be necessary to maintain *Foxg1* expression and thus retain telencephalic identity (Brown, Keynes, and Lumsden 2001). Removal of anterior neural ridge cells results in substantial loss of telencephalic territory.

### Compartmentalization of the Prosencephalon

Morphological studies originally suggested that within prosencephalic regions six compartment-like structures, called prosomeres, emerge ordered in a caudal to rostral sequence, p1–p6 (Puelles 1995). Although prosomeric organization bears some resemblance to the rhombomeric organization in the hindbrain, there is recent evidence that prosomeres, at least as originally defined, do not form true compartments and that their cell lineages do not show the same degree of restriction as is observed in rhombomeres (Braun et al. 2003; Brown, Keynes, and Lumsden 2001). Recently the prosomere model has been modified and now defines more limited compartmentalization within anterior regions than was proposed in the earlier prosomere model. The new model includes only three prosomeres confined to the diencephalic region, plus a single large anterior segment encompassing the telencephalon and the rostral diencephalon (Puelles and Rubenstein 2003). The most caudal prosomere is p1, which is located in the region of the midbrain tectum. P2 is postulated to include the region of the diencephalon that will give rise to the thalamus, an important sensory relay nucleus. P3 lies anterior to p2 and includes the prethalamus.

Recent work has documented a well-defined boundary structure that separates p2 and p3 and acts as a signaling center to provide regional identity to the structures immediately anterior and posterior to it (Kiecker and Lumsden 2004). The boundary structure is referred to as the zona limitans intrathalamica (ZLI). The ZLI is a thin band of cells that separates two regions that are defined by the expression of two different transcription factors. The region anterior to ZLI expresses *Six3*, while the posterior region expresses *Irx3*. The differential expression zones for these two transcription factors are initially established early in neural plate formation by the activity of Wnts, the potent posteriorizing agents important for setting up the initial anterior-posterior organization of the neural tube. *Irx3* expression is activated by Wnts, while *Six3* expression is suppressed. Thus the establishment of the initial position of the ZLI appears to be the product of a complex early signaling pathway involving *Wnt, Irx3,* and *Six3* (Braun et al. 2003). Another important gene expressed in the ZLI is *Shh*. Recall that Shh is a secreted molecule that is expressed in the notochord and prechordal plate mesoderm and is critical in the establishment of ventral identity along the extent of the neuraxis. The only place along the neuraxis where *Shh* extends dorsally is in the ZLI (Figure 5.9). In the ZLI, *Shh* expression stretches dorsally in a thin band separating the two major diencephalic regions, the thalamus and the prethalamus (Kiecker and

Lumsden 2004; Zeltser 2005; note that these structures are also referred to as the ventral and the dorsal thalamus, respectively). Expression of *Shh* in the ZLI regulates the development of the adjacent structures. Overexpression of *Shh* results in expansion of the posterior boundary to more anterior regions, while suppression of *Shh* has the opposite effect. Thus, like the isthmus region of the midbrain, the ZLI appears to act as a local signaling center that differentially regulates the development of adjacent brain regions both anteriorly and posteriorly and establishes differential regional identity along its borders.

## Early Patterning of the Emerging Cerebral Cortex

Although comparatively little is known about segmentation within the prosencephalon generally, considerably more work has been directed to the study of anterior-posterior patterning within the largest telen-

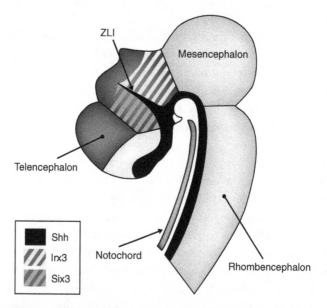

Figure 5.9. Differentiation within the prosencephalon involves a structure called the zona limitans intrathalamica (ZLI). The ZLI marks the expression boundaries of two transcription factors, Six3 is expressed anterior to the ZLI, and Irx3 is expressed posteriorly. Expression of Shh in the ZLI regulates the development of the adjacent structures. (From Kiecker and Lumsden 2004. Adapted with the permission of Nature Publishing Group.)

cephalic structure, indeed the largest brain structure, the cerebral cortex. In mammals, there are three subdivisions of the cerebral cortex. The phylogenetically older divisions are the paleocortex, which arises from the lateral portion of the early telencephalic vesicle and becomes primary olfactory cortex, and the archicortex, which derives from medial regions of the vesicle and will give rise to the hippocampus, an important memory area. The neocortex, also called the isocortex, is phylogenetically the newest cortical region and is unique to mammals. It arises out of the dorsolateral region of the telencephalic vesicle and constitutes by far the largest part of the cerebral cortex. It controls sensation, perception, cognition, and action. Within the dorsal telencephalon, the cells that will become the neocortical progenitors express the transcription factor Lhx2. Lhx2 is a unique marker because it is expressed only in cells that will become neocortical progenitors. Mutations of the *Lhx2* gene result in failure of the neocortical proliferative zone to develop (Monuki and Walsh 2001).

Across its surface extent, the mature neocortex is partitioned into well-defined structurally and functionally distinct areas. The areas are differentiated by their cellular organization and patterns of neuronal connectivity. This section will consider the initial patterning of the neocortex that results from differential signaling of populations of neural progenitor cells in the dorsal telencephalon.

## The Role of Emx2 and Pax6 in Early Neocortical Patterning

Two transcription factors, Emx2 and Pax6, play an essential role in the early patterning of the presumptive neocortex. These two transcription factors are expressed in opposing gradients along the anterior-posterior extent of the dorsal telencephalon in a process similar to that observed for dorsal-ventral patterning in the spinal cord. *Emx2* is expressed in a gradient that is highest in caudal and medial regions and lowest in rostral and lateral regions, while *Pax6* is expressed in the opposite gradient, highest in rostral and lateral regions and lowest in caudal and medial regions (Figure 5.10). These two transcription factors mutually repress each other in a graded fashion (Muzio and Mallamaci 2003), and the interaction of these two concentration gradients is thought to provide early specification of cortical regions in a concentration-dependent fashion (Bishop, Rubenstein, and O'Leary

2002; Hamasaki et al. 2004). A high concentration of Pax6 and a low concentration of Emx2 leads to induction of cells that will give rise to the motor cortex, while the opposite concentration values induce cells that will produce the visual cortex. Intermediate levels of both gene products result in formation of somatosensory cortices. Studies of mutant mice for which expression of either *Emx2* or *Pax6* is blocked show systematic shifts in the organization of cortical areas, suggesting that it is the interaction of these two gene products that induces change in the surrounding cell populations. In typically developing animals, primary sensory and motor areas are distributed along the anterior-posterior axis of the neocortex, with the motor area located in the most anterior region, the somatosensory area in the middle, and the visual area in the posterior cortex. When either *Emx2* or *Pax6* expression is blocked, the topographical relations between these cortical areas remain, but changes are observed in the size of the areas and in their locations (Figure 5.10). In *Emx2* mutants, visual areas shrink, while somatosensory and motor areas enlarge, and there is a posterior shift in their locations. Conversely, when *Pax6* is blocked, visual areas enlarge, while somatosensory and motor areas shrink, and an anterior shift in their locations is observed.

Double-knockout studies, in which activity of both *Pax6* and *Emx2* is blocked, provide evidence that these two transcription factors act as the primary functional specification signals in the developing neo-cortex (Muzio et al. 2002). The presumptive cortical regions of these mutants are reduced in size and show no evidence of the typical layered organization of the neocortex. Further, none of the genes that are typically expressed in the cortex are present, but a large number of gene markers typical of more ventral areas, specifically the lateral ganglionic eminence (LGE), are found, and the LGE is converted to a medial ganglionic eminence (Muzio and Mallamaci 2003). Thus it appears that in the absence of both Pax6 and Emx2 transcription factors, the neocortical progenitor cells are converted to ganglionic progenitors. Importantly, the presence of either Pax6 or Emx2 rescues the neocortical progenitors from the ganglionic fate, as observed in the single-gene mutant cases. Other genes can also ventralize dorsal telencephalic areas. The earlier description of *Gli3* mutants showing enhanced ventral regions via upregulation of the Shh pathway provides one example. However, these effects are not as pervasive as those observed with the double mutants, and the mechanism of change is less direct.

One difficulty with the mutant studies has been that the effects of the gene mutations are so pervasive that the dorsal telencephalon is dysmorphic, as well as dramatically reduced in size. Consequently, the animals do not survive to the time when cortical areas and their primary input pathways actually emerge. Thus, although the studies document failure of dorsal telencephalic fate induction in the absence of *Emx2* or *Pax6* expression, the data defining the role of these two transcription factors in the specification of cortical areas have been less complete. A solution to this problem was recently provided by the

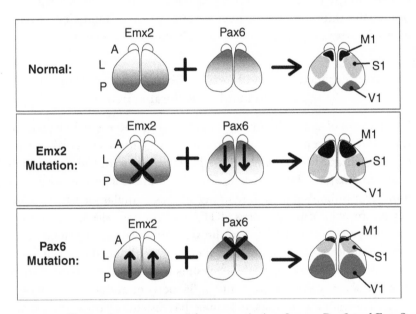

Figure 5.10. Expression patterns of the transcription factors Pax6 and Emx2. Emx2 is expressed in a gradient that is highest in caudal and medial regions and lowest in rostral and lateral regions, while Pax6 is expressed in the opposite gradient. The combination of specific concentrations of the two transcription factors gives rise to different functional areas in the neocortex. Mutation of either gene shifts the boundaries of the functional cortical areas. M1 = primary motor; S1 = primary somatosensory; V1 = primary visual; A = anterior; L = lateral; P = posterior. (From Bishop, Rubenstein, and O'Leary 2002. Adapted with the permission of the Society for Neuroscience.)

creation of a transgenic mouse model in which *Emx2* is overexpressed rather than repressed. This model provides a means of examining directly the effect of *Emx2* modulation on the emergence of cortical areas in animals that survive past birth (Hamasaki et al. 2004).

The pattern of cortical organization observed in the transgenic mice is consistent with that obtained from the *Pax6* mutants. In the case of the Pax6 mutants, blocking the expression gradient of *Pax6* allowed for the expansion of the *Emx2* expression gradient, which resulted in the enlargement of visual areas and reduction of somatosensory and motor areas, which were also displaced anteriorly. A very similar pattern of cortical reorganization was associated with the augmented expression of *Emx2* in the transgenic animals. Importantly, these animals survived postnatally, thus allowing for detailed anatomical examination of reorganized cortex, as well as assessment of behavioral function.

## Altering Pax6 or Emx2 Levels Affects Neuroanatomical Organization and Behavioral Function

Comparison of the brain anatomy in the transgenic and wild-type mice reveals no differences in total cortical size or patterns of cortical laminar organization (Hamasaki et al. 2004). The size of the dorsal thalamus, the major subcortical sensorimotor input nucleus, is normal in transgenic animals. Further, marking studies of thalamocortical axons (TCAs) reveal normal patterns of TCA pathfinding. However, anatomical differences are observed in the size and location of primary sensory and motor cortical areas. Specifically, the enhanced levels of *Emx2* expression in the transgenic mice results in a 25 percent reduction of primary sensory cortex (S1) and a 36 percent reduction in motor areas. The viability of transgenic mice has also allowed for the examination of whether change in the size of cortical areas affects behavior (Leingartner et al. 2007). These animals do not differ from wild type over a range of factors that might affect overall sensorimotor performance, such as body weight, mobility, or grip strength. However, on tests that specifically assess sensorimotor coordination and locomotor agility, their performance is significantly poorer than that of wild-type controls. The transgenic mice make more errors in foot placement when traversing a wire mesh grid and are more likely to fall from the grid. They are also less able to maintain balance and position when placed on a rotating rod. Thus, the genetically induced alteration in the size of sensorimotor cortical areas has direct consequences for later behavioral functioning. While the specific effects of cortical reduction on behavior have not been defined, possible candidate factors include alteration in the convergence of thalamocortical inputs or disruption of area-specific cortical outputs (Leingartner et al. 2007).

## Regulation of *Pax6* and *Emx2* Gene Expression

The results of the transgenic mice studies, in combination with the earlier work, have led a number of investigators to suggest that *Emx2*, and likely *Pax6*, may serve as the master genes for specification of the neocortex (Hamasaki et al. 2004; Muzio and Mallamaci 2003; Shimogori et al. 2004). However, the expression patterns of *Emx2* and *Pax6* are regulated by a complex set of factors. Patterning within the telencephalon is controlled by the expression of secreted molecules emanating from a number of signaling centers (Zaki, Quinn, and Price 2003). As discussed earlier, dorsal-ventral patterning is controlled by signals from the prechordal plate mesoderm and anterior medial telencephalic structures. The anterior medial telencephalic signaling center, in conjunction with a third center, the cortical hem, is also critical for the regulation of gene expression that establishes anterior-posterior patterning in the neocortex. The anterior medial signaling center expresses *Fgf8*, while the cortical hem expresses both *Bmps* and *Wnts*. Fgf8 is important for regulating the expression of *Emx2*. Specifically, Fgf8 appears to repress *Emx2* expression in a graded fashion along the anterior-posterior axis, but does not appear to affect *Pax6* expression (Hamasaki et al. 2004). Artificially altering the level of Fgf8 produces a pattern of results that is the mirror of manipulations of *Emx2* expression. Specifically, augmenting the amount of Fgf8 in the anterior expression site enlarges anterior cortical areas and shrinks posterior areas, while blocking *Fgf8* expression has the opposite effect (Fukuchi-Shimogori and Grove 2001; Grove and Fukuchi-Shimogori 2003). Interestingly, the introduction of Fgf8 into posterior regions where it is not normally expressed creates anomalously placed regions that express anterior identity. These findings are consistent with a model in which the graded expression of *Emx2* is regulated by the expression of signaling molecules emanating from local signaling centers. *Pax6* expression is thought to be regulated directly or indirectly by Emx2.

Finally, the expression of *Fgf8* must be further modulated to achieve appropriate cortical patterning in anterior regions. Bmps block expression of *Fgf8* within specific regions, thus setting up expression boundaries that limit the range of Fgf8 effectiveness in the downregulation of *Emx2* expression. *Wnts* are expressed in the cortical hem near the site of the developing hippocampus and are critical for its development. However, *Wnts* are blocked by Fgf8. Bmps prevent *Fgf8* expression in the cortical hem, thus protecting Wnt activity and preserving its role in hippocampal development (Shimogori et al. 2004).

This greatly simplified account includes only a fraction of the genes that are involved in patterning of the neocortex. It focuses on the major transcription factors and secreted molecules that act in concert as a regulatory network to establish the essential organizational scheme for the developing neocortex. Many other genes contribute to the establishment of local area boundaries and patterns of connectivity both within and among cortical areas.

## Clinical Correlation: Isotretinoin (Accutane) Exposure in the Early Prenatal Period

Retinoic acid (RA) is an important posteriorizing agent that acts in the developing central nervous system to regulate the expression of *HOX* genes. It has also been implicated as a critical regulator of a class of genes that is important for controlling neuron production. RA acts to upregulate genes that promote the production of neurons and downregulate genes that inhibit neuron production (Maden 2002). Because it is a regulator, RA acts in a dose-dependent fashion in the developing central nervous system. Either depletion of or overexposure to RA leads to serious defects in hindbrain patterning and in formation of the spinal column.

The distribution of RA in the central nervous system is consistent with its role in caudal specification. It is found in highest concentration in the spinal cord, with very little in forebrain, midbrain, or hindbrain. In addition, RA is found in the meninges of the central nervous system. The meninges are a set of three layered membranes that cover and protect the brain and spinal cord. RA is obtained through dietary sources and is typically derived from vitamin A (Sakai et al. 2001). As discussed earlier, the level of RA in the system is regulated by two enzymes. RALDH2 synthesizes RA, while CYP26 degrades it. Regulation of RA is controlled by the liver. RA precursors are stored in the liver, thus providing a continuing source to the system. In addition, the liver can also act as a sink, sequestering RA precursors when there is an excess. In mice, sufficient RA is stored in the liver by the end of weaning to last the lifetime of the animal (McCaffery et al. 2003).

Vitamin A was first recognized as an essential dietary element in 1933 (Hale 1933), but its potential as a teratogen, or an agent that causes abnormalities in the developing human embryo or fetus, was not recognized for 20 years (Cohlan 1953). In 1982, 13-cis retinoic acid, isotretinoin, was introduced as a treatment for serious, chronic cystic acne (McCaffery et al. 2003). Isotretinoin is an orally administered medication that is taken for a period of weeks or months to treat the underlying cause of this deforming condition. It was released under the trade name Accutane. Before its release, animal studies of prenatal isotretinoin exposure indicated that this form of RA was safe and had little effect on the developing embryo. The initial animal studies used a mouse model. Unfortunately, the product had been marketed for sale to humans for three years before additional studies with primates were completed. Those studies revealed that there are significant differences in the level of drug transfer across the placenta in mice and primates. In primates, including humans, the recommended dosage of isotretinoin is highly teratogenic.

The first detailed studies of the effects of isotretinoin exposure on developing human fetuses were completed in 1985 (Lammer et al. 1985). They reported a range of abnormal outcomes that varied from isolated cognitive impairment to death. In their sample of cases with documented prenatal exposure to isotretinoin, they found a spontaneous abortion rate of 40 percent. The rate of clinically significant malformations among children born live was 35 percent. Importantly, they found that 47 percent of children in their sample had significant cognitive deficits, scoring in the below-average range on IQ measures. Further, of that 47 percent, 25 percent of the children with serious cognitive compromise had no evidence of physical malformation. At birth, these children had been judged to be normal. The observed variability in outcome following prenatal isotretinoin exposure is likely explained by dosage effects. Although all the mothers took isotretinoin early in pregnancy, there were variations in the dosage levels, the number of days of exposure, and the exact timing of exposure, as well as individual differences in susceptibility. Finally, within the sample, males appeared to be more vulnerable than females in that the group with cognitive deficit was not evenly distributed. Rather, 68 percent of males born after isotretinoin exposure had serious cognitive compromise, while only 19 percent of females had comparable problems.

The range of physical malformations observed in the children prenatally exposed to isotretinoin was consistent with the known effects of RA. Hindbrain abnormalities were common and in some cases were accompanied by hydrocephaly. The most common type of malformation involved the cerebellum. Cranial nerve defects were also prevalent. Children with hindbrain abnormalities typically had sensory and motor delays and severe mental retardation. There were also reports of forebrain abnormalities, including microcephaly and cortical heterotopias, disorders of neural migration that result in misplaced pockets of neurons. Findings of cerebellar, hindbrain, and spinal-cord abnormalities reflect the role of RA in caudal patterning. The forebrain and some cerebellar abnormalities likely reflect the activity of RA within the meninges as a regulator of neural proliferation. One source of the neurons that make up the cerebellum is a dorsal hindbrain structure called the rhombic lip. The progenitor cells that give rise to granule neurons are initially produced in the rhombic lip. The neurons then migrate over the surface of the brain in an external cerebellar layer. As they migrate, these cells are exposed to the overlying meninges, which strongly express RALDH2, the enzyme that synthesizes RA. Thus some of the abnormalities associated with RA overexposure could derive from sources in the meninges (McCaffery et al. 2003).

Isotretinoin is still marketed for treatment of cystic acne. However, the recommendations for administration of the drug have changed dramatically in the wake of the primate and human studies. The current U.S. National Institutes of Health guidelines involve not simply informing patients of the risks surrounding isotretinoin use; they recommend monthly pregnancy tests for all female patients.

## Chapter Summary

- Dorsal-ventral specification within the spinal column is directed by opposing gradients of two secreted proteins that act as morphogens. In ventral regions, the notochord provides initial signaling to establish the floor plate in the ventral spinal column. In dorsal regions, the overlying epidermis expresses Bmps, which are secreted in a gradient that opposes the ventral Shh gradient. The interaction of these two gradients serves to induce a range of cell types that are each specified by the concentration of the signaling molecules.

- Dorsal-ventral patterning in the telencephalon begins with the emergence of the ganglionic eminences (GEs). Shh expressed in the ventral telencephalon provides preliminary specification of these structures. However, unlike the spinal column, where ventral cell-type specification depends on the concentration of Shh, specification of GE structures appears to depend on the timing of Shh exposure. Shh signaling appears to be modulated by the transcription factor Gli3, via an as-yet-unspecified factor.

- Wnt signaling is also important in dorsal-ventral patterning in the telencephalon. During the gastrula stage, Wnts were important for caudal specification. Interestingly, later in development, they appear to be important in conveying dorsal fate to neurons in the telencephalon.

- Anterior-posterior specification in the spinal cord is first marked by the formation of a series of eight longitudinal compartments, called rhombomeres. *Hox* gene expression confers positional value on cells within each rhombomere. *Hox* genes are a family of homeobox genes that are expressed in a nested pattern along the extent of the hindbrain and the spinal column. Retinoic acid is an important regulator of *Hox* gene expression. RA is expressed in a gradient along the neuraxis from the anterior hindbrain through the spinal column. Further, a temporal exposure gradient within hindbrain regions appears to modulate the concentration of RA to which hindbrain cells are exposed, altering positional value.

- The midbrain-hindbrain border is established by the interaction of a number of different genes expressed in specific spatial and temporal patterns. Two homeobox genes, *Otx2* and *Gbx2*, are expressed in opposed gradients at the isthmus; each blocks the other's activity. En1 and En2 act to establish regional identity within the midbrain and the anterior hindbrain. Their expression patterns are, in turn, regulated by *Fgf8* and *Wnt* expression.

- Specification of the telencephalic-diencephalic border centers on a boundary structure called the zona limitans intrathalamica (ZLI). The ZLI is a thin band of cells that separates two regions defined by the expression of different transcription factors, Six3 anterior to the ZLI and Irx3 posterior to it.
- The three major divisions of the telencephalon are the paleo-cortex, the archicortex, and the neocortex. Parcellation of the te-lencephalon is not well understood. Cells that will become neo-cortical progenitors all express the transcription factor Lhx2, and mutation of this gene causes failure of the neocortical prolifera-tive zone to develop.
- Initial patterning of the neocortex is regulated by the expression of two transcription factors, Emx2 and Pax6. They are expressed in opposing gradients along the anterior-posterior axis, and they mutually repress each other's expression. Double-knockout studies establish the importance of these genes as primary cor-tical specification signals. Cortical regions in mutant animals are reduced in size and show no layering; further, the cells express markers typical of ventral brain regions.
- Mutations of either *Pax6* or *Emx2* result in changes in the size and location of functional areas in the neocortex. Studies of transgenic mice have shown that these changes are associated with abnormalities in the structure and function of the neocortex and in the behaviors of the animals.

### References

Bishop, K. M., J. L. Rubenstein, and D. D. O'Leary. 2002. "Distinct actions of Emx1, Emx2, and Pax6 in regulating the specification of areas in the developing neocortex." *Journal of Neuroscience*, 22: 7627–7638.

Braun, M. M., A. Etheridge, A. Bernard, C. P. Robertson, and H. Roelink. 2003. "Wnt signaling is required at distinct stages of development for the induction of the posterior forebrain." *Development*, 130: 5579–5587.

Brown, A. L. 1975. "The development of memory: Knowing, knowing about knowing, and knowing how to know." *Advances in Child Development and Behavior*, 10: 103–152.

Brown, M., R. Keynes, and A. Lumsden. 2001. *The developing brain*. Oxford: Oxford University Press.

Cohlan, S. Q. 1953. "Excessive intake of vitamin A as a cause of congenital anomalies in the rat." *Science*, 117: 535–536.

Fukuchi-Shimogori, T., and E. A. Grove. 2001. "Neocortex patterning by the secreted signaling molecule FGF8." *Science*, 294: 1071–1074.

Gavalas, A. 2002. "ArRAnging the hindbrain." *Trends in Neurosciences*, 25: 61–64.

Gavalas, A., C. Ruhrberg, J. Livet, C. E. Henderson, and R. Krumlauf. 2003. "Neuronal defects in the hindbrain of *Hoxa1*, *Hoxb1* and *Hoxb2* mutants reflect regulatory interactions among these Hox genes." *Development*, 130: 5663–5679.

Gilbert, S. F. 2006. *Developmental biology*. 8th ed. Sunderland, MA: Sinauer Associates.

Giudicelli, F., E. Taillebourg, P. Charnay, and P. Gilardi-Hebenstreit. 2001. "Krox-20 patterns the hindbrain through both cell-autonomous and non cell-autonomous mechanisms." *Genes and Development*, 15: 567–580.

Glover, J. C., J. S. Renaud, and F. M. Rijli. 2006. "Retinoic acid and hindbrain patterning." *Journal of Neurobiology*, 66: 705–725.

Grove, E. A., and T. Fukuchi-Shimogori. 2003. "Generating the cerebral cortical area map." *Annual Review of Neuroscience*, 26: 355–380.

Gunhaga, L., T. M. Jessell, and T. Edlund. 2000. "Sonic hedgehog signaling at gastrula stages specifies ventral telencephalic cells in the chick embryo." *Development*, 127: 3283–3293.

Gunhaga, L., M. Marklund, M. Sjodal, J. C. Hsieh, T. M. Jessell, and T. Edlund. 2003. "Specification of dorsal telencephalic character by sequential Wnt and FGF signaling." *Nature Neuroscience*, 6: 701–707.

Gutin, G., M. Fernandes, L. Palazzolo, H. Paek, K. Yu, D. M. Ornitz, S. K. McConnell, and J. M. Hebert. 2006. "FGF signalling generates ventral telencephalic cells independently of SHH." *Development*, 133: 2937–2946.

Hale, F. 1933. "Pigs born without eyeballs." *Journal of Heredity*, 24: 105–106.

Hamasaki, T., A. Leingartner, T. Ringstedt, and D. D. O'Leary. 2004. "EMX2 regulates sizes and positioning of the primary sensory and motor areas in neocortex by direct specification of cortical progenitors." *Neuron*, 43: 359–372.

Kiecker, C., and A. Lumsden. 2004. "Hedgehog signaling from the ZLI regulates diencephalic regional identity." *Nature Neuroscience*, 7: 1242–1249.

———. 2005. "Compartments and their boundaries in vertebrate brain development." *Nature Reviews Neuroscience*, 6: 553–564.

Kintner, C., and A. Lumsden. 1999. "Neural induction and pattern formation." In *Fundamental neuroscience*, ed. M. J. Zigmond, F. E. Bloom, S. C. Landis, J. L. Roberts, and L. R. Squire, 417–450. San Diego, CA: Academic Press.

Kohtz, J. D., D. P. Baker, G. Corte, and G. Fishell. 1998. "Regionalization within the mammalian telencephalon is mediated by changes in responsiveness to Sonic Hedgehog." *Development*, 125: 5079–5089.

Krumlauf, R. 1993. "*Hox* genes and pattern formation in the branchial region of the vertebrate head." *Trends in Genetics*, 9: 106–112.

Lammer, E. J., D. T. Chen, R. M. Hoar, N. D. Agnish, P. J. Benke, J. T. Braun, C. J. Curry, P. M. Fernhoff, A. W. Grix Jr., I. T. Lott, J. M. Richard, and S. C. Sun. 1985. "Retinoic acid embryopathy." *New England Journal of Medicine*, 313: 837–841.

Lee, K. J., P. Dietrich, and T. M. Jessell. 2000. "Genetic ablation reveals that the roof plate is essential for dorsal interneuron specification." *Nature*, 403: 734–740.

Leingartner, A., S. Thuret, T. T. Kroll, S. J. Chou, J. L. Leasure, F. H. Gage, and D. D. O'Leary. 2007. "Cortical area size dictates performance at modality-specific behaviors." *Proceedings of the National Academy of Sciences of the United States of America*, 104: 4153–4158.

Lumsden, A., and R. Keynes. 1989. "Segmental patterns of neuronal development in the chick hindbrain." *Nature*, 337: 424–428.

Lumsden, A., and R. Krumlauf. 1996. "Patterning the vertebrate neuraxis." *Science*, 274: 1109–1115.

Maden, M. 2002. "Retinoid signalling in the development of the central nervous system." *Nature Reviews Neuroscience*, 3: 843–853.

McCaffery, P. J., J. Adams, M. Maden, and E. Rosa-Molinar. 2003. "Too much of a good thing: Retinoic acid as an endogenous regulator of neural differentiation and exogenous teratogen." *European Journal of Neuroscience*, 18: 457–472.

McGinnis, W., and R. Krumlauf. 1992. "Homeobox genes and axial patterning." *Cell*, 68: 283–302.

McKay, I. J., I. Muchamore, R. Krumlauf, M. Maden, A. Lumsden, and J. Lewis. 1994. "The kreisler mouse: A hindbrain segmentation mutant that lacks two rhombomeres." *Development*, 120: 2199–2211.

Monuki, E. S., and C. A. Walsh. 2001. "Mechanisms of cerebral cortical patterning in mice and humans." *Nature Neuroscience*, 4 (Suppl.): 1199–1206.

Muzio, L., B. DiBenedetto, A. Stoykova, E. Boncinelli, P. Gruss, and A. Mallamaci. 2002. "Emx2 and Pax6 control regionalization of the preneuronogenic cortical primordium." *Cerebral Cortex*, 12: 129–139.

Muzio, L., and A. Mallamaci. 2003. "*Emx1, Emx2* and *Pax6* in specification, regionalization and arealization of the cerebral cortex." *Cerebral Cortex*, 13: 641–647.

Nakamura, H., T. Katahira, T. Sato, Y. Watanabe, and J. Funahashi. 2004. "Gain- and loss-of-function in chick embryos by electroporation." *Mechanisms of Development*, 121: 1137–1143.

Puelles, L. 1995. "A segmental morphological paradigm for understanding vertebrate forebrains." *Brain, Behavior and Evolution,* 46: 319–337.

Puelles, L., and J. L. Rubenstein. 2003. "Forebrain gene expression domains and the evolving prosomeric model." *Trends in Neurosciences,* 26: 469–476.

Rallu, M., J. G. Corbin, and G. Fishell. 2002. "Parsing the prosencephalon." *Nature Reviews Neuroscience,* 3: 943–951.

Rallu, M., R. Machold, N. Gaiano, J. G. Corbin, A. P. McMahon, and G. Fishell. 2002. "Dorsoventral patterning is established in the telencephalon of mutants lacking both Gli3 and Hedgehog signaling." *Development,* 129: 4963–4974.

Sakai, Y., C. Meno, H. Fujii, J. Nishino, H. Shiratori, Y. Saijoh, J. Rossant, and H. Hamada. 2001. "The retinoic acid–inactivating enzyme CYP26 is essential for establishing an uneven distribution of retinoic acid along the anterio-posterior axis within the mouse embryo." *Genes and Development,* 15: 213–225.

Schilling, T. F., and R. D. Knight. 2001. "Origins of anteroposterior patterning and *Hox* gene regulation during chordate evolution." *Philosophical Transactions of the Royal Society of London,* ser. B, *Biological Sciences,* 356: 1599–1613.

Shimogori, T., V. Banuchi, H. Y. Ng, J. B. Strauss, and E. A. Grove. 2004. "Embryonic signaling centers expressing BMP, WNT and FGF proteins interact to pattern the cerebral cortex." *Development,* 131: 5639–5647.

Wurst, W., and L. Bally-Cuif. 2001. "Neural plate patterning: Upstream and downstream of the isthmic organizer." *Nature Reviews Neuroscience,* 2: 99–108.

Zaki, P. A., J. C. Quinn, and D. J. Price. 2003. "Mouse models of telencephalic development." *Current Opinion in Genetics and Development,* 13: 423–437.

Zeltser, L. M. 2005. "Shh-dependent formation of the ZLI is opposed by signals from the dorsal diencephalon." *Development,* 132: 2023–2033.

Zigmond, M. J., F. E. Bloom, S. C. Landis, J. L. Roberts, and L. R. Squire, eds. 1999. *Fundamental neuroscience.* San Diego, CA: Academic Press.

# SIX

# The Production of Brain Cells:
# Neurons and Glia

BY THE MIDDLE of the second prenatal month, the differentiation of the embryo along the anterior-posterior and dorsal-ventral axes has advanced significantly. The five secondary vesicles have emerged, and the processes of bending and folding have given the embryo its characteristic shape. Growth in anterior regions has outpaced that in posterior regions, and that expansion is particularly marked in the telencephalon. Within the central nervous system (CNS), clearly defined regional boundaries have been established, and significant and quite specific patterning within each region has emerged. Signaling centers in both dorsal and ventral regions of the CNS have expressed complex combinations of transcription factors and secreted molecules. The interactions among these gene products have begun to specify cell fates and to create more and more elaborate regional patterning. Within the telencephalon, the observed changes mark the first steps in the formation of the neocortical plate, the future neocortex.

This chapter will consider the changes that occur within the neocortex at a more microscopic level, the level of the cell. It will examine the generation of four populations of cells. The first are the multipotent neural progenitors, which will generate the remaining three types of cells: the long-range projection neurons, the local-circuit interneurons, and the neuronal support cells or glial cells. The projection neurons and interneurons will form the information-processing network of the cerebral cortex. These two classes of cells are produced in different proliferative regions. Projection neurons are initially produced exclusively in the ventricular zone (VZ), a proliferative region located at the center of the neural tube, and later in a second proliferative zone, the subventricular zone (SVZ). Production of interneurons appears to differ across mammalian species. In mice, interneurons are produced in a more caudally positioned proliferative zone in the region of the ganglionic eminences (GEs). In primates, including humans, interneurons appear to be produced in both the region of the GEs and the VZ/SVZ. Finally, the glial cells provide structure to the brain and support for the neurons. Different types of glial cells are produced in both the region of the GEs and the VZ (Kessaris et al. 2006).

The initial pool of multipotent neural progenitor cells was specified during gastrulation when the signaling molecules from the mesendoderm blocked the midline ectodermal cells from receiving signals that would have directed them to an epidermal fate. However, that original pool of neural progenitors was comparatively small, far too limited to produce the estimated 100 billion neurons that make up the CNS (Pakkenberg and Gundersen 1997; Williams and Herrup 1988). Thus, the first question to be considered in this chapter concerns the generation of a sufficiently large population of neural progenitor cells to support brain development. Next, the production of the large populations of cortical neurons will be considered. Neuronal development involves three primary steps: proliferation, migration, and differentiation. Proliferation refers to the generation of neurons. The neocortex is composed of a variety of different neuron types that are produced at different points in cortical development and from different proliferative regions. The central questions about proliferation concern how the correct number and type of cortical neurons are generated at the right time in brain development. Migration refers to the movement of newly generated neurons away from the proliferative zones. Differentiation refers to the changes in neurons that allow them to acquire the appropriate neurochemical signaling factors and to establish connections with other neurons. Together, this complex set of developmental events establishes the neural pathways that mediate all aspects of behavior, from sensation to movement to high-level cognition. This chapter will consider neuron proliferation, and Chapter 7 will discuss neuron migration and differentiation.

The final class of cells generated by progenitors is glial cells. Most glial cells are generated after neuron production is complete. The glia

serve a variety of roles in the structure and functioning of the neocortex. There are three primary classes of glia. Astrocytes provide a
support framework for neurons, modulate neural activity at the
synapse, and respond to insult or injury to the neural system. Oligodendrocytes are the myelin-forming cells in the brain. Microglia support immune functions in the brain, as well as serving as macrophages
to clear debris from the system (Bell, Anthony, and Simmonds 2006).

## The Cellular Organization of the Neocortex

To appreciate the magnitude of the task of neocortical development, it
is useful to consider the end state (Figure 6.1A). It is estimated that the
adult human neocortex contains approximately 20 billion of the 100
billion neurons that comprise the CNS. Each neuron connects to
1,000 other neurons, creating a neural network with trillions of connections. The great majority of neurons are generated during the
second trimester of pregnancy. At the peak of proliferation, it is estimated that in excess of 200,000 neurons are generated every minute.

The neocortex forms a mantle or sheet that covers the surface of the
brain, much like the rind on an orange (Figure 6.1B). In species with
small cerebral cortices, such as the rat, the cortical sheet on the surface of the brain is smooth. The dramatic evolutionary expansion of
the neocortical surface, which is especially evident in primates (including humans), required a novel adaptation to fit the greatly enlarged cortical sheet into the spatially limited cranial vault. The cortical sheet in species with large cerebral cortices is not smooth; rather,
it is folded into an intricate pattern of gyri (ridges) and sulci (valleys)
that serve to compact the surface area and allow it to fit within the cra-
nium (Figure 6.1B). The flattened, horizontal surface area of the entire mature human cerebral cortex, including the archicortex, paleocortex, and neocortex, measures approximately 2,500 cm². The area of
the human neocortex is roughly 1,850 cm² (~2.0 ft²), but, perhaps surprisingly, it measures only 2.5 mm (2 to 5 mm across regions) in its vertical thickness (Pakkenberg and Gundersen 1997). By comparison, the
surface area of a rat cerebral cortex is 6 cm², and it is 1 to 2 mm thick.
Thus, although the vertical thickness of the cerebral cortex is well conserved across species, there have been dramatic differences in horizontal surface area.

The organization of the neocortex is very uniform. Within the vertical dimension, it is composed of six layers of cells. The layers are distinguished by the types of neurons they contain and by the connections they form. There are three main types of cortical neurons: pyramidal cells, excitatory interneurons, and inhibitory interneurons. There are several different types of pyramidal cells, but they all mediate cortical output. They receive input from other pyramidal cells, thalamic afferents, and excitatory interneurons. The main class of excitatory interneurons is the spiny stellate cell. They have limited dendritic arbors (neural processes where connections are made) and mediate only local excitatory interactions. Inhibitory interneurons

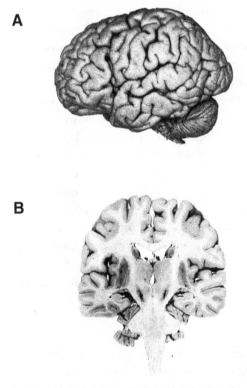

Figure 6.1. A. In the lateral (side) view of the adult brain, the convoluted pattern of gyral and sulcal folding is evident. B. In the coronal section of the adult brain, the thin mantle of the cerebral cortex and the underlying white-matter pathways are clearly defined. (From DeArmond, Fusco, and Dewey 1989. Reprinted with the permission of Oxford University Press.)

include basket, chandelier, and double-bouquet cells; each is named for its characteristic shape. All are inhibitory cells that regulate pyramidal cell function (they use GABA as their neurotransmitter substance and thus are called GABAergic cells). Each of these cell types is found in characteristic positions within the six-layered neocortex. Table 6.1 provides a summary of the distribution of cell types within the cortical layers. By convention, the cell layers are numbered 1 to 6, where layer 1 is the most superficial and layer 6 is the deepest cortical layer.

As discussed in greater detail in Chapter 7, the neocortical layers emerge in an orderly sequence during development (Marin-Padilla 1971, 1972; Meyer et al. 2000). During approximately the sixth week of gestation in humans (GW6), neurogenesis, or the production of neurons, begins. The first neurons generated in the VZ move to the far edge of the VZ to form the sparsely populated early marginal zone. The next wave of neuronal migration, at approximately GW7, moves farther away from the VZ. These neurons create a horizontal monolayer of cells called the preplate. Beginning at about GW7 to GW8, the preplate is split by the emerging cortical plate into the marginal zone and the subplate. The cortical layers form in an inside-out spatiotemporal sequence within the cortical plate. The cells from the deepest cortical layer, layer 6, form first, followed by the cells of layers 5, 4, and so on. The last cortical neurons to be generated are those that form layer 2. Layer 1 differs somewhat from the other layers. In the mature cortex, layer 1 contains mainly axons, but during development this layer serves a number of important but transient functions. The process of cortical development thus encompasses the production of an astonishing number of elements generated in a carefully choreographed temporal sequence and a well-defined spatial context.

## Neocortical Progenitor Cells

With the closure of the anterior neuropore, the neocortical progenitor cells all populate a single cell layer that lines the inner surface of the neural tube adjacent to its central opening, or lumen. The ballooning of the telencephalic vesicles expands the lumen into two large outpocketings that will eventually form the network of cerebral ventricles. The term given to the single-layered neocortical proliferative zone is the ventricular zone (VZ). Soon after the onset of neurogen-

**Table 6.1** Major cell types in different cortical layers

| Cortical Layer | Cell Type | Organization |
|---|---|---|
| 1 | Cajal-Retzius cells | • Contains very few neuronal cell bodies.<br>• Cajal-Retzius cells produce reelin and are critical in establishing laminar organization of the neocortex. |
| | GABAergic cells | • GABAergic cells play an inhibitory role in neural networks.<br>• Contains mainly axons that run laterally and synapse on apical dendrites of cells in deeper layers. |
| 2 | Small pyramidal cells | • Small pyramidal cells provide output to other cortical regions. |
| | Double-bouquet cells | • Double-bouquet cells provide inhibitory regulation. |
| 3 | Medium pyramidal cells | • Medium pyramidal cells, with layer-2 cells, provide output to both ipsilateral cortical regions and commissural projections to contralateral hemisphere. |
| | Basket cells<br>Chandelier cells<br>Double-bouquet cells | • Basket, chandelier, and double-bouquet cells are all GABAergic and provide inhibitory regulation. |
| 4 | Pyramidal cells | • Contains pyramidal cells that communicate with other layers |

Table 6.1 (*continued*)

| Cortical Layer | Cell Type | Organization |
| --- | --- | --- |
| | Spiny stellate cells | • Rich in spiny stellate cells, which are excitatory interneurons that organize local circuit networks<br>• Layer 4 of the sensory cortex receives afferent input from the thalamus.<br>• Nonsensory regions of the cortex have very few excitatory interneurons. |
| 5 | Very large pyramidal cells | • Contains the largest pyramidal cells, which give rise to the long axons that leave the cortex and extend to subcortical regions, the spinal cord, and so on. |
| | Basket cells<br>Double-bouquet cells | • Basket and double-bouquet cells are also prevalent and provide inhibitory regulation. |
| 6 | Pyramidal cells | • Contains pyramidal cells that are more variable in size and shape than pyramidal cells in other layers<br>• They project back to the thalamus and make cortico-cortical connections |

*Sources:* M. J. Gutnick and I. Mody, The cortical neuron (New York: Oxford University Press, © 1995); G. M. Shepherd, The synaptic organization of the brain, 5th ed. (Oxford: Oxford University Press, © 2004); and L. W. Swanson, Brain architecture: Understanding the basic plan (Oxford: Oxford University Press, © 2003).

esis, a secondary proliferative zone begins to form immediately adjacent to the VZ called the subventricular zone (SVZ). The VZ and SVZ are the primary sources of excitatory neurons in the developing neocortex. A third proliferative zone including the medial, lateral, and caudal ganglionic eminences (MGE, LGE, CGE) has recently been identified. In mouse models, the MGE and the LGE appear to be the source of nearly all inhibitory interneurons (Anderson et al. 2001), though, as discussed later, there may be greater variability in primates (Letinic, Zoncu, and Rakic 2002; Rakic and Zecevic 2003b).

## Progenitor Cell Division in the VZ

The VZ is composed of a single layer of dividing cells, but it appears as a multilayered structure (Figure 6.2A). The laminar appearance of the VZ is due to the process by which progenitor cells divide. Just before the onset of the mitotic cycle (the cell-division cycle), the progenitor cell is positioned at the inner margin of the VZ, near the lumen. It is attached to its neighboring cells in the vicinity of the lumen through structures called junctional complexes (Chenn et al. 1998). At the beginning of the mitotic cycle, the cell is small and elliptical in shape. As the mitotic cycle begins, the cell elongates and projects a cytoplasmic extension toward the outer margin of the VZ, where it establishes contact with the basal lamina on the external surface of the VZ (Figure 6.2B). At this point, the nucleus of the cell begins to move up within the VZ in the direction of the VZ surface through a process referred to as interkinetic migration. Later the nucleus will return to the bottom of the VZ near the lumen. The movement of the nucleus coincides with the four well-defined phases of the mitotic cell cycle (Takahashi, Nowakowski, and Caviness 1993; Figure 6.2B). The first phase is Gap 1, during which the cell elongates and makes contact with the basal lamina on the outer surface of the VZ. The second is the S phase, during which the nucleus moves toward the outer surface of the VZ and DNA synthesis commences. DNA synthesis begins when the nucleus reaches the outer margin of the VZ and continues as it begins to descend again toward the lumen. DNA synthesis continues during the Gap 2 phase. Finally, the M phase begins after the nucleus has returned to the lumen. During the M phase, the cell divides into two daughter cells, and the process begins again. The stratified appearance of the VZ derives from the fact that at any given time, different cells are in different phases of the mitotic cell cycle, and thus the nuclei are positioned at different levels within the VZ.

## Early Symmetrical Division Increases the Pool of Progenitors

Throughout the period of cortical neurogenesis, the progenitor cells divide repeatedly, but the character and outcome of cell division in the first part of the proliferative period differ from those observed later in proliferation. Neocortical progenitor cells undergo two distinct types of cell division. During the early period of proliferation, cell division is symmetrical in that each of the daughter cells that is produced during mitosis is identical to the other daughter and to the parent cell. The symmetrical division of progenitor cells thus serves to increase the size

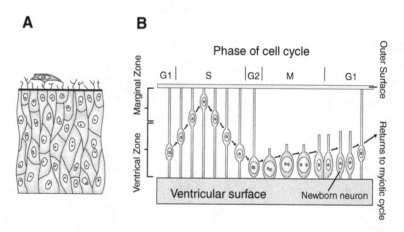

Figure 6.2. A. The ventricular zone (VZ) contains a single layer of dividing cells. The laminar appearance of the VZ derives from the process by which progenitor cells divide. B. The progenitor cell division cycle has four phases. Gap 1(G1): the cell elongates and makes contact with the outer surface of the VZ; Synthesis (S-phase): the nucleus moves toward the outer surface of the VZ, and DNA synthesis begins; Gap 2(G2): DNA synthesis continues; Mitosis (M-phase): begins after the nucleus has returned to the lumen. The cell divides into two daughter cells, and the process begins again. (A from Sadler 2006. Adapted with the permission of Lippincott Williams & Wilkins. B from Chenn and McConnell 1995. Adapted with the permission of Elsevier.)

of the proliferating cell population. With the onset of neurogenesis, a subset of the progenitor cells begin to divide asymmetrically. Asymmetrical cell division produces two daughter cells that differ both in the cell-intrinsic fate-determining molecules they contain and in their capacity to receive extrinsic signaling from other cells (Chenn and McConnell 1995; Fishell and Kriegstein 2003; Haydar, Ang, and Rakic 2003; Petersen et al. 2006; Wodarz and Huttner 2003). Within the VZ and during most of the period of neurogenesis, asymmetrical cell division produces one daughter cell that remains in the proliferative cycle and continues to divide and reproduce and one that exits the cycle, stops mitotic division, and migrates away from the VZ. In the early phase of asymmetrical cell division, the postmitotic cells are the young neurons. Later this population will also include glial cells.

Symmetrical cell division provides a mechanism for rapidly increasing the pool of progenitor cells necessary for neocortical genesis. Within the pool of proliferating cells, a single round of symmetrical cell division doubles the number of available progenitors. Thus the pool of proliferating neural progenitors increases exponentially over a series of symmetrical mitotic cycles. Indeed, it has been argued that the prolongation of symmetrical cell division for even a few mitotic cycles could account for the dramatic increases in the size of the neocortex that are observed across mammalian neocortical evolution (Caviness, Takahashi, and Nowakowski 1995; Finlay, Hersman, and Darlington 1998; Rakic 1995). Mitotic cell division of progenitors in the VZ is entirely symmetrical until GW7. After that time, a small number of progenitors begin to divide asymmetrically. Over the period of neurogenesis, the proportion of asymmetrically dividing progenitors gradually increases such that by the later period of neurogenesis, more than half the progenitors divide asymmetrically (Takahashi, Nowakowski, and Caviness 1996).

The production of neurons in the VZ begins in humans in GW7, and the period of neurogenesis extends for approximately 100 days (Bayer et al. 1993; Rakic 1995). The estimates are approximate because there is considerable regional variability in the length of the neurogenic period (Dehay et al. 1993). Along the extent of the neuraxis, the duration of neurogenesis is longer as one movies from caudal to more rostral regions, with the most extended periods observed in the rostral telencephalon (Finlay, Hersman, and Darlington 1998). Further, within the telencephalon, there is variation in the onset and duration of neurogenesis. In the telencephalon, development proceeds in a rostrolateral-to-caudal-medial sequence (Anthony et al. 2004).

## Fate Restriction in Progenitors

All neural progenitor cells derive from the multipotent neural progenitors that were produced during gastrulation. However, it is less clear whether a single progenitor cell type produces all of the neural elements of the cerebral cortex, or if there are several different progenitor cell types that are more or less restricted in their capacity to generate different types of cells (e.g., multipotent progenitors, neural-restricted progenitors, glial-restricted progenitors). It was recently documented that with the onset of neurogenesis, the neural progenitor cells in the VZ undergo a series of changes including the expression of astroglial markers. The appearance of these changes marks the transformation of neural progenitor cells into radial glial (RG) cells (Gotz and Huttner 2005). Radial glial cells were originally thought to serve only a supporting role in cortical development by providing a kind of cellular scaffolding for support and guidance of new neurons migrating from the VZ to the developing neocortex (Rakic 2003). However, recent work in mice has shown that RG cells are the primary neural progenitor cell line, with estimates that 95 percent of cortical neurons derive either directly or indirectly from RG cells (Anthony et al. 2004; Fishell and Kriegstein 2003; Malatesta et al. 2003; Noctor et al. 2001, 2002). These findings led to the suggestion that RG cells may be the sole class of neural progenitor cells in the murine brain.

Studies from primate species, including humans, confirmed the role of RG cells in neuronal and later glial production but also suggest that there may be greater diversity in the range of progenitor cell lines (Gotz and Huttner 2005; Howard, Chen, and Zecevic 2006; Rakic 2006; Zecevic, Chen, and Filipovic 2005). This divergence in findings led to the suggestion that there may be species differences in the range of neuro-generative cell lines. However, very recent work has now documented multiple progenitor cell lines in the mouse (Gal et al. 2006).

Within the human telencephalon, RG cells first appear at approximately GW7 (Howard, Chen, and Zecevic 2006), coinciding with the onset of neurogenesis. However, before that time, cells expressing neural but not glial molecular markers can be detected in the telencephalic VZ, suggesting the presence of an early line of neural-fate-restricted progenitor cells (Howard, Chen, and Zecevic 2006). Later in development, there is evidence that there may be different subclasses of RG cells, as indexed by differences in the types of transcription factors they express. RG cells also produce a different type of progenitor cell, called the intermediate, or basal, progenitor cell. These cells are generated in the VZ but migrate to the SVZ where they then divide symmetrically, producing either two neurons or two progenitor cells (Martinez-Cerdeno, Noctor, and Kriegstein 2006; Noctor et al. 2004). Finally, as discussed later, there is evidence that different subpopulations of neural progenitors may be restricted in the type of glial lineage they can produce. In different regions of the fetal telencephalon, progenitors appear to be restricted to the generation of only one glial cell line and are thus capable of generating neurons and astrocytes or neurons and oligodendrocytes (Liu and Rao 2004; Sun, Martinowich, and Ge 2003).

## Neuronal Proliferation

The first cortical neurons begin to be produced in GW7 by a small subset of dividing progenitor cells. The neurons are distinct from the progenitor cells in that they are postmitotic; that is, they are no longer capable of dividing. Specifying the neuronal fate of the newly produced cell involves two related sets of signaling processes. The first is the processes that result in the differentiation of the new neuron from the neuroprogenitor cell. This critical step in the neural differentiation process involves the shift from symmetrical to asymmetrical progenitor cell division. The second set of processes controls the generation of specific neural identities. A salient feature of the emerging laminar organization of the developing cerebral cortex is the presence of different types of neurons within the different layers. Neurons from different layers of the neocortex are generated within the VZ/SVZ and then migrate to appropriate laminar positions. One important question is how and when the specific neural fates are determined.

## Asymmetrical Cell Division and the Differentiation of Progenitors and Neurons

Asymmetrical cell division produces two daughter cells that differ in their generative roles and their specified fate. One daughter cell reenters the mitotic cycle, while the other, in an event referred to as the neuronal cell birthday, exits the proliferative cycle and migrates away from the VZ. The cells also differ in their intrinsic cell-fate determinants and in their capacity to respond to extrinsic signals (Chenn et al. 1998; Huttner and Brand 1997; Wodarz and Huttner 2003). The intrinsic cell-fate determinants include a variety of proteins and signaling molecules in the cytoplasm and membranes of progenitor cells. The membranes of the cells are also sites of contact with other cells, thus providing a mechanism for extrinsic signaling. During symmetrical cell division, the cells cleave such that both the intrinsic determinants and the contact sites are divided equally between the two daughter cells. However, during asymmetrical cell division, the plane of cell cleavage is rotated, and the determinants are distributed differently in the two daughter cells. It is thought that the differential distribution of determinants provides two distinct sets of signals to the daughter cells. One cell receives signals to remain in the mitotic cycle and continue as a progenitor, while the other receives signals to leave the proliferative cycle and differentiate into a neuron (Wodarz and Huttner 2003). The symmetrical or asymmetrical distribution of cell-intrinsic and cell-extrinsic factors derives from the basic morphological properties of the neural progenitor cell.

Neural progenitor cells belong to a very large class of cells called epithelial cells, and thus they are often referred to as neuroepithelial cells. Like all epithelial cells, neuroepithelial cells have a characteristic polarized organization, referred to as apical-basal polarity. Rather than being uniform in the shape and distribution of cellular materials, neuroepithelial cells have a apical-to-basal organization (Huttner and Brand 1997). The apical portion of the neural progenitor cell is attached to the ventricular surface of the VZ, near the lumen, while the basal portion of the cell extends and makes a connection with the basal lamina on the external surface of the VZ (Figure 6.3). The apical and basal regions of the cell contain varying concentrations of different signaling molecules, and the surface membranes of the two ends of the cell establish contact with a different group of external cells. If cell division occurs along the vertical meridian of the cell (Figure 6.3A), each daughter cell receives an equal portion of all the signaling molecules and the membrane surface components in both the apical and basal regions. Thus division along the vertical axis results in symmetrical cell division. However, if cell division occurs along the horizontal meridian,

then each daughter cell receives very different sets of signaling molecules and membrane surface components, resulting in asymmetrical
cell division (Figure 6.3B).

A number of studies have documented these differential planes of cell
division in neural progenitors of the developing mammalian VZ. These
studies show that the activities of the two daughter cells differ depending on whether cell division occurs along the vertical on the horizontal cell axis (Chenn and McConnell 1995). The activities of the two
daughter cells produced by vertical cell division are very similar. After

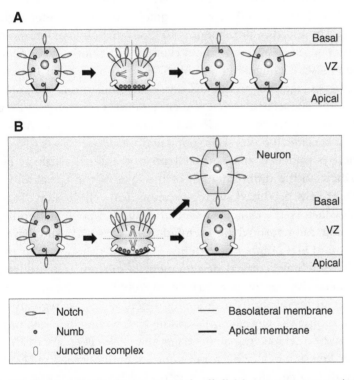

Figure 6.3. Symmetrical and asymmetrical cell division among progenitor
cells in the VZ. A. When cell division occurs along the vertical meridian,
each daughter cell receives an equal portion of all the signaling molecules,
and cell division is symmetrical. B. When cell division occurs along the horizontal meridian, each daughter cell receives different signaling molecules,
and cell division is asymmetrical. (From Huttner and Brand 1997. Adapted
with the permission of Elsevier.)

cell division, the two siblings remain in close proximity. Both remain attached to the ventricular surface, and both establish polarity by slowly elongating and eventually making contact with the outer surface of the VZ at the basal membrane. By contrast, the activities of the two daughter cells produced by horizontal cell division are very different. The sibling that inherits the apical cell characteristics acts much like the daughter cells observed during symmetrical cell division; it maintains contact with the ventricular surface and elongates to make contact with the outer surface of the VZ. The sibling that acquires the basal characteristic acts very differently. It fails to establish contact with the ventricular surface, moves several cell widths away from its sibling, and extends a thick process. Then the whole cell moves very quickly toward the outer region of the VZ. The speed of movement is 10 times that observed in the other sibling. The shape and movement characteristics of the basal daughter cell are those of a migrating neuron. These very different patterns of activity suggest that horizontal cell division produces one daughter cell with apical characteristics that remains a neural progenitor and returns to the mitotic cell-division cycle and a second cell with basal characteristics that becomes a postmitotic young neuron.

There is evidence that both cell-intrinsic and cell-extrinsic factors contribute to the differentiation of the fates of the apical and basal daughter cells produced during asymmetrical cell division. Two cell-intrinsic factors, the proteins Notch and Numb, were first identified as important for neuronal differentiation in *Drosophila* and have now been found in a number of vertebrate species. Although their precise role in vertebrate cortical development is still not fully understood (Castaneda-Castellanos and Kriegstein 2004), the Notch protein is thought to be involved in inducing a neural fate by regulating the cell's response to external signals, while Numb regulates Notch activity (Chenn 2005; Hatakeyama and Kageyama 2006; Petersen et al. 2004; also see Petersen et al. 2006 for evidence of multiple roles of Notch signaling during cell division). In the period between mitotic cell divisions, both are distributed throughout the cell; thus the cell retains its status as a mitotic neocortical progenitor. However, during mitosis, Notch becomes concentrated in the basal region of the cell (Chenn and McConnell 1995), while Numb is distributed in the apical region (Zhong et al. 1996). When the axis of cell cleavage is vertical, Notch and Numb are distributed evenly between the two daughter cells, and the neural progenitor fate is retained for both siblings (Figure 6.3). However, when the axis of cell division is horizontal, the two cell-fate determinants are unequally distributed between the two daughter cells, and division is asymmetrical. The daughter cell that is derived from the apical half of the mother cell (containing Numb) becomes a neuron-generating neuroepithelial cell, a neural progenitor. The daughter cell derived from the basal portions of the progenitor becomes a neuron (Huttner and Brand 1997).

Extrinsic signals emanating from the sites of cell contact may also contribute to differentiation of neuronal cell fate. The apical membranes of progenitors form structures called junctional complexes that serve to attach the cell to adjacent cells, thus supporting the structural integrity of the VZ structure. However, the apical membranes also contain molecules, including cadherins and catenins, that are involved in cell-cell signaling. Cadherins regulate both cell proliferation and differentiation. Beta-catenin is a component of junctional complexes and part of a Wnt signaling pathway that is necessary to establish the appropriate orientation of cell cleavage (Chenn et al. 1998). Control of cleavage orientation is central to the determination of whether cell division will be symmetrical or asymmetrical and, by extension, whether cell division will augment the progenitor pool or produce a neuron. Overexpression of Beta-catenin has been shown to enhance the likelihood of cells taking on progenitor fates and thus should increase the size of the cortical sheet. Mouse mutant models that have enhanced *Beta-catenin* expression demonstrate just this effect. Examination of the brains of *Beta-catenin*-enhanced mutants reveals dramatic enlargement of the cortical sheet. The surface of a normal mouse brain is smooth, lacking noticeable gyral or sulcal folding. By contrast, the brain of *Beta-catenin*-enhanced mutants, examined at late neurogenesis (E15.5), exhibited significant expansion of the cortical sheet evidenced by marked folding throughout the cerebral cortex (Figure 6.4; Chenn and Walsh 2002). Assessment of the organization of the cortices in these animals revealed relatively normal thickness and laminar organization. This suggests that enhancement of Beta-catenin does not interrupt the normal developmental sequence but appears to act in a more limited fashion that has the effect of expanding the pool of neural progenitors. These data confirm that Beta-catenin plays an important role in regulating whether a cell will reenter the cell-division cycle. Thus the signaling molecules concentrated in the junctional complexes may play an important role in regulating the ability of daughter cells to respond to external signaling cues (Chenn et al. 1998; Wodarz and Huttner 2003).

Finally, recent evidence suggests that late in neurogenesis, another shift in the profile of cell cleavage within the VZ may emerge (Haydar, Ang, and Rakic 2003). Studies using real-time imaging techniques have recorded patterns of cell cleavage across the entire period of neurogenesis. These studies confirm the previously reported shift in the proportion of vertical versus horizontal cell divisions from the early to the middle phases of neurogenesis. However, they also observed an unexpected change during late neurogenesis. At the end of neurogenesis, the proportion of vertically aligned cell divisions within the VZ increased, and vertically aligned cell division became the overwhelmingly predominant mode of cell cleavage. In addition, as was the case with symmetrical cell division in the earlier phases of neurogenesis, the activity of the two daughter cells produced by the vertical cleavage was similar. However, the profile of activity for the two siblings was not that of a progenitor. Rather, the activity of both daughter cells was characteristic of migrating neurons. Thus, unlike the early period of neurogenesis, when symmet-

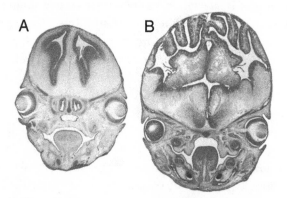

Figure 6.4 Beta-catenin influences the shift from symmetrical to asymmetrical cell division in the VZ. A. The surface of a normal mouse brain is smooth, lacking noticeable gyral or sulcal folding. B. The brain of Beta-catenin-enhanced mutants (E15.5) shows significant expansion of the cortical sheet. (From Chenn and Walsh 2002. Reprinted with the permission of AAAS.)

rical cell division serves to increase the progenitor pool, symmetrical cell division in late neurogenesis increases the rate of neuron production. This late shift to symmetrical cell division is also accompanied by a reduction in the progenitor pool. These data suggest that the model of neuronal fate determination may be more complex than originally proposed. If apical-basal distribution of different fate-determining factors in VZ progenitors is the basis for creating daughter cells with divergent fates, one neural and one progenitor, then it is difficult to explain within a simple model how symmetrical neuronal production could emerge late in neurogenesis. It has been suggested that the distribution of fate-determining molecules may change later in development, or that alternative signaling pathways may emerge that allow for a neurogenic, as opposed to progenitor-generating, pattern of symmetrical cell division.

Patterns of progenitor cell division within the SVZ are predominantly symmetrical. The intermediate or basal progenitor cells that populate the SVZ are derived from the RG cells of the VZ (Gotz and Huttner 2005; Haubensak et al. 2004; Miyata et al. 2004). They migrate to the SVZ, where they divide symmetrically to produce either two progenitor cells or two neurons. However, while both types of symmetrical cell division are observed, the great majority of intermediate progenitor cell division (89.5 percent) produces neurons (Noctor et al. 2004). Thus, it is thought that the intermediate progenitor pool may serve to amplify the supply of cortical neurons in mammals. In fact, there is evidence that by late corticogenesis, the intermediate progenitors of the SVZ may be the source of the majority of neurons that form the upper layers of cortex (Haubensak et al. 2004; Noctor et al. 2004; Quinn et al. 2007; Smart et al. 2002).

## Differentiation of Layer-Specific Neuronal Types

As discussed earlier, the mammalian cerebral cortex is a six-layered structure defined by the neuronal subtypes and patterns of neuronal connectivity. During development, the cortical layers emerge in an inside-out spatiotemporal sequence such that the deep cortical layers form first, followed by progressively more superficial layers. Thus in the typical course of development, there is a close correspondence between the time that a neuron is generated and the cortical layer to which it migrates. Two models of layer-specific neuronal production are possible. First, there may be a specific subpopulation of neural progenitors that generate the neurons for each cortical layer. Cell-intrinsic factors could then specify the emerging cell subtypes. This model is unlikely, however, because studies using techniques to label all the neurons that are produced by a particular progenitor cell show that neurons generated by the same progenitor migrate to different layers of the cerebral cortex (Reid, Liang, and Walsh 1995). A second model posits that progenitors may be capable of producing different neuronal cell types at different points in development. Within this model, the signal to change neuron subtype production could be internal to the cell, or it could be extrinsic. One suggestion of a potential cell-intrinsic signal is a kind of "counting" mechanism where the number of sequential cell divisions dictates the point at which the shift to a new neuronal subtype is initiated. Alternatively, there could be some factor in the cell that becomes diluted during sequential divisions. Here the signal to shift subtype production is derived from the changing concentration of the factor. It is also possible that the signal to generate different neuron subtypes may arise from a source external to the cell, either within the VZ itself or from cells in the developing cortical plate (Desai and McConnell 2000).

In an elegant series of studies, McConnell and colleagues used progenitor cell transplantation techniques to explore the potential of neural progenitor cells to generate neuron subtypes appropriate for the different layers of the developing cerebral cortex (Desai and Mc-Connell 2000; Frantz and McConnell 1996; McConnell and Kaznowski 1991). In all the studies, dividing progenitor cells from a donor animal were transplanted into the ventricular region of a host animal. If neuronal subtype is determined entirely by cell-intrinsic factors, then the transplantation should not affect the type of neurons produced by the donated progenitor cells; they should be appropriate to the developmental stage of the donor animal. However, if cell-extrinsic factors influence the determination of neuronal subtype, and if the transplanted progenitors are sensitive to those signals, then the neurons produced should be appropriate for the developmental stage of the host animal. The animal model used in these studies was the ferret. Gestation time in the ferret is 41 days. Early neurogenesis, the period when layer-6 neurons are being generated, occurs in the ferret at approximately E30. Middle neurogenesis, corresponding to the generation of layer-4 neurons, occurs on E36, and late neurogenesis, corresponding to generation of the most superficial cortical layers, 2 and 3, occurs on the second postnatal day (P2).

In the first of three studies, McConnell (McConnell 1992) transplanted dividing progenitor cells from the VZ of a young donor animal into the ventricle of an older host. The transplanted cells were incorporated into the VZ of the host animal. The donor progenitor cells in this study were obtained on E30. They were dividing asymmetrically and would have produced cells appropriate for cortical layer 6 in the donor animal. The host received the transplant on P2, when it was generating layer-2 and 3 cells. The central question of the study was whether the transplantation of younger donor progenitor cells into the VZ of an older host would alter the fate of the neurons produced by the transplanted progenitor cells. Progenitor cells that were transplanted as they were about to undergo mitotic cell division (cells in the M phase, Figure 6.2B) generated cells appropriate for the donor, that is, layer-6 cells. However, progenitor cells that were transplanted when they were synthesizing DNA (cells in the S phase) produced cells appropriate for the host, layer-2 and 3 cells. This study demonstrates that at least early in neurogenesis, neural progenitor cells are multipotent, that is, they are capable of producing a range of neuron types. Further, some kind of cell-extrinsic factor must be playing a role in signaling differentiation of particular neuronal subtypes, and the progenitors must be sensitive to that signaling pathway.

A second study asked the same question in reverse by implanting progenitor cells from an older P2 donor into a younger E30 host. This study addressed the question whether progenitor cells retain their multipotent capacity throughout neurogenesis. Unlike the findings of the earlier study, the transplanted, late-stage, S-phase progenitor cells did not produce cells characteristic of the host. Rather, they generated cells appropriate for the older animal, layer-2 and 3 cells. This finding suggests that with development, progenitor cells become restricted in their capacity to produce the full range of neuronal cell types, but the question remains how this process of restriction emerges. A simple progressive restriction model would predict that the signal to the progenitor to begin to generate a new neuronal subtype would be accompanied by loss of ability to generate earlier-produced subtypes. This finding would be consistent with cell-intrinsic signaling models that rely either on a count of cell divisions or on the concentration level of a regulatory factor, in combination with sensitivity to external signaling. Alternatively, the process of restriction could be more complex, suggesting a larger role for extrinsic factors. To address this question, the third study asked whether the restriction was gradual and yoked to the timing of subtype signaling or emerged only late in development.

In this study, McConnell and colleagues (Desai and McConnell 2000) transplanted progenitor cells from midneurogenesis donors (E36) into the ventricles of both younger (E30) and older (P2) host animals. The transplantation to the older host replicated the findings from the first study. Midneurogenesis progenitors transplanted during the S phase generated neurons appropriate for the late-neurogenesis host, layer-2 and 3 neurons. However, the findings for the transplantation to the younger host were somewhat different from what would be predicted from findings of the second study. The simple progressive restriction model predicts that since the midneurogenesis transplants would have produced layer 4 in the donor animal, they should have lost the capacity to produce cells typical of earlier phases of development and so should produce only layer-4 cells in the host. However, while the transplanted midneurogenesis progenitors did not produce layer-6 cells (the cells characteristic of the host), they did produce cells appropriate for layers 5, 4, and even 2 and 3, all in significant numbers. This finding is not consistent with either of the cell-intrinsic models, at least as sole accounts of fate restriction for neural progenitors. McConnell has proposed that external signaling must also play a role in regulating the potential of progenitors to generate neural types. She has hypothesized that a signaling pathway from the neurons that have migrated to the developing cortical layers may play a significant role in restricting the range of cell types produced in the VZ. Specifically, she has proposed that at the completion of cortical-layer formation, the newly consolidated layer of cells inhibits the further production of cells for that layer. However, when layers are still forming, the signaling pathway is not yet established, and the progenitor is capable of receiving signals specifying a range of neuronal fates. When the midneurogenesis progenitors were transplanted to the young host, signals from the layer-6 neurons in the host inhibited the production of that neuron type. However, the young-host environment did not provide signals to the transplanted progenitors specifying layer-4 subtype production. In the absence of that signal, the multipotent progenitors produced a range of neuronal subtypes (Desai and McConnell 2000).

In summary, these studies suggest that neural progenitor cells are multipotent in that they are capable of generating a range of neuronal types. With development, the range of cell types that can be produced becomes more and more restricted and in late neurogenesis is limited to production of cells appropriate to the most superficial layers of the cortex. Further, both cell-intrinsic and cell-extrinsic signals appear to play important roles in the differentiation of neuronal cell types. This series of studies focused on the role of external signaling pathways in determining neuronal fate. However, it is likely that this external signaling pathway works in concert with cell-intrinsic signaling. A large number of "proneural" genes have been identified that play a role in specifying both progenitor-neural differentiation and neuronal subtypes. The specific pathways by which these genes act to orchestrate neural differentiation are only beginning to be understood (Bertrand, Castro, and Guillemot 2002).

## The Production of Interneurons

For many years, it was thought that all the neurons that compose the cortical plate arise from the VZ/SVZ. However, more recent work has demonstrated that one major class of neurons, the interneurons, appears to be generated in another proliferative zone in the ventral telencephalic region, the ganglionic eminences (GEs). Animal models of interneuron production have identified ventral proliferative regions that contribute interneurons to different regions of the cerebral cortex. They are the medial ganglionic eminence (MGE), the lateral ganglionic eminence (LGE), and the caudal ganglionic eminence (CGE) (Figure 6.5). The MGE and the LGE will give rise later in development to the basal ganglia, and the CGE will form part of the limbic system amygdaloid complex (Anderson et al. 2001; Corbin, Nery, and Fishell 2001). During neurogenesis, progenitors from each of these regions generate inhibitory, GABAergic interneurons that migrate dorsally and become integrated into different cortical structures. Early in neurogenesis, the MGE interneurons migrate to the developing cortical plate and invade the emerging structures derived from the preplate, the marginal zone, and the subplate (see the discussion of neuronal migration in Chapter 7). During midneurogenesis, the MGE becomes the principal source of cortical interneurons migrating to both the deep embryonic cortical plate structures (subventricular zone, intermediate zone, and subplate) and the emerging cortex. At this same time, interneurons from the LGE migrate to the olfactory bulb but do not at this point in development invade the cortex. Late in neurogenesis, migrating interneurons from both the MGE and the LGE migrate to the developing cortical plate (Corbin, Nery, and Fishell 2001).

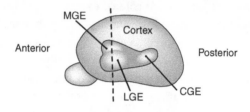

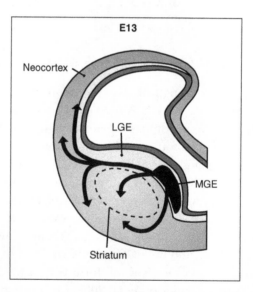

Figure 6.5. A proliferative zone in the ventral telencephalic region of the ganglionic eminences (GEs) has been identified as the site of production of GABAergic interneurons and glial cells. There are three subregions of the GEs within each cerebral hemisphere. The medial ganglionic eminence (MGE) and the lateral ganglionic eminence (LGE) will give rise to the basal ganglia. The caudal ganglionic eminence (caudal to the MGE and LGE, not shown in the coronal figure) will form part of the limbic system.

Throughout both middle and late neurogenesis, progenitor cells in both the MGE and the LGE also generate the projection neurons for the developing basal ganglia. In addition, these structures appear to be a major source of oligodendrocytes, the glial cells that form the myelin sheath on cortical axons later in development. Less is known about the timing or progress of cells generated in the CGE. However, this structure appears to be a primary source of interneurons for structures of the amygdaloid region of the limbic system (Nery, Fishell, and Corbin 2002), and contributes a subset of interneurons to the hippocampus and to some cortical regions (Alifragis, Liapi, and Parnavelas 2004; Corbin, Nery, and Fishell 2001; Xu et al. 2004).

The GE structures were identified as principal sources of interneurons by a variety of techniques, including mutant mouse models. In mice, the transcription factors Dlx1 and Dlx2 are initially expressed exclusively in the three subregions of the GEs and only later in more dorsal telencephalic regions (Corbin, Nery, and Fishell 2001; Parnavelas 2002; Parnavelas, Alifragis, and Nadarajah 2002). They, along with another transcription factor, Mash1, are thought to regulate the differentiation of GABAergic neurons (Anderson et al. 2002; Casarosa, Fode, and Guillemot 1999). Mice that fail to express *Dlx1* and *Dlx2* show dramatic loss of interneurons throughout the developing cortex and hippocampus. The selective contributions of the individual subregions to different brain structures have also been demonstrated with specific gene mutation studies. Loss of the transcription factor Nkx2.1 results in the respecification of the MGE to an LGE fate. The mutation results in a 50 percent reduction in cortical interneurons and a loss of striatal neurons, but interneuron populations in the olfactory bulb are normal. By contrast, loss of transcription factor Gsh2 results in the repatterning of the boundaries of the LGE and a reduction in olfactory bulb interneurons (Marin and Rubenstein 2001).

Across a range of mammalian species, including both the mouse and the ferret, it has been estimated that virtually all cortical interneurons are derived from the ventral telencephalon GE structures (Anderson et al. 2001; Letinic, Zoncu, and Rakic 2002; Marin and Rubenstein 2001, 2003; Parnavelas 2002; Parnavelas, Alifragis, and Nadarajah 2002). It is thus surprising that recent evidence suggests that in humans both dorsal and ventral telencephalic proliferative zones contribute to the cortical interneuron population (Letinic, Zoncu, and Rakic 2002).

It is estimated that 65 percent of cortical interneurons in humans are generated in the dorsal VZ/SVZ, with the remaining obtained from the ventral ganglionic eminence structures. A subset of progenitor cells in the VZ/SVZ, like those in the GEs, express MASH1, one of the transcription factors associated with the differentiation of GABAergic cell fates, and GABAergic daughter cells from these progenitors have been identified within the VZ/SVZ. These data suggest that in humans, there may be multiple proliferative sources of interneurons for the developing neocortex. The first is the evolutionarily well-conserved source in the ventral telencephalon, and the second is a novel source within the dorsal telencephalic proliferative zone. This quite dramatic expansion of progenitor resources may reflect the demands that the greatly enlarged telencephalon places on both the volume of neuronal production and the distances over which neurons must migrate to reach their cortical target locations (Letinic, Zoncu, and Rakic 2002; Rakic and Zecevic 2003b; Tan 2002). These data are not the only evidence that suggests novel or multiple proliferative populations within the developing human nervous system. There is evidence of a novel contribution of cells from the GEs to the developing human thalamus that is not found in other species (Letinic and Rakic 2001).

## Gliogenesis: Production of the Brain's Support Cells

Glial cells are far more numerous than neurons, constituting approximately 90 percent of the cells in the mature brain, and because they are smaller than neurons, they compose about half of the brain's volume. In most regions of the brain, neurons are produced before glia. The exceptions to this rule include the SVZ and the hippocampus, where neurogenesis persists throughout the lifespan (Sun, Martinowich, and Ge 2003). The durations of neurogenesis and gliogenesis are also markedly different. While neurogenesis is largely complete in the prenatal period, gliogenesis persists long after neurogenesis. Astrocytes (Lee, Mayer-Proschel, and Rao 2000) and possibly oligodendrocytes (Ligon et al. 2006) are produced throughout the lifespan.

Two of the three major classes of glial cells, astrocytes and oligodendrocytes, are generated from the same multipotent neural progenitor cells that produce neurons (microglia are produced outside the CNS in the bone marrow). Thus neural progenitors generate the vast majority of both neural and nonneural cells that constitute the CNS. The capacity of neural progenitors to produce the range of neuron types necessary for cortical plate formation was discussed earlier. These same multipotent neural progenitors can also receive signals that induce a shift to glial cell production, that is, to gliogenesis (Sun, Martinowich, and Ge 2003). There is evidence that at the end of neurogenesis, neural progenitor cells alter their mode of cell division from asymmetrial to symmetrical. As discussed earlier, for some cells, this is a new form of cell division in which two neuronal daughter cells are produced. However, for other progenitors, the return to symmetrical cell division appears to be a means of increasing the progenitor pool in preparation for glial production (Sun, Martinowich, and Ge 2003).

The factors that signal progenitor cells to shift from neuron to glial production are not well understood. Specific genes have been identified that are closely associated with neurogenesis and gliogenesis. During neurogenesis, high levels of proneural genes, such as *Bhlh* and *Socs2*, are expressed in progenitors. Bhlh promotes neuron production, while Socs2 acts by blocking expression of a gene that blocks *Bhlh* expression. Another signaling molecule, *Egf*, is expressed late in neurogenesis and serves to promote gliogenesis. However, it is unclear whether Egf acts to signal the shift to gliogenesis or to block neurogenesis (Sauvageot and Stiles 2002; Sun, Martinowich, and Ge 2003).

It has long been thought that the two major glial cell types are generated from the same neural progenitors (O-2A cells), and indeed, when studied in culture, these progenitor cells produce both astrocytes and oligodendrocytes. However, there is more recent evidence that neural progenitors may further differentiate early in development, before the onset of gliogenesis, such that specific progenitors become limited to the production of either astrocytes or oligodendrocytes (Sun, Martinowich, and Ge 2003; Wakamatsu 2004). First, there is evidence that astrocyte and oligodendrocyte progenitors spatially segregate and populate different parts of the neuroepithelium. Further, the timing of astrocyte and oligodendrocyte production differs significantly. In rats, the peak of neuron production is E14, the peak of astrocyte production is P0–P2, and the peak of oligodendrocyte production is P14 (Sauvageot and Stiles 2002). Progenitors within these different spatial regions and timescales appear to be restricted to the generation of only one glial cell line and are thus capable of generating neurons and astrocytes or neurons and oligodendrocytes (Liu and Rao 2004; Sun, Martinowich, and Ge 2003). Indeed, there is evidence that some cells may further differentiate, becoming glial-restricted progenitor (GRP) cells that are capable of producing only glia (Liu and Rao 2004). Furthermore, there appear to be distinct signals that direct astrocyte or oligodendrocyte differentiation. Shh activates *Olig2* to direct oligodendrocyte development. By contrast, Bmps and Wnt suppress oligodendrocyte development and promote astrocyte development (Ligon et al. 2006).

Astrocytes make up 20 to 50 percent of most brain areas (Liu and Rao 2004). The extent of diversity in the astrocyte population is unclear, though at least two distinct classes have been identified by differences in their morphology. Astrocytes participate in a wide range of functions within the CNS. For many years, they were thought to participate mainly in housekeeping functions within the brain: providing structural support, participating in metabolic exchange, acting as macrophages to clear debris, or responding to brain insult or injury. They were also known to contribute to the maintenance of the blood-brain barrier by surrounding brain capillaries and lining the pial surface of the brain. More recently it has been documented that astrocytes participate in a much broader range of functions. Most important, they play a central role in establishing information-processing networks in the brain by regulating synapse formation (Ehlers 2005) and modulating neural activity at the synapse (Newman 2003; Perea and Araque 2006). The source of astrocyte progenitor cells is not well understood, but they appear to be of dorsal origin, generated within the cortical SVZ (Lee, Mayer-Proschel, and Rao 2000; Liu and Rao 2004; Sauvageot and Stiles 2002). A number of fate-restricted progenitor lineages, all derived from multipotent neural progenitor cells, have been identified as astrocyte progenitors, including GRPs. There is also substantial evidence that astrocytes mature from radial glial cells after the period of neurogenesis (Liu and Rao 2004).

The principal function of oligodendrocytes is formation of myelin in the CNS. In order to establish connections, neurons extend axonal processes that can reach over considerable distances in the brain. Efficient transmission of neuron signals requires the "insulation" of the axonal processes. Oligodendrocytes extend a cytoplasmic tongue that surrounds the axon, spiraling and ensheathing it in multiple layers of tissue. In the peripheral nervous system, members of a second class of

cells, Schwann cells, provide the myelin sheath. In addition to producing myelin, oligodendrocytes function to maintain axon integrity
and participate in signaling networks (Ligon et al. 2006). The origin of
the progenitor cells that will give rise to oligodendrocyte progenitors
(OLPs) differs from that of astrocytes and appears to be somewhat
more complex. Studies of both mice and humans have provided evidence that OLPs arise in multiple proliferative sites within the ventral
and dorsal telencephalon (Kessaris et al. 2006; Rakic and Zecevic
2003a). Within ventral regions, OLPs arise in the medial, lateral, and
caudal GEs and later migrate to cortical regions. Within dorsal regions,
they are generated in the cortical SVZ. Recent studies suggest that the
timing of the contribution of cells from the different regions may
change over the course of development. OLPs from each of the proliferative regions express distinctive markers that make it possible to
identify the origin of the cell after it has migrated to the cortex. Marker
studies have shown that the dominant populations of OLPs in the
cortex derive from different sources at different points in pre- and postnatal development. In mice, OLPs appear in the MGE on approximately E12 and arrive at the cortex by E16; at that point they make up
the entire population of OLPs in the cortex. By P10, this early population of MGE-derived OLPs is gone from the cortex and is replaced by
OLPs originating in the LGE, the CGE, and the cortex (Kessaris et al.
2006). The functional consequences of the shifting pool of OLPs
within the cortex are unclear. Knockout studies that eliminated systematically one of the three sources of OLPs showed little effect associated
with loss of any single population. Rather, cells from one of the other
two sources filled in and replaced the missing population (Kessaris
et al. 2006). In humans, OLPs are present in the SVZ by GW19 to
GW20. The early cells produced are concentrated in the SVZ but extend up to the cortical plate (Jakovcevski and Zecevic 2005), suggesting
the extension of proliferative oligodendrocyte regions to the forebrain
from early in development. By late gestation, a second population of
OLPs is present in the subplate.

## Clinical Correlation: Autosomal Recessive Primary
## Microcephaly (MCPH), a Disorder of Neuron Production

During infancy and early childhood, the occipital-frontal circumfer-
ence (OFC) measurement of the head provides a useful estimate of

brain size. During the prenatal and early postnatal period, the skull enlarges because of pressure exerted by the growing brain (Woods 2004). During the first year, the human brain typically doubles in size from approximately 400 grams at birth to 900 grams at age one. Microcephaly is a clinical finding defined by a reduction in OFC. The reduction is clinically significant when OFC is found to be three standard deviations (SD) below that of an age- and sex-matched control population (Menkes, Sarnat, and Maria 2006). There are two broad categories of microcephaly, primary and secondary. Primary microcephaly is a static neurological condition of prenatal onset. Primary microcephaly has for many years been assumed to be a disorder associated with disruption of neuron production, though until recently, specific links to neuroproliferative processes have been limited. Secondary microcephaly is a distinct disorder from primary microcephaly. It is a progressive, neurodegenerative condition that begins in the postnatal period. It is thought to be associated with near-normal neural numbers but progressive loss of connectivity and brain activity (Woods 2004). Genetic and nongenetic causes have been identified for both primary and secondary microcephaly. Over the past several years, considerable progress has been made in understanding the underlying pathology in primary microcephaly, largely because of advances in defining a critical set of genes associated with this disorder.

One important form of primary microcephaly is autosomal recessive primary microcephaly (MCPH). The initial definition of this disorder included three diagnostic critiera: congenital microcephaly with OFC 4 SD below average; mental retardation but no progressive neurological condition; and normal height, weight, chromosomal analysis, and brain scan (Woods, Bond, and Enard 2005). MCPH fits the classification as a primary microcephaly because of its prenatal origin and nonprogressive course. Prenatal ultrasonography suggests that head growth in cases of MCPH is normal through approximately the first 20 gestational weeks (GW) but then begins to decline, with significant reductions in head size observed by GW 31 (Woods, Bond, and Enard 2005). After birth, OFC ranges from 3 to 12 SDs below normal. MRI studies report reductions in CNS volume, with the greatest reduction in the cerebral cortex, but gyral patterning is normal and there is no evidence of migration deficits. Children with MCPH typically fall within the mild to moderate range of mental retardation. They exhibit no motor deficits and often excel in sports and other motor activities. Delays are typically observed in cognitive, linguistic, and social development, though by adolescence they are described as cheerful and compliant (Woods, Bond, and Enard 2005). Incidence of the disorder differs by population group, with higher frequencies noted in Asian and Arab populations where consanguineous marriage practices are common. For example, the incidence rate in Japan is estimated at 1/30,000, while in Britain it is 1/1 million.

Four related genes have been associated with MCPH. The genes were first identified in other animals and each was given a unique name, but the human forms have been renamed for uniformity (Evans et al. 2005). The first two genes to be identified were microcephalin (*MCPH1;* Jackson et al. 2002) and abnormal spindle-like microcephaly associated (*ASPM,* now termed *MCPH5;* Bond et al. 2002). More recently, cyclin dependent kinase 5 regulatory associated protein 2 (*CDK5RAP2,* now termed *MCPH3*) and centromere associated protein J (*CENPJ,* now termed *MCPH6*) have been recognized. Microcephalin is expressed in the forebrain during neurogenesis. It is thought to participate in regulation of the cell cycle and in DNA repair. *ASPM* is expressed within the VZ at sites of active neurogenesis. *ASPM* was first identified in *Drosophila,* where it was found to be involved in regulation of the cell cycle and in specifying spindle orientation during asymmetrical cell division.

The identification of specific genes associated with MCPH has helped define more precisely both the cause and the locus of the neurodevelopmental disorder that results in this form of primary microcephaly. All the genes thus far identified are expressed during neurogenesis, and their expression patterns generally target the neural proliferative zones. These findings narrow the focus of the disorder to the disruption of neurogenesis rather than anomalies involving other aspects of neural development, such as migration, programmed cell death, or neuron differentiation. The precise functions of these genes have not yet been documented. However, their involvement in the shift from symmetrical to asymmetrical cell division suggests that they may play an important role in controlling the size of neuroprogenitor populations and thus the size of the neuronal population. Their role in controlling the cell-cycle parameters suggests a second avenue for control of neuronal numbers. All these functions are consistent with the primary characteristics of the disorder. The hallmark of primary microcephaly is a reduction in the number of neurons in the cerebral cortex in the context of otherwise comparatively normal brain organization. The identification of a set of genes whose functions appear to target neural proliferation is therefore consistent with the principal deficits of this serious neurodevelopmental disorder.

## Chapter Summary

- The neocortex is a uniform, six-layered structure, with layers defined by neuron type and pattern of connections. The thickness of the neocortex is well conserved across species, but dramatic differences are found in the horizontal extent of the cortex. Neocortical layers emerge in an orderly inside-out sequence in development.

- There are three stages in neuronal development: production, migration, and differentiation.

- After the closure of the neural tube, the neural progenitor cells form a single-layered proliferative zone at the center of the tube near the lumen, called the ventricular zone (VZ). The subventricular zone (SVZ) is a secondary proliferative zone that forms adjacent to the VZ soon after the onset of neurogenesis. The VZ/SVZ is the source of all projection neurons in the neocortex and, in primates, a subset of the inhibitory interneurons. An additional proliferative zone has been identified in the region of the ventral ganglionic eminences (GEs). The GEs are the source of inhibitory interneurons and glial cells.

- During the period of neurogenesis, progenitor cells divide repeatedly. Initially, cell division is symmetrical; that is, each daughter cell is identical to both the sibling and the parent. Symmetrical cell division provides a mechanism for rapidly expanding the pool of neural progenitors. Later, progenitors begin to divide asymmetrically. Asymmetrical cell division produces two daughter cells that differ both in the cell-intrinsic, fate-determining molecules they contain and in their capacity to receive extrinsic signaling from other cells.

- Neurons are produced during asymmetrical cell division. They are postmitotic cells, no longer capable of dividing. Soon after cell division, they migrate away from the proliferative zone and take up their position in the developing neocortex.

- Neuronal cell type is specified by both cell-intrinsic factors and external signaling. Progenitors are capable of producing a range of different neuron types across the period of neurogenesis, but the range of expression becomes progressively more restricted with development. Signaling from neurons in established cortical layers is hypothesized to provide a signal to progenitor cells to stop generating earlier neuron types.

- Glial cells are derived from the multipotent neural progenitor cells. Throughout most regions of the brain, glia are produced after neurons. There are two primary classes of glia, astrocytes and oligodendrocytes, that are produced in different regions of the neuroepithelium and at different times in fetal development. Astrocytes perform a wide range of functions in the brain, from neuron maintenance to modulation of synapses. The primary role of oligodendrocytes is to provide the myelin sheets that surround the axons of neurons.

### References

Alifragis, P., A. Liapi, and J. G. Parnavelas. 2004. "Lhx6 regulates the migration of cortical interneurons from the ventral telencephalon but does not specify their GABA phenotype." *Journal of Neuroscience*, 24: 5643–5648.

Anderson, S. A., C. E. Kaznowski, C. Horn, J. L. Rubenstein, and S. K. McConnell. 2002. "Distinct origins of neocortical projection neurons and interneurons in vivo." *Cerebral Cortex*, 12: 702–709.

Anderson, S. A., O. Marin, C. Horn, K. Jennings, and J. L. Rubenstein. 2001. "Distinct cortical migrations from the medial and lateral ganglionic eminences." *Development*, 128: 353–363.

Anthony, T. E., C. Klein, G. Fishell, and N. Heintz. 2004. "Radial glia serve as neuronal progenitors in all regions of the central nervous system." *Neuron*, 41: 881–890.

Bayer, S. A., J. Altman, R. J. Russo, and X. Zhang. 1993. "Timetables of neurogenesis in the human brain based on experimentally determined patterns in the rat." *Neurotoxicology*, 14: 83–144.

Bell, J. E., I. C. Anthony, and P. Simmonds. 2006. "Impact of HIV on regional and cellular organisation of the brain." *Current HIV Research*, 4: 249–257.

Bertrand, N., D. S. Castro, and F. Guillemot. 2002. "Proneural genes and the specification of neural cell types." *Nature Reviews Neuroscience,* 3: 517–530.

Bond, J., E. Roberts, G. H. Mochida, D. J. Hampshire, S. Scott, J. M. Askham, K. Springell, M. Mahadevan, Y. J. Crow, A. F. Markham, C. A. Walsh, and C. G. Woods. 2002. "ASPM is a major determinant of cerebral cortical size." *Nature Genetics,* 32: 316–320.

Casarosa, S., C. Fode, and F. Guillemot. 1999. "Mash1 regulates neurogenesis in the ventral telencephalon." *Development,* 126: 525–534.

Castaneda-Castellanos, D. R., and A. R. Kriegstein. 2004. "Controlling neuron number: Does Numb do the math?" *Nature Neuroscience,* 7: 793–794.

Caviness, V. S., Jr., T. Takahashi, and R. S. Nowakowski. 1995. "Numbers, time and neocortical neuronogenesis: A general developmental and evolutionary model." *Trends in Neurosciences,* 18: 379–383.

Chenn, A. 2005. "The simple life (of cortical progenitors)." *Neuron,* 45: 817–819.

Chenn, A., and S. K. McConnell. 1995. "Cleavage orientation and the asymmetric inheritance of Notch1 immunoreactivity in mammalian neurogenesis." *Cell,* 82: 631–641.

Chenn, A., and C. A. Walsh. 2002. "Regulation of cerebral cortical size by control of cell cycle exit in neural precursors." *Science,* 297: 365–369.

Chenn, A., Y. A. Zhang, B. T. Chang, and S. K. McConnell. 1998. "Intrinsic polarity of mammalian neuroepithelial cells." *Molecular and Cellular Neurosciences,* 11: 183–193.

Corbin, J. G., S. Nery, and G. Fishell. 2001. "Telencephalic cells take a tangent: Non-radial migration in the mammalian forebrain." *Nature Neuroscience,* 4 (Suppl.): 1177–1182.

DeArmond, S. J., M. M. Fusco, and M. M. Dewey. 1989. *Structure of the human brain: A photographic atlas.* 3rd ed. New York: Oxford University Press.

Dehay, C., P. Giroud, M. Berland, I. Smart, and H. Kennedy. 1993. "Modulation of the cell cycle contributes to the parcellation of the primate visual cortex." *Nature,* 366: 464–466.

Desai, A. R., and S. K. McConnell. 2000. "Progressive restriction in fate potential by neural progenitors during cerebral cortical development." *Development,* 127: 2863–2872.

Ehlers, M. D. 2005. "Synapse formation: Astrocytes spout off." *Current Biology,* 15: R134–R137.

Evans, P. D., S. L. Gilbert, N. Mekel-Bobrov, E. J. Vallender, J. R. Anderson, L. M. Vaez-Azizi, S. A. Tishkoff, R. R. Hudson, and B. T. Lahn. 2005. "Microcephalin, a gene regulating brain size, continues to evolve adaptively in humans." *Science,* 309: 1717–1720.

Finlay, B. L., M. N. Hersman, and R. B. Darlington. 1998. "Patterns of vertebrate neurogenesis and the paths of vertebrate evolution." *Brain, Behavior and Evolution,* 52: 232–242.

Fishell, G., and A. R. Kriegstein. 2003. "Neurons from radial glia: The consequences of asymmetric inheritance." *Current Opinion in Neurobiology,* 13: 34–41.

Frantz, G. D., and S. K. McConnell. 1996. "Restriction of late cerebral cortical progenitors to an upper-layer fate." *Neuron,* 17: 55–61.

Gal, J. S., Y. M. Morozov, A. E. Ayoub, M. Chatterjee, P. Rakic, and T. F. Haydar. 2006. "Molecular and morphological heterogeneity of neural precursors in the mouse neocortical proliferative zones." *Journal of Neuroscience,* 26: 1045–1056.

Gotz, M., and W. B. Huttner. 2005. "The cell biology of neurogenesis." *Nature Reviews Molecular Cell Biology,* 6: 777–788.

Hatakeyama, J., and R. Kageyama. 2006. "*Notch1* expression is spatiotemporally correlated with neurogenesis and negatively regulated by *Notch1*-independent *Hes* genes in the developing nervous system." *Cerebral Cortex,* 16 (Suppl. 1): i132–i137.

Haubensak, W., A. Attardo, W. Denk, and W. B. Huttner. 2004. "Neurons arise in the basal neuroepithelium of the early mammalian telencephalon: a major site of neurogenesis." *Proceedings of the National Academy of Sciences of the United States of America,* 101: 3196–3201.

Haydar, T. F., E. Ang Jr., and P. Rakic. 2003. "Mitotic spindle rotation and mode of cell division in the developing telencephalon." *Proceedings of the National Academy of Sciences of the United States of America,* 100: 2890–2895.

Howard, B., Y. Chen, and N. Zecevic. 2006. "Cortical progenitor cells in the developing human telencephalon." *Glia,* 53: 57–66.

Huttner, W. B., and M. Brand. 1997. "Asymmetric division and polarity of neuroepithelial cells." *Current Opinion in Neurobiology,* 7: 29–39.

Jackson, A. P., H. Eastwood, S. M. Bell, J. Adu, C. Toomes, I. M. Carr, E. Roberts, D. J. Hampshire, Y. J. Crow, A. J. Mighell, G. Karbani, H. Jafri, Y. Rashid, R. F. Mueller, A. F. Markham, and C. G. Woods. 2002. "Identification of microcephalin, a protein implicated in determining the size of the human brain." *American Journal of Human Genetics,* 71: 136–142.

Jakovcevski, I., and N. Zecevic. 2005. "Sequence of oligodendrocyte development in the human fetal telencephalon." *Glia,* 49: 480–491.

Kessaris, N., M. Fogarty, P. Iannarelli, M. Grist, M. Wegner, and W. D. Richardson. 2006. "Competing waves of oligodendrocytes in the forebrain and postnatal elimination of an embryonic lineage." *Nature Neuroscience,* 9: 173–179.

Lee, J. C., M. Mayer-Proschel, and M. S. Rao. 2000. "Gliogenesis in the central nervous system." *Glia*, 30: 105–121.

Letinic, K., and P. Rakic. 2001. "Telencephalic origin of human thalamic GABAergic neurons." *Nature Neuroscience*, 4: 931–936.

Letinic, K., R. Zoncu, and P. Rakic. 2002. "Origin of GABAergic neurons in the human neocortex." *Nature*, 417: 645–649.

Ligon, K. L., S. P. Fancy, R. J. Franklin, and D. H. Rowitch. 2006. "*Olig* gene function in CNS development and disease." *Glia*, 54: 1–10.

Liu, Y., and M. S. Rao. 2004. "Glial progenitors in the CNS and possible lineage relationships among them." *Biologie Cellulaire*, 96: 279–290.

Malatesta, P., M. A. Hack, E. Hartfuss, H. Kettenmann, W. Klinkert, F. Kirchhoff, and M. Gotz. 2003. "Neuronal or glial progeny: Regional differences in radial glia fate." *Neuron*, 37: 751–764.

Marin, O., and J. L. Rubenstein. 2001. "A long, remarkable journey: Tangential migration in the telencephalon." *Nature Reviews Neuroscience*, 2: 780–790.

———. 2003. "Cell migration in the forebrain." *Annual Review of Neuroscience*, 26: 441–483.

Marin-Padilla, M. 1971. "Early prenatal ontogenesis of the cerebral cortex (neocortex) of the cat *(Felis domestica):* A Golgi study. I. The primordial neocortical organization." *Zeitschrift für Anatomie und Entwicklungsgeschichte*, 134: 117–145.

———. 1972. "Prenatal ontogenetic history of the principal neurons of the neocortex of the cat (Felis domestica): A Golgi study. II. Developmental differences and their significances." *Zeitschrift für Anatomie und Entwicklungsgeschichte*, 136: 125–142.

Martinez-Cerdeno, V., S. C. Noctor, and A. R. Kriegstein. 2006. "The role of intermediate progenitor cells in the evolutionary expansion of the cerebral cortex." *Cerebral Cortex*, 16 (Suppl. 1): i152–i161.

McConnell, S. K. 1992. "The control of neuronal identity in the developing cerebral cortex." *Current Opinion in Neurobiology*, 2: 23–27.

McConnell, S. K., and C. E. Kaznowski. 1991. "Cell cycle dependence of laminar determination in developing neocortex." *Science*, 254: 282–285.

Menkes, J. H., H. B. Sarnat, and B. L. Maria. 2006. *Child neurology*. 7th ed. Philadelphia: Lippincott Williams & Wilkins.

Meyer, G., J. P. Schaaps, L. Moreau, and A. M. Goffinet. 2000. "Embryonic and early fetal development of the human neocortex." *Journal of Neuroscience*, 20: 1858–1868.

Miyata, T., A. Kawaguchi, K. Saito, M. Kawano, T. Muto, and M. Ogawa. 2004. "Asymmetric production of surface-dividing and non-surface-dividing cortical progenitor cells." *Development*, 131: 3133–3145.

Nery, S., G. Fishell, and J. G. Corbin. 2002. "The caudal ganglionic eminence is a source of distinct cortical and subcortical cell populations." *Nature Neuroscience*, 5: 1279–1287.

Newman, E. A. 2003. "New roles for astrocytes: Regulation of synaptic transmission." *Trends in Neurosciences*, 26: 536–542.

Noctor, S. C., A. C. Flint, T. A. Weissman, R. S. Dammerman, and A. R. Kriegstein. 2001. "Neurons derived from radial glial cells establish radial units in neocortex." *Nature*, 409: 714–720.

Noctor, S. C., A. C. Flint, T. A. Weissman, W. S. Wong, B. K. Clinton, and A. R. Kriegstein. 2002. "Dividing precursor cells of the embryonic cortical ventricular zone have morphological and molecular characteristics of radial glia." *Journal of Neuroscience*, 22: 3161–3173.

Noctor, S. C., V. Martinez-Cerdeno, L. Ivic, and A. R. Kriegstein. 2004. "Cortical neurons arise in symmetric and asymmetric division zones and migrate through specific phases." *Nature Neuroscience*, 7: 136–144.

Pakkenberg, B., and H. J. Gundersen. 1997. "Neocortical neuron number in humans: Effect of sex and age." *Journal of Comparative Neurology*, 384: 312–320.

Parnavelas, J. G. 2002. "The origin of cortical neurons." *Brazilian Journal of Medical and Biological Research*, 35: 1423–1429.

Parnavelas, J. G., P. Alifragis, and B. Nadarajah. 2002. "The origin and migration of cortical neurons." *Progress in Brain Research*, 136: 73–80.

Perea, G., and A. Araque. 2006. "Synaptic information processing by astrocytes." *Journal of Physiology, Paris*, 99: 92–97.

Petersen, P. H., H. Tang, K. Zou, and W. Zhong. 2006. "The enigma of the Numb-Notch relationship during mammalian embryogenesis." *Developmental Neuroscience*, 28: 156–168.

Petersen, P. H., K. Zou, S. Krauss, and W. Zhong. 2004. "Continuing role for mouse Numb and Numbl in maintaining progenitor cells during cortical neurogenesis." *Nature Neuroscience*, 7: 803–811.

Quinn, J. C., M. Molinek, B. S. Martynoga, P. A. Zaki, A. Faedo, A. Bulfone, R. F. Hevner, J. D. West, and D. J. Price. 2007. "Pax6 controls cerebral cortical cell number by regulating exit from the cell cycle and specifies cortical cell identity by a cell autonomous mechanism." *Developmental Biology*, 302: 50–65.

Rakic, P. 1995. "A small step for the cell, a giant leap for mankind: A hypothesis of neocortical expansion during evolution." *Trends in Neurosciences*, 18: 383–388.

———. 2003. "Elusive radial glial cells: Historical and evolutionary perspective." *Glia*, 43: 19–32.

———. 2006. "A century of progress in corticoneurogenesis: From silver impregnation to genetic engineering." *Cerebral Cortex*, 16 (Suppl. 1): i3–i17.

Rakic, S., and N. Zecevic. 2003a. "Early oligodendrocyte progenitor cells in the human fetal telencephalon." *Glia*, 41: 117–127.

———. 2003b. "Emerging complexity of layer I in human cerebral cortex." *Cerebral Cortex*, 13: 1072–1083.

Reid, C. B., I. Liang, and C. Walsh. 1995. "Systematic widespread clonal organization in cerebral cortex." *Neuron*, 15: 299–310.

Sadler, T. W. 2006. *Langman's medical embryology.* 10th ed. Philadelphia: Lippincott Williams & Wilkins.

Sauvageot, C. M., and C. D. Stiles. 2002. "Molecular mechanisms controlling cortical gliogenesis." *Current Opinion in Neurobiology*, 12: 244–249.

Smart, I. H., C. Dehay, P. Giroud, M. Berland, and H. Kennedy. 2002. "Unique morphological features of the proliferative zones and postmitotic compartments of the neural epithelium giving rise to striate and extrastriate cortex in the monkey." *Cerebral Cortex*, 12: 37–53.

Sun, Y. E., K. Martinowich, and W. Ge. 2003. "Making and repairing the mammalian brain—Signaling toward neurogenesis and gliogenesis." *Seminars in Cell and Developmental Biology*, 14: 161–168.

Takahashi, T., R. S. Nowakowski, and V. S. Caviness Jr. 1993. "Cell cycle parameters and patterns of nuclear movement in the neocortical proliferative zone of the fetal mouse." *Journal of Neuroscience*, 13: 820–833.

———. 1996. "Interkinetic and migratory behavior of a cohort of neocortical neurons arising in the early embryonic murine cerebral wall." *Journal of Neuroscience*, 16: 5762–5776.

Tan, S. S. 2002. "Developmental neurobiology: Cortical liars." *Nature*, 417: 605–606.

Wakamatsu, Y. 2004. "Understanding glial differentiation in vertebrate nervous system development." *Tohoku Journal of Experimental Medicine*, 203: 233–240.

Williams, R. W., and K. Herrup. 1988. "The control of neuron number." *Annual Review of Neuroscience*, 11: 423–453. Revised 1998–2001 HTML edition posted on http://www.nervenet.org/papers/NUMBER_REV_1988.html.

Wodarz, A., and W. B. Huttner. 2003. "Asymmetric cell division during neurogenesis in *Drosophila* and vertebrates." *Mechanisms of Development*, 120: 1297–1309.

Woods, C. G. 2004. "Human microcephaly." *Current Opinion in Neurobiology*, 14: 112–117.

Woods, C. G., J. Bond, and W. Enard. 2005. "Autosomal recessive primary microcephaly (MCPH): A review of clinical, molecular, and evolutionary findings." *American Journal of Human Genetics*, 76: 717–728.

Xu, Q., I. Cobos, E. De La Cruz, J. L. Rubenstein, and S. A. Anderson. 2004. "Origins of cortical interneuron subtypes." *Journal of Neuroscience*, 24: 2612–2622.

Zecevic, N., Y. Chen, and R. Filipovic. 2005. "Contributions of cortical subventricular zone to the development of the human cerebral cortex." *Journal of Comparative Neurology*, 491: 109–122.

Zhong, W., J. N. Feder, M. M. Jiang, L. Y. Jan, and Y. N. Jan. 1996. "Asymmetric localization of a mammalian numb homolog during mouse cortical neurogenesis." *Neuron*, 17: 43–53.

# SEVEN

# Neuronal Migration and
# Neuronal Differentiation

THE ONSET OF asymmetrical cell division in the proliferative regions of the brain marks the shift to neuron production, but the newly born neurons do not remain in the proliferative zones. Soon after they are born, these postmitotic cells begin to move away from the region in which they were produced toward the positions they will assume in the developing cortex. The general term *migration* is used to refer to neuronal movement away from the proliferative zones, but the character of cell movement varies depending on cell type, position, and the distances over which a cell must travel. In some cases, particularly early in development, the distances are as small as a few microns (one millionth of a meter). However, because of the size of the mammalian cortex, in most cases neurons must migrate over considerable distances to their target locations within the cortical plate (CP). Radially migrating neurons must migrate as far as 2 cm, while tangentially migrating cells may migrate as far as 15 cm before reaching their destination (Tsai and Gleeson 2005). Several modes of neuronal migration have been documented in the neocortex, including somal translocation, radial glial-guided locomotion, and tangential migration. Each is important for different subsets of neurons at different points in neocortical development. In humans, the major period of neuronal migration is during midgestation, between approximately 7 and 20 gestational weeks (GW) (Volpe 2001).

Neuron differentiation refers to the acquisition of appropriate neurochemical signaling factors and the establishment of connections with other neurons. Once neurons reach their destination in the neocortex, they develop the structural and molecular elements that will allow them to connect with other neurons (Mrzljak et al. 1990). This requires change both in the shape of the cells and in their capacity to send and receive molecular signals. Three primary changes are observed for most new neurons. First, all neurons undergo neuritogenesis, in which they extend neuronal processes, axons and dendrites, that allow them to establish connections with other neurons. Second, the movement of axons is guided by a structure that forms at their tip called the growth cone. Growth cones establish contact with the surrounding environment, allowing them to respond to signaling cues in the local environment. Finally, neurons must acquire the signaling molecules, the neurotransmitters, that will allow them to communicate with other neurons. This complex set of developmental events establishes the neural pathways that mediate all aspects of behavior, from sensation to movement to high-level cognition.

## Forms of Neuronal Migration

Soon after they are born, new neurons begin to move away from their place of origin in either the VZ/SVZ or the ganglionic eminences in a process called neuronal cell migration. This section will consider three distinct modes of neuronal migration that have been identified within the developing nervous system. Two of them reflect the radially directed outward movement of the new neuron as it goes from the VZ/SVZ to the overlying cortical plate (CP). These two forms of radial migration are referred to as locomotion along radial glial guides and somal translocation of radially oriented neurons. The third mode of migration involves cell movement that is orthogonal to the first two and is referred to as tangential migration. Tangentially migrating cells move across the horizontal extent of the developing brain to reach their target location in the CP. Neurons adopt different modes of migration depending on both where and when they are generated.

## Somal Translocation

Neurons generated early in corticogenesis need to traverse relatively small distances to exit the VZ. These cells appear to use a mode of migration referred to as somal translocation (Figure 7.1A; Nadarajah et al. 2003). When these cells are born in the VZ, they extend a long basal process and attach it to the pial surface, which is the outer surface of the developing brain (Miyata et al. 2001). The cell nucleus then translocates into the cytoplasm of the basal process in a single smooth and continuous movement (Nadarajah et al. 2003; Nadarajah and Parnavelas 2002). As the nucleus advances, the basal process becomes shorter and thicker and remains attached to the outer surface (Nadarajah et al. 2003; Nadarajah and Parnavelas 2002). This mode of migration is observed more frequently among the early-migrating neurons that will form the preplate layer of the developing cortex and much less frequently among neurons that migrate in mid-to-late corticogenesis. This simpler mode of migration requires a less complex signaling system than glial-guided locomotion and is sufficient for establishing the earliest layers of the neocortex (Weissman et al. 2003). The complex molecular signaling pathways that direct somal translocation are just beginning to be understood (Nadarajah et al. 2003).

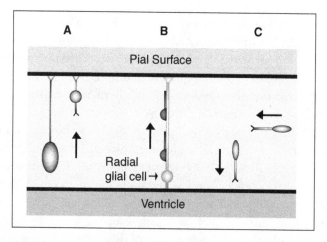

Figure 7.1. Modes of neuronal migration in the developing nervous system. A. During somal translocation, the cell extends a process to the pial surface, and the cell nucleus moves radially away from the VZ. B. Radial glial guides provide a scaffold for neuron migration away from the VZ. C. Tangentially migrating cells move across the plane of the developing brain to reach their target location in the cortical plate. (From Nadarajah et al. 2003. Adapted with the permission of Oxford University Press.)

## Locomotion along Radial Glial Guides

As the CP begins to expand, the distances over which neurons must migrate require the establishment of a more complex guidance network. Thus throughout much of corticogenesis, the predominant mode of neuronal migration from the dorsal telencephalic proliferative zone, that is, the VZ, involves cell movement along intricate and radially oriented cellular scaffolding. This mode of neuronal migration was first identified and described in the early 1970s (Rakic 1972). The cells that form the scaffold express a protein, glial fibrillary acidic protein (Gfap), that identifies their glial origin, and thus they were called radial glial (RG) cells (Rakic 2003b). As discussed in Chapter 6, a number of investigators have confirmed that in addition to their role in guiding the migration of new neurons, the RG cells are also capable of generating neurons. Indeed, some investigators have suggested that the RG cells may be the sole class of progenitor cells within the dorsal telencephalic VZ (Noctor et al. 2002; Parnavelas, Alifragis, and Nadarajah 2002; Weissman et al. 2003), while others have argued that they may be one of several classes of progenitors (Rakic 2003b). Whether or not RG cells are the exclusive source of neurons in the VZ, it is now clear that they perform two critical roles in neurogenesis, the generation of neurons and the guidance of neurons to target locations within the developing CP.

Beyond the earliest phase of neurogenesis, the rapid expansion and curvature of the developing cortex complicates the task of directing the migrating neurons to the correct target locations within the CP. RG cells create a kind of cellular scaffold that provides a pathway over which the migrating neurons can traverse the distance between the VZ and their target locations within the CP. The apical end of the RG cell attaches to the ventricular surface by a single endfoot. It extends a single process toward the pial surface of the developing cortex, where it attaches, often with several endfoot terminals. As the width of the developing CP expands and the surface begins to curve, the RG cell lengthens and bends, creating a single continuous radial fiber that connects the proliferative zone with the cortex (Rakic 2003a). The newly born neuron extends a leading process that contacts the adjacent RG fiber. The process extends, aligning the neuron radially along the surface of the RG cell (Figure 7.1B). The leading process of the neuron slowly and continuously extends, and periodically the nucleus of the cell rapidly translocates into the cytoplasm of the leading process. The rapid, intermittent movement of the nucleus gives the cell the appearance of moving in a saltatory, or stepwise, manner along the RG fiber.

Cells that are migrating along glial guides require a complex signaling pathway. The new neuron must first recognize and establish contact with the glial guide and then adhere to it and determine the direction of the movement. Finally, it must recognize when to stop its migration and detach from the glial fiber (Nadarajah and Parnavelas 2002). Neuregulin *(Nrg)* has been associated with neuron-glial interactions, and astrotactin *(astn)* has been shown to be involved in establishing the bond that allows the neuron to adhere to the glial fiber. As discussed later, reelin (Reln), a secreted molecule that is expressed in neurons of the preplate, is critical for providing the stop signals for neuron migration.

## Tangential Migration

The migratory path for cells leaving the VZ/SVZ is radial and is accomplished via either somal translocation or glial-guided locomotion. However, as discussed in Chapter 6, there is good evidence that a subset of cells that make up the developing cortex originates in a separate proliferative zone in the ventral telencephalon, the ganglionic eminences (GEs). These cells must travel long distances, traversing the cortical mantle using a mode of migration that has been called tangential migration (Nadarajah et al. 2003). This form of migration is observed throughout corticogenesis, and multiple migratory pathways have been identified (Nadarajah and Parnavelas 2002; Figure 7.1C). The signaling pathways that guide the movement of tangentially migrating cells differ from those involved in radial migration. Three sets of factors are needed to regulate tangential migration: factors that trigger the movement of the cell, those that establish the migratory substrate, and those that serve as guidance signals for the migrating cell (Marin and Rubenstein 2001). A number of neurotrophic factors, including brain-derived neurotrophic factor (Bdnf) and neurotrophin 4 (Nt4), as well as hepatocyte growth factor / scatter factor (Hgf), appear to stimulate movement of interneurons in the GEs. Experimentally induced augmentation of the concentrations of these factors increases the number of cells migrating from the GE regions, creating abnormal and inappropriately positioned accumulations of cells. Little is known about the guidance pathways for tangentially migrating neurons. There is some evidence that these cells may use the axons of the earlier established corticofugal projection pathway for guidance. Migration is disrupted when the expression of molecules that allow the interneurons to adhere to cells of the established pathway is blocked. Finally, guidance molecules can direct the movement by establishing signaling pathways that either attract or repel the migrating cells. Although the set of factors is not well understood, members of one class of chemorepellent molecules, semaphorin 3a (Sema 3a) and 3f (Sema 3f), have been shown to direct migrating interneurons away from ventral regions (Marin and Rubenstein 2001). In addition, slit is a secreted molecule that is expressed in the GEs and also provides repulsive cues to GABAergic interneurons to leave the GEs (Parnavelas 2000). Stromal cell-derived factor 1 (Sdf1) is a potent chemoattractant molecule that is expressed in a gradient from the meninges that overlie the developing CP. Interneurons that migrate from the ventral to the dorsal telencephalon strongly express the receptor for the Sdf1 protein. Thus *Sdf1* expression is thought to direct the migration of interneurons dorsally toward the CP (Stumm et al. 2003).

## Formation of the Cortical Plate

As discussed earlier, the first phase of corticogenesis involves the symmetrical division of neural progenitor cells. The symmetrical division serves to increase the size of the progenitor pool that will later give rise to the neurons and glial cells of the cerebral cortex (Figure 7.2A). During GW6, a subset of progenitor cells shifts from a symmetrical to an asymmetrical mode of cell division, thus generating the first population of neurons. The first neurons to exit the VZ during GW6 in humans form a sparse, superficial layer. As neuronal migration proceeds (GW7), a horizontal layer called the primordial plexiform layer, or the preplate (PP), forms (Figure 7.2B; Marin-Padilla 1971, 1972; Meyer et al. 2000). Cells entering this layer are thought to exit the VZ via somal translocation. Axons of the preplate neurons, together with the axons growing into the cortex from subcortical areas, form the intermediate zone (IZ), which separates the VZ from the preplate (Figure 7.2C). These axons will provide the initial connections between the cortex and the major subcortical relay nucleus, the thalamus. As the pace of neuron production increases (beginning at approximately GW7 to GW8), progenitor cells produce neurons destined for cortical layers. These cells migrate through the IZ and form the cortical plate (CP) by splitting the preplate into two subdivisions, the marginal zone (MZ), which is located along the pial surface, and the subplate, which is located below the newly forming CP (Figure 7.2D). The MZ will become cortical layer 1. It contains a class of cells, the Cajal-Retzius cells, that will provide critical signals to migrating neurons about their future position in the cortex. The subplate is a transient embryonic structure that plays a critical role in the early development of neocortical circuitry (Arber 2004; Kostovic and Rakic 1990; Figure 7.2D). Beginning soon after the onset of neurogenesis, a second zone of mitotically active cells forms between the VZ and the IZ, called the subventricular zone (SVZ; Figure 7.2D). This is a cell-dense zone containing mitotically active, dividing cells. It is a secondary proliferative layer that in humans gives rise to neurons, interneurons and glial cells (Letinic, Zoncu, and Rakic 2002; Rakic 2006; Zecevic, Chen, and Filipovic 2005). The progenitor cells in the SVZ, which are referred to as intermediate or basal progenitor cells, are generated by radial glia in the VZ and then migrate to the SVZ (Britz et al. 2006; Noctor et al. 2004). Initially the SVZ is thinner than the VZ, but it gradually enlarges and by late in gestation becomes considerably thicker (Figure 7.2E). Nearly all the embryonic cellular zones are unique to the developing brain. Only the CP and the underlying white matter have counterparts in the adult brain (Figure 7.2F).

## Establishing the Laminar Organization of the Neocortex

With the exception of the cells that form the preplate (the future MZ and subplate layer), the projection neurons that migrate from the VZ/SVZ to form the CP locomote along radial glial guides. The main layers of the CP are formed in an inside-out spatiotemporal sequence, with the cells that form the deepest layers of the cortex migrating first and those in the most superficial layers migrating last. The signal to neurons to stop is critical to this orderly process of cortical layer, or lamina, formation. The signal is regulated by reelin (Reln), a secreted protein that is expressed by an important class of neurons located in the MZ, the Cajal-Retzius (C-R) cells. The C-R cells migrate to the preplate from subcortical regions (Bielle et al. 2005) and make up a significant proportion of cells in the MZ. The critical protein expressed by C-R cells, Reln, is an extracellular protein that acts by binding to transmembrane receptors of the migrating neuron. The Reln signal induces a complex cell-internal program in the migrating neuron that instructs the cell to stop migrating just below the MZ and take up its position in the developing CP (Tissir and Goffinet 2003). Reelin is secreted by the C-R cells into extracellular space, creating a signaling pathway that regulates final cell position, but not cell migration per se. As the CP grows, the reelin-containing zone moves farther away from the ventricular surface,

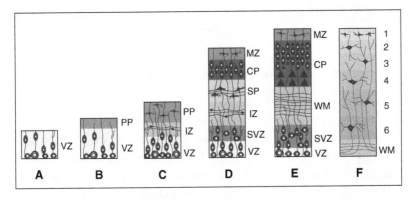

Figure 7.2. Cortical plate formation. A schematic representation of human neocortical development. A. The VZ before the onset of neuronal migration contains symmetrically dividing progenitor cells. B. The first neurons to leave the VZ form a sparse preplate layer at the edge of the VZ (GW<7). C. Axons of the preplate neurons, along with the axons projecting from subcortical areas, form the intermediate zone. D. The preplate is split into an outer MZ and a deeper subplate zone by the developing cortical plate (beginning GW7–8). E. The SVZ gradually enlarges, and by late gestation it becomes thicker than the VZ. F. In the mature cortex, only the six cortical layers and the underlying white matter pathways are evident. VZ=ventricular zone; MZ=marginal zone; PP=preplate; SP=subplate; IZ=intermediate zone; SVZ=subventricular zone; CP=cortical plate; WM=white matter.

and the migrating neurons receive the Reln signal at distances progressively farther away from the VZ/SVZ, thus creating the inside-out organization of the cortical layers. Mice with mutations of the *Reln* gene have profoundly disorganized cortices. A reeler mutant strain of mise arose spontaneously in the 1950s, and at that time both behavioral and neurological deficits were noted (Rice and Curran 2001). Examination of the reeler mutant brain revealed a specific set of abnormalities. Although all the major classes of neural cells are present and appear at the appropriate times in development, the splitting of the preplate is abnormal, and the typical inside-out laminar organization is disrupted (Figure 7.3; Rice and Curran 2001). Rather than the normal subdivision of the preplate into an MZ and a subplate, reeler mutants have a single superficial structure called a superplate (SPP) that contains both C-R and subplate neurons. The migrating CP neurons fail to receive the appropriate positioning signals and accumulate in a disorganized agglomeration, ordered roughly in a reversed sequence, below the superplate.

## Tangential Migration of Ventrally Generated Interneurons

There is recent evidence that the migration pathways into the CP for tangentially migrating interneurons may be somewhat more varied than those of the radially migrating VZ/SVZ projection neurons. A subset of interneurons from the GEs migrates tangentially to the region of the VZ and then uses the glial guides to migrate radially into the cortical layers. These interneurons manifest the same inside-out organization relative to the time of their birth as the projection neurons (Metin et al. 2006). Specifically, once the early-born interneurons have migrated tangentially to the VZ, they travel along radial guides and occupy deep cortical layers; later-born interneurons occupy more superficial layers. However, another subset of interneurons has also been identified. These cells migrate tangentially to the MZ layer of the cortex and are initially interspersed with the C-R cells. They then migrate radially along glial guides, but the direction of their movement is inward toward the deeper cortical layers (Hevner et al. 2004). The positioning of these cells does not appear to be affected by Reln signaling; in mice with *Reln* mutations, these cells migrate to appropriate cortical layers. Interestingly, these inwardly migrating interneurons move to cortical layers that are consistent with their birthdays, just as cells migrating in an outward direction from the VZ/SVZ. It is thought that the cells that undergo this inward pattern of radial migration may receive positioning signals from projection neurons within the emerging cortical layers that have the same birthdays as the inwardly migrating interneurons. Recent data suggest that signaling may be reciprocal (Metin et al. 2006).

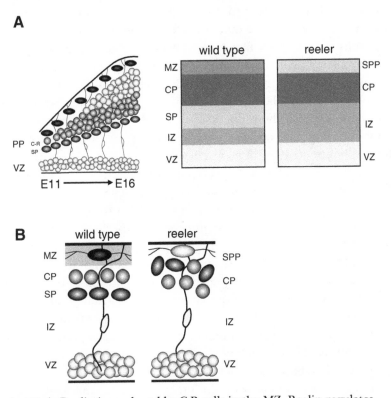

Figure 7.3. A. Reelin is produced by C-R cells in the MZ. Reelin regulates neuron migration and creates the inside-out organization of the cortical layers. B. Mice with mutations of the *reelin* gene have profoundly disorganized cortices (Rice and Curran 2001). All the major classes of neural cells are present and appear at the appropriate times in development, but the splitting of the preplate is abnormal, and laminar organization is disrupted. Reeler mutants have a single superficial structure, called a superplate (SPP), that contains both C-R and subplate neurons. (From Rice and Curran 2001. Adapted with the permission of Annual Reviews.)

## Formation of the Subplate

The subplate is a transient embryonic structure that plays a critical role in establishing early patterns of connectivity in the brain. As will be discussed in greater detail in Chapter 8, the subplate neurons play an important role in directing the formation of the major sensory and motor pathways in the developing brain, the thalamocortical and corticothalamic pathways. During the preplate stage, it is the axons of the future subplate cells that invade the IZ and send pioneering projections to the thalamus. In humans, axons projecting dorsally from the thalamus to the cortex first enter the subplate during approximately GW18. The axons remain in the subplate for several weeks before entering the CP at approximately GW26 (Kostovic et al. 2002). During the period when thalamic axons wait in the subplate, subplate neurons and neurons from the input layer of the developing cortex (layer 4) establish reciprocal connections (Kostovic et al. 2002; Kostovic and Rakic 1990; Shatz 1994). Later in development, the thalamic axons will invade the cortex at layer 4 and replace the subplate connections. But experimental evidence demonstrates that the early, transient connections between subplate neurons and layer-4 neurons are essential for establishing thalamocortical connections. Experimental ablation of the subplate results in significant disruption of later cortical organization and functioning. In these animals, organization of the thalamus is normal, and the basic thalamocortical connections form. However, the patterns of connectivity fail to mature normally (Kanold et al. 2003). Within the primary visual cortex, for example, salient features of organization, such as ocular dominance and orientation-specific columns, fail to form. Subplate ablation also triggers a cascade of abnormal gene signaling. Expression of neurotrophic factors is disrupted; *Bdnf* is overexpressed and neurotrophin 3 *(Ntf3)* is underexpressed. There is also overexpression of an enzyme that regulates GABA synthesis in interneurons. These data suggest that the role of the subplate in early cortical development involves preparing the developing input layers of the cortex for future connections with the thalamus and other pathways, including the corpus callosum (Kostovic et al. 2002). Once it has fulfilled its function, the subplate gradually disappears such that by the early postnatal period only cellular remnants of the structure can be discerned (Kostovic and Jovanov-Milosevic 2006). However, there is evidence that even those remaining cells may continue to participate in endogenous signaling and help establish cortico-cortical connectivity in the developing brain (Kostovic and Jovanov-Milosevic 2006).

## Differentiation of Neurons

The process of neuronal differentiation results in the complex mix of highly specialized neuronal subtypes that compose the cerebral cortex. The processes involved in establishing specific neuronal identity begin very early in development, prior to neuron production. During the first month postconception, the initial patterning of the embryo emerges. Within the nervous system, neural progenitor cells establish regional identities along the dorsal-ventral, anterior-posterior, and right-left axes of the embryo. As discussed earlier, secreted molecules, such as Shh, Bmp, and Fgf8, and transcription factors, such as Pax6 and Emx2, play important roles in this early process of regionalization by signaling the differential, site-specific fates for the progenitor cells. This early signaling provides the preliminary specification of neuronal identity within particular brain regions. Further neuronal specialization is observed during the development of the CP as proliferative-zone progenitors receive temporally varying signals to produce neurons appropriate to different cortical layers. However, this initial specification is both incomplete and mutable. The postmitotic neurons will undergo significant and highly specific changes in both their morphology and their molecular signaling capabilities before achieving their mature and stable state (Mrzljak et al. 1988).

As they mature, the young neurons become part of information-processing networks in which highly orchestrated electrochemical signals are relayed along complex interconnected neural pathways. The process of neuronal differentiation begins as the immature neurons start to migrate away from the VZ/SVZ to target sites in the developing cortex. Once young neurons reach their target destinations in the developing neocortex, they begin to develop the structural and molecular elements that will allow them to establish connections with other neurons in the network. This requires a series of changes in the morphology of the cells and in their capacity to send and receive molecular signals. The next three sections will discuss three primary sets of morphological and molecular change that are observed for most new neurons. First, all neurons undergo neuritogenesis, whereby the neuronal processes, axons and dendrites, are extended. The neuronal processes provide the primary means through which cells establish contact with other cells. Second, neurite extension is guided by a structure that forms at the tip of the growing neurite called the growth cone. Growth cones establish contact with the surrounding environment and serve both to anchor the extending neurite and to respond to directional signaling cues in the local environment. Growth-cone development is particularly crucial for axons. Axons carry outgoing information from the cell body toward target cells. Thus axons must often extend over considerable distances, sometimes by indirect pathways, to reach their targets. The axonal growth cones direct this movement. Finally, when the axon reaches its target, signaling between the cells is established at the synapse. The formation of synapses requires the cell to express specific and sometimes changing types of signaling molecules, neurotransmitters, as well as to acquire the receptors necessary to receive signals.

## Neuritogenesis

The term *neurite* is used to refer collectively to the two basic types of neuronal processes, dendrites and axons. The typical mature neuron has one axon and many dendrites. Axons relay information from the cell to other cells; dendrites typically receive input from other cells. In the early phase of neurite generation, the neuron generates many processes that grow at approximately the same rate. The growth of one of the processes eventually exceeds that of the other processes, and that process becomes the axon of the cell. The designation of a particular process as the axon does not appear to be prespecified. If the emerging axon is eliminated early in development, another developing neurite will become the axon (Brown, Keynes, and Lumsden 2001).

The polarity of developing neurons is defined in part by the differentiation of axons and dendrites. A shift in the site of expression of growth-associated protein 43 (Gap43) to the axons of neurons is an important marker of this polarity. *Gap43* is initially expressed in all the emerging neurites of the cell. A decline in Gap43 in dendrites, coupled with an increase in the axon, signals the differentiation of the axon. With development, *Gap43* becomes maximally expressed in axons, with the highest intensity of expression in the growth cones at the leading edge of the neurite (Brown, Keynes, and Lumsden 2001). The redistribution of Gap43 is thought to play an important role in axon extension, neurotransmitter formation, and the establishment of synapses (Oestreicher et al. 1997). Overexpression of *Gap43* leads to excessive sprouting and extension of axons, while interference with expression leads to a reduction in axonal growth. Further, distribution of Gap43 within the axon can be modulated by extrinsic signaling factors. For example, Piontek and colleagues (2002) have shown that contact with astroglial cells in the vicinity of the extending axon leads to the redistribution of Gap43 in the regions of the growth cone, altering the morphology of the cell.

It is estimated that the typical neuron receives from 1,000 to 10,000 synaptic inputs. Most of the input is received via the dendrites. The generation and maturation of dendrites begin soon after neurons reach the CP, prior to the arrival of afferent input (Mrzljak et al. 1990). The maturation of dendrites is marked by the extension and complex branching of the neurite processes into what has been described as the dendritic arbor and by the formation of dendritic spines. Dendritic spines are mushroom-shaped protrusions that extend from the dendrites. They are the primary sites of contact for incoming axons. The formation of dendritic arbors is influenced by both cell-intrinsic and cell-extrinsic factors. Early in development, arbor formation appears to be regulated by cell-intrinsic factors. Cells placed in culture develop relatively normal dendritic arbors (Brown, Keynes, and Lumsden 2001). In addition, experiments with mice in which extrinsic signaling, including both excitatory input and neurotrophic factor expression, is blocked report relatively normal early development of the dendritic tree (Adcock, Metzger, and Kapfhammer 2004). Furthermore, there is considerable conservation of the morphology of dendritic arbors within cell type across species (Libersat and Duch 2004). Thus, although the nature of the intrinsic signaling pathway is not well defined, it is clear that initial specification of the dendritic architecture is under genetic control.

However, there is substantial evidence that the growth and elaboration of dendritic arbors, and thus the available synaptic space, are highly influenced by cell-extrinsic factors as well. These include both the excitatory input to the cell and the influence of neurotrophic factors (Adcock, Metzger, and Kapfhammer 2004; Cline 2001; Libersat and Duch 2004). Both spontaneous firing of cells and activity-dependent firing in response to sensory or motor input influence the formation of dendritic arbors. In many parts of the nervous system, the onset of activity-dependent activation is correlated with growth of dendritic arbors (Libersat and Duch 2004). These effects extend even to adult animals (Greenough, Hwang, and Gorman 1985). There is also evidence that dendritic arbor elaboration is enhanced by introduction of neurotrophic factors, including Bdnf, Ntf3, and Ntf4 (McAllister 2002). As will be discussed at length in Chapter 8, neurotrophic factors are essential substances that are necessary for survival and growth of neurons. They are produced by presynaptic neurons and secreted into the extracellular space at the site of synapses where they can be taken up by postsynaptic neurons. Further, the quantity and action of available neurotrophic factors are enhanced by activation of the cell. There is evidence that both spontaneous and input-dependent activation of a neuron may trigger a calcium-dependent gene expression pathway that results in upregulation of *Bdnf* expression within the neurons, thus increasing the available quantity of the neurotrophic factor (Libersat and Duch 2004). Consistent with this, recent work suggests that *Bdnf* expressed in the cell body and dendrites of neurons induces branching of the dendritic arbors of nearly all cells while having little effect on dendritic spine formation or axon extension (Horch and Katz 2002).

## Growth Cones and Axon Extension

At the tip of the outgrowing axon, a cone-shaped protrusion is formed by the plasma membrane of the cell. These structures were first recognized by Ramon y Cajal in 1893. He speculated that they are the regions where axon extension occurs and thus referred to them as growth cones. That original idea was later confirmed and extended to dendrites, as well as axons. Axons can grow at a rate of many microns per hour (several millimeters per day). Growth cones are both the site of axon extension and the source of directional guidance as axons navigate through tissue. Axon guidance is achieved via signals received from the local environment by the growth cones. This signaling pathway directs the forward extension of the axon through the developing brain tissues. Upon reaching their target sites, growth-cone structures facilitate target recognition, halt further axonal growth, and may provide primitive signaling at newly formed synapses.

### The Structure of the Growth Cone

The growth cone consists of a central region (Figure 7.4A) filled with microtubules, which are thin tubes of protein that are bundled together to provide structure for the axon. Microtubules also participate in axon extension. One end of the microtubule bundle is anchored in the axon shaft; the other end extends forward into the peripheral regions of the growth cone. The peripheral regions of the growth cone consist of the filopodia and the lamellipodia. The filopodia are long, thin spikes of membrane on the leading edge of the growth cone. They act as sensory receivers that sample the extracellular space for guidance signals in the local environment of the advancing growth cone. They convert the external directional signals into internal signals that direct the movement of the growth cone (Price and Willshaw 2000). The lamellipodia are the thin, weblike membranes that connect the filopodia. Filopodia contain high concentrations of F-actin, a filament-shaped protein, and G-actin, the subunits that combine (polymerize) to create the F-actin filaments. The ongoing polymerization, or assembly, of the smaller G-actin subunits to form F-actin filaments and the subsequent depolymerization, or breakdown, of F-actin into G-actin subunits are critical for axon extension.

### Axon Extension

Axon extension occurs by the addition of the cellular components at the border between the axon and the growth cone. As the leading edge of the growth cone advances, the base of the growth cone becomes transformed into the neurite. Thus extension of the axon does not involve axon movement, but rather continuous lengthening of the distal extremity of the axon. The materials necessary for axon growth are transported through the central zone of the axon to the growth cone. Growth cones, however, appear to contain all the machinery needed for axon lengthening, since growth cones disconnected from the rest of the cell body continue to extend the axon for a period of time (Brown, Keynes, and Lumsden 2001). Growth-cone extension occurs in the filopodia in the leading edge of the growth cone. The mechanism of extension is the continuous polymerization of F-actin

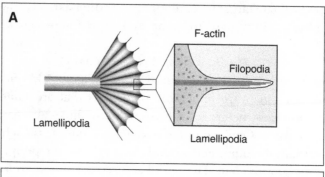

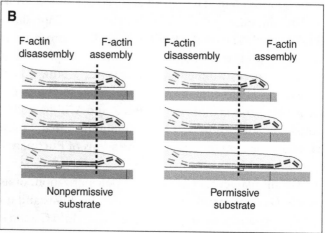

Figure 7.4 A. Growth cones are composed of lamellipodia and filopodia. They are filled with actin, which provides structure for the growth cone and is essential for axon extension. B. Axon extension occurs by the addition of the cellular components at the border between the axon and the growth cone. The ongoing formation and breakdown of F-actin filaments are critical for axon extension. Axon extension relies on cell adherence to the extracellular surface. The growth cone needs a permissive surface that it can adhere to in order to advance. Growth cones cannot advance if the surface is nonpermissive. Dotted lines indicate the position of the growth cone on permissive versus nonpermissive surfaces.

filaments from G-actin subunits. The assembly of actin filaments is balanced by the ongoing depolymerization of these filaments into G-actin at the other end of the filopodium. These cycles of construction and deconstruction are linked by a continuous retrograde flow of actin back from the leading edge of the filopodia toward the central core of the growth cone. The force that extends the axon derives from this

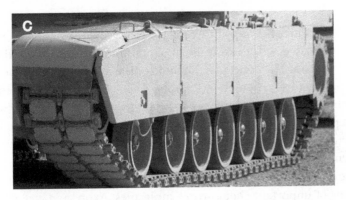

Figure 7.4 *(continued)*. C. The process of growth-cone extension has been likened to the movement of a tank tread. (Photo Courtesy of U.S. Army. Photo taken by Staff Sgt. Suzanne Day.)

backward flow of actin within the growth cone (Figure 7.4B). However, axon extension also depends critically upon whether the growth cone can adhere to the extracellular surface.

When the growth cone contacts a nonpermissive surface, one to which it cannot adhere, the retrograde flow of actin simply returns actin to the central core of the growth cone, and the axon does not advance. When the growth cone contacts a permissive surface, one to which it can adhere, the combination of the adhesion and the retrograde flow of actin prevents the return of actin to the central core and forces the forward extension of the growth cone and the lengthening of the axon (Figure 7.4B). This process has been likened to the movement of a tank tread (Figure 7.4C) in that if the wheel assembly is lifted from the ground or placed in thick mud (a nonpermissive surface), the vehicle makes no forward progress, but when the tread contacts hard ground (a permissive surface), it moves ahead. The adhesion of the advancing growth cones to the surrounding cells or to the extracellular substrate is achieved via classes of molecules referred to as cell adhesion molecules (Cadms). Cell-cell or cell-surface adhesion occurs by binding of a Cadm produced in the cell to the same Cadm on an adjacent cell or surface. There are different families of neural adhesion molecules involved in axonal extension. Specific molecules arise on the surface of growing neurons at different times and locations in development (Brown, Keynes, and Lumsden 2001).

## Axon Guidance

The advancement of growth cones is orchestrated by a complex and highly regulated set of extracellular signals in a process referred to as chemotropism. The concept of chemotropism as a mechanism for axon guidance was first proposed by Ramon y Cajal (1890). He suggested that diffusible molecules produced by the target cells of advancing axons might provide crucial guidance cues. Since then a number of guidance molecules have been identified. They include both chemoattractants, molecules that promote the advancement of growth cones, and chemorepellents, molecules that direct movement away. Table 7.1 lists a number of important chemotropic molecules. Axon guidance involves the coordinated action of both attractant and repellent cues, and each class of guidance cues can involve either direct contact with growth cones in the immediate cell environment or signals from a more distant source. Contact-dependent attraction and repulsion involve the modulation of the adhesion of the growth cone to the extracellular matrix and to other cells. Upon contact with chemorepulsive cues, the growth cone collapses and the filopodia and lamellipodia retract. Growth cones can also be guided by chemoattractive gradients of diffusible factors emanating from their targets, or they can be directed away from a site by the expression of chemorepulsive gradients (Levitan and Kaczmarek 2002).

Axons do not typically branch before reaching their initial target locations. Once they arrive there, branching is observed, and different axonal branches form synapses on different target cells. Some branches extend outside the target region. These branches form new growth cones and extend to other target sites (Brown, Keynes, and Lumsden 2001).

## Synapse Formation

The final step in differentiation requires the formation of synapses and the synthesis and storage of specific neurotransmitters. This section begins with a summary of the basic structure of a synapse and a description of the two principal synapse types, symmetrical and asymmetrical. Next, a brief overview of the very large topic of neurotransmitter acquisition will be provided. By far the most abundant neurotransmitters in the brain are the excitatory neurotransmitter glutamate and the inhibitory neurotransmitter GABA. Both are expressed from early in development. Finally, in addition to their role in neural signaling path-

Table 7.1   Guidance molecules

Semaphorins:
- Can exist as (1) fixed-membrane proteins or (2) secreted proteins
- Can provide either attractant or repulsive cues
- Family of proteins: nine subclasses
- Present on a subset of axons and nonneuronal cells along which growth cones travel
- Alter the direction of advancing growth cones by local activation of receptors on neurons

Netrins:
- Secreted proteins
- Provide attractant cues
- Some alter the direction of advancing growth cones by local activation of receptors on neurons
- Others bind to receptors on other cells along which axons grow

Nogos:
- Fixed-membrane proteins
- Provide strong repulsive cues
- Major repulsive factor produced by oligodendrocytes

Ephrins:
- Membrane proteins
- Can provide either attractant or repulsive cues
- Gradients of ephrins can shape the pattern of synapse formation and may represent the first step in synapse formation.
- Others bind to receptors on other cells along which axons grow

*Source:* I. B. Levitan and L. K. Kaczmarek, *The neuron: Cell and molecular biology,* 3rd ed. (Oxford: Oxford University Press, © 2002).

ways, neurotransmitters play a role in modulating a wide variety of basic functions including the shift from symmetrical to asymmetrical cell division in the VZ, modulation of cell-cycle duration, and guidance of migrating neurons.

### The Structure of a Synapse

Synapses are highly specialized points of contact between a presynaptic nerve terminal and a postsynaptic neuron (Figure 7.5). Within the presynaptic side of the synapse are small capsulelike structures, called vesicles, that contain neurotransmitters. Within the presynaptic membrane are voltage-gated calcium ($Ca^{2+}$) channels and receptor sites for recovery of neurotransmitters. Transmitter-specific receptors are localized in the postsynaptic membrane. In a chemical synapse, an action potential propagating through the presynaptic cell initiates a sequence of events that results in the release of the neurotransmitter. The action potential changes the electrical balance between the inside and the outside of the cell, depolarizing the membrane. This depolarization causes the voltage-gated calcium channels in the presynaptic membrane to open and $Ca^{2+}$ to enter the cell. The influx of $Ca^{2+}$ initiates the process of exocytosis, in which the vesicles fuse with the presynaptic membrane and release their neurotransmitter into the space between the pre- and postsynaptic membranes called the synaptic cleft. The neurotransmitter then diffuses across the synaptic cleft and binds to the receptors in the postsynaptic membrane, initiating a signaling cascade within the postsynaptic cell. There are two broad classes of postsynaptic receptors, ionotropic and metabotropic. Ionotropic receptors use ion channels to convert the chemical signal from the neurotransmitter directly and very quickly (in less than a millisecond) into a postsynaptic electrical signal. Metabotropic receptors act by relaying neurotransmitter signals to second messenger mole-

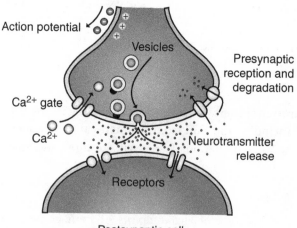

Figure 7.5. Schematic representation of a chemical synapse.

cules within the postsynaptic cells that in turn transmit the signal; thus their signaling is much slower, typically taking tens of milliseconds (Herlenius and Lagercrantz 2004). After the signal is transmitted, the neurotransmitter is either degraded by a process called hydrolysis and enzymatically converted to an inactive form or taken back up into presynaptic cells by transporter molecules.

Two types of synapses have been identified. Type 1, or asymmetric, synapses contain round or spherical vesicles, and the postsynaptic membrane appears thickened. These synapses are excitatory in activity and are the most abundant synapse type. Type 2, or symmetric, synapses contain flattened vesicles, and their pre- and postsynaptic membranes are parallel and of equal density. They are inhibitory in their activity and account for approximately 15 to 20 percent of synapses in the cerebral cortex. By far the greatest proportion of synapses are axodendritic, meaning that the axon contributes the presynaptic component and the dendrite the postsynaptic component. However, many other variants do occur, though less frequently; these include axo-axonic, somato-axonic, somato-dendritic, and dendro-dendritic.

## Acquisition of Neurotransmitters

The acquisition of cell-specific neurotransmitters and their receptors involves a complex cascade of events that includes both cell-intrinsic and cell-extrinsic factors. A great deal of work has elucidated the role of cell-intrinsic factors in specification of transmitter type. These studies suggest unique acquisition pathways for each of the major types of neurotransmitters, requiring the expression of cell-specific transcription factors. The two most abundant neurotransmitters are glutamate and gamma-aminobutyric acid (GABA). Glutamate is the primary excitatory neurotransmitter. It is expressed in half of all neurons in the cerebral cortex, including most pyramidal cells (Herlenius and Lagercrantz 2004). Subtypes of receptors for glutamate can be detected very early in development during early CP formation (Lujan, Shigemoto, and Lopez-Bendito 2005). GABA is the primary inhibitory neurotransmitter. It is expressed in 25 to 40 percent of neurons and in most inhibitory interneurons of the neocortex (Owens and Kriegstein 2002). GABA expression can be detected very early in CP development, during the formation of the preplate, GW6 to GW9 in humans; Verney 2003). Extensive work has identified patterns of expression of both neurotransmitters and their receptors. Glutamate has three sub-classes of ionotropic receptors, AMPA, NMDA, and kainate receptors, as well as eight subtypes of metabotropic receptors. Eight subtypes of ionotropic receptors have been identified for GABA, as well as three metabotropic subtypes. In addition to these most widely expressed neurotransmitters, a number of other very important but less extensively expressed neurotransmitters and their receptors have also been identified. A few of the best understood include acetylcholine, the monoamines (dopamine, serotonin, norepinephrine, epinephrine, and histamine), nitric oxide, and carbon monoxide (for recent reviews, see Herlenius and Lagercrantz 2004; Verney 2003). The expression patterns for a wide range of neurotransmitters and receptors have been well studied (Bloom 1988; Roth et al. 1998). The findings are complex, and a complete discussion of them is well beyond the scope of this book. However, it is important to note that the expression patterns for neurotransmitters and their receptors are not constant across development. The expression patterns and the composition of the receptors during the prenatal period are different from those observed in adulthood, suggesting that different components of the signaling system are more critical for establishing neural connectivity than for maintaining the neural circuitry in the more stable adult state (Lujan, Shigemoto, and Lopez-Bendito 2005; Van Eden et al. 1995). Mature patterns of neurotransmitter expression are not observed until adolescence for many classes of neurotransmitters (de Graaf-Peters and Hadders-Algra 2006; Uylings 2006). Levels of most neurotransmitters increase with synapse formation and later level off. While some neurotransmitters, such as serotonin, reach their stable adult state in early postnatal development, others, such as dopamine, undergo a protracted period of development that extends well into adolescence (de Graaf-Peters and Hadders-Algra 2006).

The determination of neurotransmitter expression is not entirely set by cell-internal programs. Recent work has shown that the level of intracellular $Ca^{2+}$ can alter the expression of neurotransmitter type (Borodinsky et al. 2004). For a transient period during early development, the embryo spontaneously generates $Ca^{2+}$-dependent action potentials that depolarize the neuronal membrane and result in an influx of $Ca^{2+}$ to the cells. This spontaneous activity plays an important role in determining the neurotransmitter expressed by the neurons.

Experimentally induced enhancement or suppression in the level of activity (and thus the levels of intracellular $Ca^{2+}$) results in alteration of the neurotransmitters that are expressed.

Overall, within an assembly of neurons, suppression of activity leads to an increase in the number of neurons expressing excitatory neurotransmitters and a decrease in the number of neurons expressing inhibitory neurotransmitters. Conversely, enhancement of activity leads to the opposite pattern, a decrease in the number of neurons expressing excitatory neurotransmitters and an increase in the number expressing inhibitory neurotransmitters (Borodinsky et al. 2004). It is notable that shifts in transmitter expression reflect the baseline expression patterns for the neurons. For example, in the suppression condition, within an assembly of cells, the normally excitatory neurons continue to express typical excitatory neurotransmitters, while a shift occurs in neurons that normally express inhibitory factors. These findings suggest a constrained but dynamic system that is seeking a homeostatic balance of activity. Early regional signaling of the neural progenitors, in concert with transcription-factor expression within the neuronal populations, establishes the preliminary specification of neurotransmitter type. Transient activity of the neurons alters the level of intracellular $Ca^{2+}$, further influencing the expression of transcription factors that require activity to initiate their expression. These findings suggest that activity can override developmental cues and provide a very early mechanism for activity-dependent modulation of neural signaling (Spitzer, Root, and Borodinsky 2004).

### Other Functions of Neurotransmitters

Finally, in addition to their role as signaling molecules at chemical synapses, neurotransmitters have recently been shown to serve a number of other important functions in early brain development. They have been shown to play a modulatory role in cell proliferation, migration, and differentiation. Both glutamate and GABA are expressed in early-migrating neurons, long before the formation of cortical synapses. Glutamate, and specifically the expression of certain of its receptors, the AMPA receptor and the NMDA receptors, is thought to play a role in signaling the shift from symmetrical to asymmetrical cell division. Within the VZ, glutamate can inhibit DNA synthesis when AMPA receptors are activated. This glutaminergic signal can induce daughter cells to shift to a postmitotic state. Within the GEs in ventral proliferative regions, glutamate activation of NMDA receptors has the opposite effect, promoting progenitor proliferation (Lujan, Shigemoto, and Lopez-Bendito 2005).

Exogenous application of either glutamate or GABA has been shown to modulate the length of the mitotic cycle. Within the dorsal VZ regions, overexpression of either neurotransmitter shortens the cell cycle, while in the dorsal SVZ, the cell cycle is lengthened (Lujan, Shigemoto, and Lopez-Bendito 2005; Represa and Ben-Ari 2005). Both of these neurotransmitters thus appear to participate in control of cell proliferation by modulating the rate of cell division. During radial migration, glutamate, but not GABA, has been identified as a chemoattractant providing directional cues for migrating neurons. GABA receptors appear to play a different signaling role during migration. Two GABA receptors, $GABA_B$ and $GABA_C$, stimulate neuron migration away from the VZ/SVZ to the IZ, while a third receptor, $GABA_A$, helps stop the migration of cells as they reach their target locations. Both neurotransmitters participate in neuronal differentiation. Glutamate appears to induce selective inhibition of dendrite growth in pyramidal neurons, while GABA promotes neurite outgrowth in interneurons (Lujan, Shigemoto, and Lopez-Bendito 2005).

The mechanism for early GABA signaling has recently been identified. GABA is the first neurotransmitter to become active in the developing brain. However, its action early in development emerges before synapse formation, and in contrast to its function in the mature brain as an inhibitor, in the early stages of brain development GABA serves an excitatory role (Owens and Kriegstein 2002; Represa and Ben-Ari 2005). The mechanism of early GABA signaling appears to be fundamentally different from that of the chemical synapse described earlier and perhaps reflects a more primitive, nonsynaptic signaling system (Owens and Kriegstein 2002). Early in development, the intracellular concentration of chlorine ions ($Cl^-$) is much higher than it is in adults. The early-emerging $GABA_A$ receptor serves as a chlorine ion-channel gate. When GABA opens the $Cl^-$ gate at the $GABA_A$ receptor, the resulting efflux of $Cl^-$ results in membrane depolarization and the propagation of an action potential. The depolarization of the membrane is sufficient to open $Ca^{2+}$ channels, resulting in an increase of $Ca^{2+}$ levels within the cell. The elevation in $Ca^{2+}$ initiates a wide range of intracellular cascades involved in neuronal growth and differentiation (Owens and Kriegstein 2002). Later in development, the intracellular concentration of Cl⁻ drops, and when the $GABA_A$ receptor is opened, Cl⁻ enters the cell and the effect is the opposite: hyperpolarization of the cell membrane (Miles 1999).

## Clinical Correlation: Disorders of Neuronal Migration

The laminar organization of the developing neocortex is critical for the establishment of functional cortical networks. Disruption of neuronal migration interferes with the orderly inside-out emergence of the cortical layers and causes severe disruption of cortical organization. In humans, both genetic and environmental factors can interfere with the processes of neuronal migration, with consequences ranging from mild to extreme depending on the timing and extent of disruption. Considerable progress has been made recently in defining the genetic causes of one of the major human neuronal migration disorders, classical lissencephaly. This section will review the evidence for the role of two genes, *LIS1* and doublecortin (*DCX*), in human neuronal migration and in lissencephaly.

The term *lissencephaly*, or "smooth brain," refers to the appearance of the cortical surface, which in the most severe cases lacks gyral and sulcal patterning and thus has a smooth, nonconvoluted appearance. There are a number of types of lissencephaly that may involve a variety of noncortical structures (cerebellum, corpus callosum, brain stem) in addition to the cortex. The current discussion will focus on the spectrum of disorders that fall within the category of classical lissencephaly / subcortical band disorder (Barkovich et al. 2001). Classical lissencephaly represents a spectrum of disorders that includes six grades that vary in severity (Kato and Dobyns 2003). At all levels of severity, the cortex is abnormally thick (10 to 20 mm, compared to 3 to 5 mm in the typical cortex), and in all but the mildest forms of the disorder, cortical lamination is abnormal. The cortex in classical lissencephaly has four layers. Layer 1 corresponds to the MZ, layer 2 is a narrow, cell-rich layer containing pyramidal cells that normally belong to deeper cortical layers, layer 3 is cell sparse (probably a persistent subplate zone), and layer 4 is thick and extends nearly to ventricles from which it is separated by a band of white matter.

Variation in the severity of lissencephaly is quantified by a six-point grading system in which grade 1 is the most severe and grade 6 is the least. Within the grading scheme there can be overlap of severity and specific brain malformation. The most severe cases of lissencephaly (grades 1 to 3) involve agyria, in which there is an absence of cortical folds. Pachygyria designates cases where small numbers of broad convolutions are observed (grades 3 to 5). All cases of classical lissencephaly involve agyria or pachygyria. A third milder form of migration disorder, subcortical band heterotopia (SBH) (grades 5 and 6), is also included in the lissencephalic spectrum. The term *heterotopia* describes groups of neurons that are misplaced within either the gray or white matter. SBH is defined by a characteristic pattern of heterotopia in which a thin band of white matter just below the CP forms a boundary that separates the plate from a heterotopic band of gray matter. The heterotopic band can vary in thickness and extension, and the severity of the disorder associated with SBH is correlated with the thickness of the band. Unlike the more severe forms of the disorder, gyral patterning in SBH is normal or simplified, and the CP appears normal (Gleeson 2001).

Two types of classical lissencephaly have been identified, Miller-Dieker syndrome (MDS) and isolated lissenencephaly sequence (ILS). MDS typically involves a very severe form of lissencephaly and is accompanied by a range of facial deformities (Sheen et al. 2006). ILS is more variable in severity and is not typically associated with other malformations. Virtually all cases of MDS and approximately 65 percent of cases of ILS are associated with mutations of the *LIS1* gene (Reiner and Coquelle 2005). The deletions observed in MDS are large, often encompassing adjacent regions of the chromosome and affecting a broader range of genes (Dobyns et al. 1993; Guerrini 2005). These additional deletions are thought to be associated with the more severe form of lissencephalic disorder (Figure 7.6A). In cases of *LIS1*-associated ILS disorder (Figure 7.6B), the gene deletions are smaller and more variable, ranging from full gene deletion (60 percent of cases) and serious mutation (6 percent) to truncations (26 percent) and single codon abnormalities (6 percent). This variability in gene abnormality is thought to account for the range of deficits observed in this group (Guerrini 2005). Lissencephalic disorders often present with graded severity along the anterior-posterior axis. In *LIS1*-associated lissencephaly, cortical malformations are typically more severe in posterior than in anterior regions (Figure 7.6A and B). Very recent work suggests that at least in the more severe forms of the disorder, such as MDS, the gene mutation may interfere with proliferative as well as migratory processes (Sheen et al. 2006).

A second gene, doublecortin *(DCX)*, has been associated with X-linked ILS (Gupta, Tsai, and Wynshaw-Boris 2002). Mutations of the *DCX* gene do not lead to MDS; rather, they are associated with either less severe forms of classical lissencephaly or SBH (Gleeson 2000). The distribution of disorder severity is unequal across genders. Females tend to present with SBH (Figure 7.6D), while males with *DCX* mutations present with classical lissencephaly (Figure 7.6C). This X-linked difference in the severity of the disorder likely comes about because females have one normal and one defective copy of the *DCX* gene. If one copy was randomly deactivated during mitosis for each new neuron, half the cells in the migrating neuronal population would receive the unaffected gene and thus appropriate signaling, and half would receive the mutated gene (Gleeson 2000). This would account for both the rel-

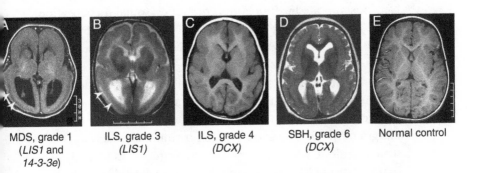

| MDS, grade 1 | ILS, grade 3 | ILS, grade 4 | SBH, grade 6 | Normal control |
| (*LIS1* and | (*LIS1*) | (*DCX*) | (*DCX*) | |
| 14-3-3e) | | | | |

Figure 7.6. The severity of lissencephalic disorders ranges through six grades, where grade 1 is the most severe. A. The most severe form of lissencephaly is Miller-Dieker syndrome (MDS). B. Isolated lissenencephaly sequence (ILS) is more variable in severity and is not typically associated with other malformations. Forms of lissencephaly associated with the *LIS1* gene are typically more severe in posterior than in anterior regions (see arrows). C. Males with *DCX* gene mutations usually present with classic lissencephaly, often of greater severity than disorders observed in females. *DCX*-associated disorders are typically more severe in anterior than in posterior regions. D. Females with *DCX* gene mutations usually present with subcortical band heterotopias (SBHs). E. Typical control brain. (From Kato and Dobyns 2003. Adapted with the permission of Oxford University Press.)

atively normal appearance of the CP and the underlying heterotopic band that is typical of SBH. In *DCX*-associated lissencephaly, cortical malformations are typically more severe in anterior than in posterior regions (Figure 7.6C).

The prevalence of classical lissencephaly is approximately 1 per 85,000 births. Affected children are initially delayed in their development and are eventually profoundly mentally retarded. Most children die in early childhood, though there are reported cases of individuals living until their early 20s. Seizures occur in more than 90 percent of the population, most beginning within the first six months of life. The effects of SBH are both milder and more variable. Cognitive functioning ranges from severe retardation to normal and is associated with the thickness and extent of the heterotopic band of cells. Most children have epilepsy, and it is severe in about 65 percent of cases (Guerrini 2005).

## Chapter Summary

- Neurons migrate by three different modes, somal translocation, radial glial locomotion, and tangential migration. Each mode of migration is appropriate to both when and where a neuron is produced. Somal translocation is observed early in development, when distances to be traversed are small. RG cells provide the structural scaffold for most neuronal migration. The radial glia are located in the VZ and extend processes that attach to the margin of the developing CP, thus providing a radially aligned structure along which neurons can migrate. It was recently determined that the RG cells are in fact neural progenitor cells. Tangential migration is the primary mode of migration used by cells migrating from the GEs.
- The cortical plate is a highly organized structure. During embryonic development, a number of transient structures serve to guide the migration of neurons and to establish early signaling pathways.
- In order to become part of functional cortical circuits, neurons must send out processes that allow them to communicate with other cells and acquire appropriate neurotransmitter substances.

- The establishment of connections requires the generation of an axon and dendrites. The process of axon and dendrite formation is called neuritogenesis. The cell axon provides the primary outgoing signal from the cell, while the dendrites are the primary signal receivers.

- Axons must often extend for long distances in the neural tissue to reach their targets. Growth cones on the tips of the axons direct their movement. Growth cones have structures called filopodia and lamellipodia that both act as sensors of the local signaling environment and serve to propel the advancement of the axon. Guidance molecules for axons can be either chemoattractant or chemorepellent.

- Critical for the advancement of axons is their ability to adhere to the tissue substrate. Cell adhesion molecules (Cadms) serve to anchor the axon to the substrate.

- Formation of synapses requires appropriate internal and external signaling. There is considerable evidence that specification of neurotransmitter type relies on cascades of transcription factors. However, there is also evidence that external $Ca^{2+}$ signaling is an important factor in modulation of neurotransmitter expression.

- Neurotransmitters have also been shown to play a neurotrophic role in early development. GABA, a normally inhibitory neurotransmitter, acts as an excitatory factor in early development, before the establishment of synapses. These kinds of early modulatory roles are thought to be important to the establishment of early signaling in the developing neocortical circuitry.

### References

Adcock, K. H., F. Metzger, and J. P. Kapfhammer. 2004. "Purkinje cell dendritic tree development in the absence of excitatory neurotransmission and of brain-derived neurotrophic factor in organotypic slice cultures." *Neuroscience*, 127: 137–145.

Arber, S. 2004. "Subplate neurons: Bridging the gap to function in the cortex." *Trends in Neurosciences*, 27: 111–113.

Barkovich, A. J., R. I. Kuzniecky, G. D. Jackson, R. Guerrini, and W. B. Dobyns. 2001. "Classification system for malformations of cortical development: Update 2001." *Neurology*, 57: 2168–2178.

Bielle, F., A. Griveau, N. Narboux-Neme, S. Vigneau, M. Sigrist, S. Arber, M. Wassef, and A. Pierani. 2005. "Multiple origins of Cajal-Retzius cells at the borders of the developing pallium." *Nature Neuroscience,* 8: 1002–1012.

Bloom, F. E. 1988. "Neurotransmitters: Past, present, and future directions." *FASEB Journal,* 2: 32–41.

Borodinsky, L. N., C. M. Root, J. A. Cronin, S. B. Sann, X. Gu, and N. C. Spitzer. 2004. "Activity-dependent homeostatic specification of transmitter expression in embryonic neurons." *Nature,* 429: 523–530.

Britz, O., P. Mattar, L. Nguyen, L. M. Langevin, C. Zimmer, S. Alam, F. Guillemot, and C. Schuurmans. 2006. "A role for proneural genes in the maturation of cortical progenitor cells." *Cerebral Cortex,* 16 (Suppl. 1): i138–i151.

Brown, M., R. Keynes, and A. Lumsden. 2001. *The developing brain.* Oxford: Oxford University Press.

Cline, H. T. 2001. "Dendritic arbor development and synaptogenesis." *Current Opinion in Neurobiology,* 11: 118–126.

de Graaf-Peters, V. B., and M. Hadders-Algra. 2006. "Ontogeny of the human central nervous system: What is happening when?" *Early Human Development,* 82: 257–266.

Dobyns, W. B., O. Reiner, R. Carrozzo, and D. H. Ledbetter. 1993. "Lissencephaly: A human brain malformation associated with deletion of the *LIS1* gene located at chromosome 17p13." *JAMA,* 270: 2838–2842.

Gleeson, J. G. 2000. "Classical lissencephaly and double cortex (subcortical band heterotopia): LIS1 and doublecortin." *Current Opinion in Neurology,* 13: 121–125.

———. 2001. "Neuronal migration disorders." *Mental Retardation and Developmental Disabilities Research Reviews,* 7: 167–171.

Greenough, W. T., H. M. Hwang, and C. Gorman. 1985. "Evidence for active synapse formation or altered postsynaptic metabolism in visual cortex of rats reared in complex environments." *Proceedings of the National Academy of Sciences of the United States of America,* 82: 4549–4552.

Guerrini, R. 2005. "Genetic malformations of the cerebral cortex and epilepsy." *Epilepsia,* 46 (Suppl. 1): 32–37.

Gupta, A., L. H. Tsai, and A. Wynshaw-Boris. 2002. "Life is a journey: A genetic look at neocortical development." *Nature Reviews Genetics,* 3: 342–355.

Herlenius, E., and H. Lagercrantz. 2004. "Development of neurotransmitter systems during critical periods." *Experimental Neurology,* 190 (Suppl. 1): S8–S21.

Hevner, R. F., R. A. Daza, C. Englund, J. Kohtz, and A. Fink. 2004. "Post-natal shifts of interneuron position in the neocortex of normal and reeler mice: Evidence for inward radial migration." *Neuroscience*, 124: 605–618.

Horch, H. W., and L. C. Katz. 2002. "BDNF release from single cells elicits local dendritic growth in nearby neurons." *Nature Neuroscience*, 5: 1177–1184.

Kanold, P. O., P. Kara, R. C. Reid, and C. J. Shatz. 2003. "Role of subplate neurons in functional maturation of visual cortical columns." *Science*, 301: 521–525.

Kato, M., and W. B. Dobyns. 2003. "Lissencephaly and the molecular basis of neuronal migration." *Human Molecular Genetics*, 12 (Spec. no. 1): R89–R96.

Kostovic, I., and N. Jovanov-Milosevic. 2006. "The development of cerebral connections during the first 20–45 weeks' gestation." *Seminars in Fetal and Neonatal Medicine*, 11: 415–422.

Kostovic, I., M. Judas, M. Rados, and P. Hrabac. 2002. "Laminar organization of the human fetal cerebrum revealed by histochemical markers and magnetic resonance imaging." *Cerebral Cortex*, 12: 536–544.

Kostovic, I., and P. Rakic. 1990. "Developmental history of the transient subplate zone in the visual and somatosensory cortex of the macaque monkey and human brain." *Journal of Comparative Neurology*, 297: 441–470.

Letinic, K., R. Zoncu, and P. Rakic. 2002. "Origin of GABAergic neurons in the human neocortex." *Nature*, 417: 645–649.

Levitan, I. B., and L. K. Kaczmarek. 2002. *The neuron: Cell and molecular biology*. 3rd ed. Oxford: Oxford University Press.

Libersat, F., and C. Duch. 2004. "Mechanisms of dendritic maturation." *Molecular Neurobiology*, 29: 303–320.

Lujan, R., R. Shigemoto, and G. Lopez-Bendito. 2005. "Glutamate and GABA receptor signalling in the developing brain." *Neuroscience*, 130: 567–580.

Marin, O., and J. L. Rubenstein. 2001. "A long, remarkable journey: Tangential migration in the telencephalon." *Nature Reviews Neuroscience* 2: 780–790.

Marin-Padilla, M. 1971. "Early prenatal ontogenesis of the cerebral cortex (neocortex) of the cat *(Felis domestica)*: A Golgi study. I. The primordial neocortical organization." *Zeitschrift für Anatomie und Entwicklungsgeschichte*, 134: 117–145.

———. 1972. "Prenatal ontogenetic history of the principal neurons of the neocortex of the cat (Felis domestica): A Golgi study. II. Developmental differences and their significances." *Zeitschrift für Anatomie und Entwicklungsgeschichte*, 136: 125–142.

McAllister, A. K. 2002. "Neurotrophins and cortical development." *Results and Problems in Cell Differentiation*, 39: 89–112.

Metin, C., J. P. Baudoin, S. Rakic, and J. G. Parnavelas. 2006. "Cell and molecular mechanisms involved in the migration of cortical interneurons." *European Journal of Neuroscience*, 23: 894–900.

Meyer, G., J. P. Schaaps, L. Moreau, and A. M. Goffinet. 2000. "Embryonic and early fetal development of the human neocortex." *Journal of Neuroscience*, 20: 1858–1868.

Miles, R. 1999. "Neurobiology: A homeostatic switch." *Nature*, 397: 215–216.

Miyata, T., A. Kawaguchi, H. Okano, and M. Ogawa. 2001. "Asymmetric inheritance of radial glial fibers by cortical neurons." *Neuron*, 31: 727–741.

Mrzljak, L., H. B. Uylings, I. Kostovic, and C. G. Van Eden. 1988. "Prenatal development of neurons in the human prefrontal cortex. I. A qualitative Golgi study." *Journal of Comparative Neurology*, 271: 355–386.

Mrzljak, L., H. B. Uylings, C. G. Van Eden, and M. Judas. 1990. "Neuronal development in human prefrontal cortex in prenatal and postnatal stages." *Progress in Brain Research*, 85: 185–222.

Nadarajah, B., P. Alifragis, R. O. Wong, and J. G. Parnavelas. 2003. "Neuronal migration in the developing cerebral cortex: Observations based on real-time imaging." *Cerebral Cortex*, 13: 607–611.

Nadarajah, B., and J. G. Parnavelas. 2002. "Modes of neuronal migration in the developing cerebral cortex." *Nature Reviews Neuroscience*, 3: 423–432.

Noctor, S. C., A. C. Flint, T. A. Weissman, W. S. Wong, B. K. Clinton, and A. R. Kriegstein. 2002. "Dividing precursor cells of the embryonic cortical ventricular zone have morphological and molecular characteristics of radial glia." *Journal of Neuroscience*, 22: 3161–3173.

Noctor, S. C., V. Martinez-Cerdeno, L. Ivic, and A. R. Kriegstein. 2004. "Cortical neurons arise in symmetric and asymmetric division zones and migrate through specific phases." *Nature Neuroscience*, 7: 136–144.

Oestreicher, A. B., P. N. De Graan, W. H. Gispen, J. Verhaagen, and L. H. Schrama. 1997. "B-50, the growth associated protein-43: Modulation of cell morphology and communication in the nervous system." *Progress in Neurobiology*, 53: 627–686.

Owens, D. F., and A. R. Kriegstein. 2002. "Is there more to GABA than synaptic inhibition?" *Nature Reviews Neuroscience*, 3: 715–727.

Parnavelas, J. G. 2000. "The origin and migration of cortical neurones: New vistas." *Trends in Neurosciences*, 23: 126–131.

Parnavelas, J. G., P. Alifragis, and B. Nadarajah. 2002. "The origin and migration of cortical neurons." *Progress in Brain Research*, 136: 73–80.

Piontek, J., A. Regnier-Vigouroux, and R. Brandt. 2002. "Contact with astroglial membranes induces axonal and dendritic growth of human

CNS model neurons and affects the distribution of the growth-associated proteins MAP1B and GAP43." *Journal of Neuroscience Research,* 67: 471–483.

Price, D. J., and D. J. Willshaw. 2000. *Mechanisms of cortical development.* Oxford: Oxford University Press.

Rakic, P. 1972. "Mode of cell migration to the superficial layers of fetal monkey neocortex." *Journal of Comparative Neurology,* 145: 61–83.

———. 2003a. "Developmental and evolutionary adaptations of cortical radial glia." *Cerebral Cortex,* 13: 541–549.

———. 2003b. "Elusive radial glial cells: Historical and evolutionary perspective." *Glia,* 43: 19–32.

———. 2006. "A century of progress in corticoneurogenesis: From silver impregnation to genetic engineering." *Cerebral Cortex,* 16 (Suppl. 1): i3–i17.

Ramon y Cajal, S. 1890. "Sur l'origine et les ramifications des fibres nerveuses de la moelle embryonnaire." *Anatomischer Anzeiger,* 5: 609–613.

Reiner, O., and F. M. Coquelle. 2005. "Missense mutations resulting in type 1 lissencephaly." *Cellular and Molecular Life Sciences,* 62: 425–434.

Represa, A., and Y. Ben-Ari. 2005. "Trophic actions of GABA on neuronal development." *Trends in Neurosciences,* 28: 278–283.

Rice, D. S., and T. Curran. 2001. "Role of the reelin signaling pathway in central nervous system development." *Annual Review of Neuroscience,* 24: 1005–1039.

Roth, B. L., S. A. Berry, W. K. Kroeze, D. L. Willins, and K. Kristiansen. 1998. "Serotonin 5-HT2A receptors: Molecular biology and mechanisms of regulation." *Critical Reviews in Neurobiology,* 12: 319–338.

Shatz, C. J. 1994. "Role for spontaneous neural activity in the patterning of connections between retina and LGN during visual system development." *International Journal of Developmental Neuroscience,* 12: 531–546.

Sheen, V. L., R. J. Ferland, M. Harney, R. S. Hill, J. Neal, A. H. Banham, P. Brown, A. Chenn, J. Corbo, J. Hecht, R. Folkerth, and C. A. Walsh. 2006. "Impaired proliferation and migration in human Miller-Dieker neural precursors." *Annals of Neurology,* 60: 137–144.

Spitzer, N. C., C. M. Root, and L. N. Borodinsky. 2004. "Orchestrating neuronal differentiation: patterns of $Ca^{2+}$ spikes specify transmitter choice." *Trends in Neurosciences,* 27: 415–421.

Stumm, R. K., C. Zhou, T. Ara, F. Lazarini, M. Dubois-Dalcq, T. Nagasawa, V. Hollt, and S. Schulz. 2003. "CXCR4 regulates interneuron migration in the developing neocortex." *Journal of Neuroscience,* 23: 5123–5130.

Tissir, F., and A. M. Goffinet. 2003. "Reelin and brain development." *Nature Reviews Neuroscience,* 4: 496–505.

Tsai, L. H., and J. G. Gleeson. 2005. "Nucleokinesis in neuronal migration." *Neuron,* 46: 383–388.

Uylings, H. B. M. 2006. "Development of the human cortex and the concept of 'critical' or 'sensitive' periods." *Language Learning,* 56: 59–90.

Van Eden, C. G., R. Parmar, W. Lichtensteiger, and M. Schlumpf. 1995. "Laminar distribution of $GABA_A$ receptor alpha 1, beta 2, and gamma 2 subunit mRNAs in the granular and agranular frontal cortex of the rat during pre- and postnatal development." *Cerebral Cortex,* 5: 234–246.

Verney, C. 2003. "Phenotypic expression of monoamines and GABA in the early development of human telencephalon, transient or not transient." *Journal of Chemical Neuroanatomy,* 26: 283–292.

Volpe, J. J. 2001. *Neurology of the newborn.* 4th ed. Philadelphia: W. B. Saunders.

Weissman, T., S. C. Noctor, B. K. Clinton, L. S. Honig, and A. R. Kriegstein. 2003. "Neurogenic radial glial cells in reptile, rodent and human: From mitosis to migration." *Cerebral Cortex,* 13: 550–559.

Zecevic, N., Y. Chen, and R. Filipovic. 2005. "Contributions of cortical subventricular zone to the development of the human cerebral cortex." *Journal of Comparative Neurology,* 491: 109–122.

# EIGHT

# Shaping the Emerging Cortical Network: The Role of Intrinsic and Extrinsic Factors

BY MIDGESTATION, NEURONAL production is essentially complete, and the generation of glial cells is in progress. Cortical network formation is under way, marking the beginning of a process that will extend well into the postnatal period. This chapter will consider work that has resulted from a central debate in the field concerning the role of intrinsic versus extrinsic factors in establishing the primary areal organization of the neocortex. The protomap view argues that spatially specific molecular signaling of neural progenitor cells in the proliferative zone establishes both the spatial location and the basic function of neurons within the primary subdivisions of the cortex. By contrast, the protocortex view asserts that early in development, the neocortex is comparatively homogeneous, and that the assignment of functional roles for neurons is dependent on input to and activity of neurons. Recent work suggests that spatially specific molecular signaling is essential in establishing the initial interareal divisions within the neocortex, but that those early areas are malleable, and the final organization of the neocortex relies upon activity-dependent signaling.

The second major topic that will be covered in this chapter concerns two somewhat counterintuitive processes that are an integral part of brain development, specifically, programmed cell death and synaptic exuberance and elimination. The hallmark of a developing biological system is the proliferation and integration of new elements. In the early prenatal period, dramatic changes in the size and shape of cortical structures reflect the prodigious rates of neuronal production. Indeed, in many regions of the developing neocortex, the pace of prenatal neurogenesis far exceeds the needs of the mature system, and many of the early generated neurons will die via the process of apoptosis, or programmed cell death. Apoptosis is a well-understood and highly regulated developmental process that serves to eliminate excess cells from the developing system. In contrast to cellular necrosis, it is not a pathological event. Rather, apoptosis is a critical regulatory function that plays an important role in establishing the optimal balance between neural subunits within the developing cortical systems. Early neural connectivity also follows a profile of initial exuberance and subsequent elimination of synapses. Many more connections are formed between neurons than will be present in the mature system. Furthermore, many of the early transient patterns of connectivity have no counterpart in the adult organism. Cells compete for both synaptic space at the connection site and neurotrophic factors. Those cells that are most successful in establishing stable connections retain them, while those that are not successful retract their neural process. The stabilization of particular synaptic pathways appears to be, at least in part, activity dependent. Cells that fail to establish active connections typically lose the competition for resources at the synaptic site, and those connections are pruned away.

## Arealization of the Developing Neocortex

The mature neocortex forms a thin mantle of cells on the surface of the brain. In its vertical dimension (i.e., its thickness), the neocortex is uniform in that it is composed of six layers that are distinguished by the cells they contain and the connections they form. Neurons within the cortical mantle are complexly connected. Some form connections with neurons in subcortical regions, establishing the basis for basic input-output pathways; others form connections with cells in distal regions of the cortex, setting up long-distance signaling centers; and yet others form connections with nearby cortical cells, creating local circuits. Although macroscopically the horizontal surface of the mature neocortex appears to be a fairly uniform structure, microscopic examination reveals that it is composed of well-defined, histologically (that is, cellularly) distinct areas. In the early 1900s, Korbinian Brodmann (1909) published a comprehensive and still widely used map of the

cytoarchitectonic areas of the human brain (Figure 8.1A) that identified 47 areas of the human cortex. Other classic neuroanatomical
studies were in basic agreement with overall partitioning but estimated
different numbers of areas. Von Economo and Kostinas identified 46
zones consisting of 107 cortical fields (von Economo and Kostinas
1925). Vogt, elaborating on Brodmann's original work, estimated more
than 200 areas. The cytoarchitectonic differences observed at area
boundaries can be pronounced. For example, the laminar organization
of primary visual cortex (Brodmann area 17, BA17) is distinct from that
of the adjacent extrastriate visual area BA18 (Figure 8.1B), and the
most notable difference between the two areas is seen in layer 4. As is
the case in most primary sensory areas, layer 4 of primary visual cortex
(BA17) is the primary input layer. It receives most of the input from the
major visual pathway that extends first from the retina to the visual nucleus of the thalamus (the lateral geniculate nucleus) and then from
the thalamus to BA17 in the cortex. One important question that arises
is when and how the complex pattern of areal differentiation emerges
in the developing cortex. This question has been at the center of a
long-standing debate in the field of developmental neurobiology.

## Protomap versus Protocortex

The classical debate over the origins of areal specification pitted two
strong views against one another: the protomap view and the protocortex view. The protomap view contended that the neural progenitor
cells of the VZ provide molecular signals to their neural progeny that
specify their areal fate, that is, their position in the cortex and their associated function (Rakic 1988). The protomap model suggested that
neuronal migration from the VZ is orderly and maintains the basic topography of the VZ progenitors (Figure 8.2). A small number of
neural progenitors from a local region of the VZ contribute to the
pool of neurons that migrate along common or closely positioned
radial glial guides. As these neurons reach the cortical plate, the
inside-out pattern of glial-guided migration results in their arrangement in a vertical column, referred to as a cortical column. Neurons
within a column thus have a common lineage that specifies their location in the cortex and their areal fate. Thus the protomap view emphasized the role of intrinsic cues derived from molecular signaling by

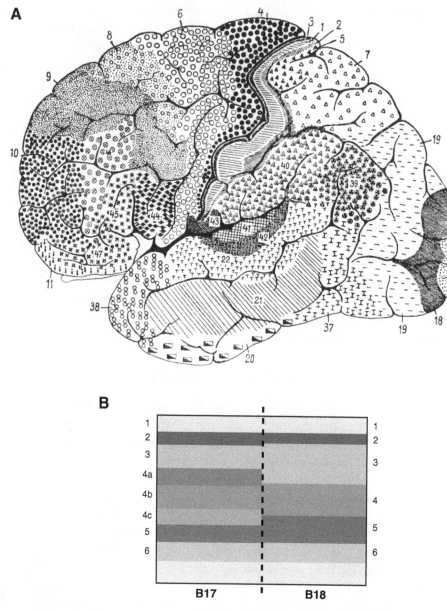

Figure 8.1. The neocortex is composed of histologically distinct areas.
A. Brodmann's map of the cytoarchitectonic areas of the human brain.
B. Laminar organization of the primary visual cortex, BA17, and the
adjacent visual area, BA18. The most notable difference is seen in layer 4,
which is markedly thicker in BA17. (A from Brodmann 1909.)

neural progenitors in the VZ in establishing the areal organization of
the developing neocortex.

By contrast, the protocortex view suggests that the initial organization of the cortical mantle is comparatively undifferentiated (O'Leary,
Schlaggar, and Tuttle 1994). Signaling in the VZ results in the basic

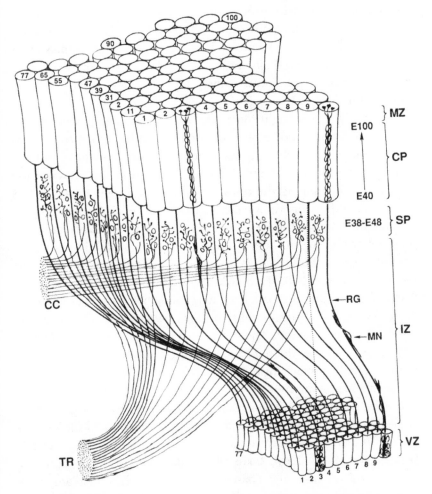

Figure 8.2. Rakic's protomap model of corticogenesis. MZ = marginal zone;
CP = cortical plate; SP = subplate; IZ = intermediate zone; VZ = ventricular
zone; RG = radial glia; MN = migrating neuron; CC = contralateral cortico-
cortical bundles; TR = thalamic radiation. (From Rakic 1988. Reprinted
with the permission of AAAS.)

six-layered organization that is characteristic of the entire neocortex. However, differences among cortical areas develop from a very different signaling pathway. By the protocortex view, the principal sources of areal specification depend on activity within the developing neural system and are thus derived from differential input. The major source of input to the developing brain is the primary input pathway that transmits information between the relay nuclei in the thalamus and the cortex, the thalamocortical (TC) pathway. The major output pathway is the corticothalamic (CT) pathway that sends signals from the cortex back to the thalamus. Thus, by the protocortex view, areal specification is the product of activity-dependent factors in the developing brain.

Recent work has brought some resolution to the debate over the origins and development of neocortical areas (Chambers and Fishell 2006; Sur and Rubenstein 2005). As discussed in Chapter 5, studies of molecular signaling in the primitive VZ have provided strong evidence for early patterning among the dorsal telencephalic progenitors. Graded expression of the transcription factors Pax6 and Emx2, supported by regional expression of the secreted molecule Fgf8, establishes anterior-posterior patterning in the VZ progenitors that is transmitted to their neural progeny (Bishop, Rubenstein, and O'Leary 2002; Grove and Fukuchi-Shimogori 2003; Hamasaki et al. 2004; O'Leary and Nakagawa 2002). These expression patterns emerge long before the development of the TC pathways, suggesting that initial patterning does not rely on activity-dependent factors. These data establish that the initial interareal differences in the developing neocortex are the product of intrinsic molecular signaling mechanisms that operate within the VZ (Vanderhaeghen and Polleux 2004).

However, it is also clear that these early-defined neocortical areas are malleable, and that the specification of intra-areal organization is protracted and involves extrinsic, as well as intrinsic, signaling (Lopez-Bendito and Molnar 2003; Rakic 2001). Chapter 10 will consider the extensive data on postnatal changes in the neocortex that are input dependent and rely on the specific experience of the individual. Those data reflect the plasticity of the developing neurocognitive system. However, essential patterns of connectivity among brain regions begin to emerge in the prenatal period. Thus one important question concerns the mechanisms that direct the initial formation of these early-developing pathways. The next section will consider the development of two of the most critical of those early pathways, the thalamocortical (TC) and the corticothalamic (CT) pathways.

## The Development of the TC and CT Pathways

The TC and CT pathways provide the essential connections between the neocortex and subcortical sensory and motor relay nuclei. The TC pathway is the major subcortical input pathway that projects from the principal subcortical sensorimotor relay nucleus, the thalamus, to the neocortex. The CT pathway is the major cortical output pathway that projects from the deep layers of the neocortex down to the thalamus. One important issue concerns whether the establishment of these critical pathways is dependent on molecular signaling primarily from the neocortex, or whether there are other signaling centers that also contribute to their formation.

The thalamus is a diencephalic structure that plays a critical role in a variety of neural pathways. It is divided into two major segments, the dorsal and the ventral thalamus, each containing a number of smaller nuclei. Only the neurons in the dorsal thalamus project to the cortex (Lopez-Bendito and Molnar 2003). The nuclei of the dorsal thalamus relay specific information to the primary sensory areas of the neocortex. The timing of neurogenesis in the thalamus coincides with that in the neocortex.

The axons of the thalamic neurons that form the TC pathway exit the dorsal thalamus and project ventrally (Figure 8.3). At the diencephalic-telencephalic border (DTB), the fibers abruptly change course and turn dorsolaterally, entering the ventral telencephalon (VT) within a region that will become the internal capsule. The internal capsule (IC) is the major fiber pathway that connects the cortex with the diencephalon and the brainstem; the TC and CT pathways are major constituents of the mature IC. Upon entering the IC, the TC fibers make contact with a transient cell population in the IC and pause their advance to the cortex. After a delay that varies across species (two days in the hamster and the rat; somewhat longer in the cat), TC axons advance toward the dorsal-ventral telencephalic border (DVTB), change course again, and move dorsally into the cortex. When TC axons first arrive at the cortex, they initially invade a transient but important embryonic cortical layer, the subplate (Catalano and Shatz 1998). In most species, TC axons remain in the subplate for a waiting period before projecting to their final targets in layer 4 of the cortex; in humans this waiting period extends from GW22 to GW26 (Kostovic and Jovanov-Milosevic 2006). During this time, TC axons form active synaptic connections with subplate neurons.

*The Role of the Subplate in Establishing the TC and CT Pathways*
Subplate neurons play an important role in the early formation of the TC and CT pathways. In addition to interacting with TC axons as they enter the subplate layer, subplate neurons also project to and receive input from neurons in layer 4 of the developing sensory cortices. That

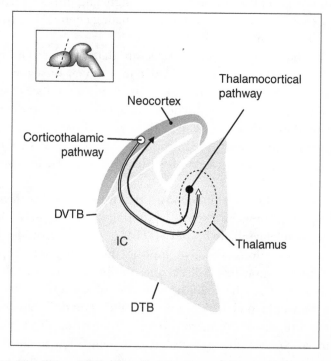

Figure 8.3. The TC and CT pathways. The TC pathway extends dorsally from the dorsal thalamus through the IC to the cortex. The CT pathway projects ventrally from the cortex through the IC to the dorsal thalamus. IC=internal capsule; DVTB=dorsal-ventral telencephalic border; DTB=diencephalic-telencephalic border.

is, they connect with the same population of neurons that will later receive the primary sensory input from the TC pathway. It is thought that this early pattern of connectivity between subplate and cortical neurons may serve to "instruct" the incoming TC axons. Connections between TC axons and subplate neurons are normally active. However, when this activity is experimentally blocked, the orderly pattern of connectivity between TC axons and layer-4 neurons is disrupted (Catalano and Shatz 1998). Thus one function of the subplate is to mediate dynamic interactions between the TC axons and the cortex.

In addition to their role in establishing the TC pathway, subplate neurons are also critical in the development of the CT pathway. Subplate neurons send what have been termed "pioneering" projections to the thalamus in advance of the projections emanating from the cells in the deep cortical layers (5 and 6) that will later constitute the mature CT pathway. The pioneering axons of subplate neurons reach the IC just before the TC axons reach the cortex (Miller, Chou, and Finlay 1993). Like the TC axons, the CT axons pause before proceeding toward the thalamus. CT axons from cortical layers 5 and 6 invade the thalamus considerably after the arrival of the subplate axons. It is thought that the subplate "pioneers" may provide guidance for the CT pathway axons that develop later.

### Guidance Cues for TC and CT Pathfinding

The dorsal thalamus is divided into a number of specific nuclei. For example, the lateral geniculate nucleus (LGN) mediates visual information, while the medial geniculate nucleus (MGN) mediates auditory information. Neurons in each nucleus receive input from a primary sensory receptor system, such as the retina of the visual system or the cochlea of the auditory system, and they relay that information to primary sensory areas of the cortex. The general topography of nuclei positions within the thalamus approximates the organization of cortical sensory areas (Vanderhaeghen and Polleux 2004) such that, for example, the more posteriorly positioned thalamic nuclei project to sensory areas in posterior cortical areas (e.g., the LGN and the primary visual cortex), while more rostrally positioned nuclei project to rostral cortical areas. One important question then concerns the guidance cues that direct the TC and CT axons to the appropriate targets in the cortex and the thalamus, respectively.

A number of candidate signaling centers have been proposed. One likely source of signaling molecules for TC axons is the targets in the developing neocortex itself. Several studies support this view. Recall that mutations of the *Emx2* gene in mice result in a shift in the expression gradients of *Emx2* and *Pax6* within the neocortical progenitor cell population. That shift is associated with modifications in the anterior-posterior organization of the neocortex and specifically in the positioning of the primary sensory areas. The alteration of expression patterns for *Emx2* is accompanied by a shift in positional targeting of the sensory TC input pathway axons as they enter the primitive cortex (Bishop, Goudreau, and O'Leary 2000; O'Leary and Nakagawa 2002). However, although *Emx2* is expressed in neural progenitors, it is not expressed by their neural offspring. Thus the source of the positional signaling within the developing cortex has been unclear. Recent studies have shown, however, that the early-migrating neurons that will form the preplate maintain close neighborhood relationships with the progenitor cells that generated them. This preservation of spatial proximity between the Emx2-producing progenitors and the neuronal progeny that will form the subplate suggests that Emx2 may indirectly signal positional and areal identity for the major sensory areas of the cortex via intermediate signaling to subplate neurons (O'Leary and Borngasser 2006). It is also postulated that molecular signaling within the subplate may provide molecular guidance for the invading TC axons (Bishop et al. 2003). Other evidence for cortical cuing of incoming TC axons comes from experiments in which sections of tissue from the frontal cortex were grafted to occipital regions of host animals, thus creating animals with two potential "frontal" signaling sites. In these animals, TC axons projected both to their normal targets in frontal regions and to the posteriorly displaced graft, suggesting some as-yet-unidentified molecular signal emanating from the grafted cortical tissue (Frappe, Roger, and Gaillard 1999).

It has been suggested that the developing TC and CT pathways themselves may provide reciprocal guidance cues. During pathway formation, both TC and CT axons pause in the IC of the VT. When each set of axons later proceeds toward its respective target, it remains in proximity to the fiber pathway previously established by the other. This pattern of proximal association between these two reciprocally advancing pathways has led to the postulation of the "handshake hypothesis" (Molnar and Blakemore 1995), which stipulates that reciprocal interaction between the two developing pathways is necessary for the development of both. Support for the handshake hypothesis comes from findings from animals with a genetic mutation that destroys subplate neurons. In these animals, the early pioneering CT pathway does not develop, and significantly, TC axons fail to find their way through the IC to the cortex (Zhou et al. 1999). This leads to the conclusion that the presence of the CT pathway is necessary for TC axons to find their way to the cortex. However, it is possible that this kind of defect may be attributed to failure of a remote signaling system rather than failure of the CT pathway per se. Furthermore, although the fiber tracts of the two pathways invade similar territories, detailed examination of their positions in the IC reveals that the two fiber bundles maintain both radial and tangential separation from each other (Auladell et al. 2000; Miller, Chou, and Finlay 1993). Thus, while the data on the handshake hypothesis are intriguing, it has not yet been demonstrated that the two pathways depend upon each other for guidance. That is, it is not known whether the interaction between the pathways is necessary for pathway formation, or if the data reflect the fact that both pathways depend autonomously on the same sets of cues emanating from the cortex and the thalamus (Lopez-Bendito and Molnar 2003).

Whether or not the fiber pathways themselves play a role in guidance, there is evidence that TC and CT axon guidance requires complex signaling involving multiple extracortical signaling centers in addition to cortical signaling. Data from studies of selective gene mutation suggest that important signaling may emanate from the VT (Hevner, Miyashita-Lin, and Rubenstein 2002). The chemoattractant netrin1 (Ntn1) appears to play an important role in directing axons from both the cortex and the thalamus to the VT regions. *Ntn1* is expressed in both the MGE and the LGE (Hevner, Miyashita-Lin, and Rubenstein 2002). Mutation of the *Ntn1* gene causes disruption of the TC pathway (Braisted et al. 2000). Ntn1 appears to act in concert with a number of other signaling molecules to direct the movement of TC and CT axons to their target locations. Mutation of the genes for the transcription factors Ebf1 and Dlx1/2 have also been shown to disrupt the organization of the TC pathway. These transcription factors are expressed primarily in the VT and to a lesser extent in the thalamus, pointing to the importance of extracortical sources of signaling in the establishment of the major sensory pathways. Furthermore, studies of animals with specific gene mutations suggest that there may be multiple cues emanating from different cortical and extracortical sources that direct axon guidance. For example, the transcription factor Tbr1 is expressed only in the cortex, Gbx2 only in the thalamus, while Pax6 and Emx2 are expressed in both structures. In animals with mutations of any one of these genes, TC and CT pathfinding is disrupted within the VT, suggesting that signaling in this region may contribute importantly to axon guidance (Vanderhaeghen and Polleux 2004).

Recent work examining chemorepulsive effects emanating from the VT also support the multisite model of axon guidance. Ephrins are membrane-bound proteins that act as a chemorepulsive factor in axon guidance. Ephrins exert their chemorepulsive function by acting as ligands that bind to specific receptors, thus transmitting a repulsive signal. *Ephrin-As* is expressed in a high-caudal–low-rostral gradient within the VT. A complementary low-caudal–high-rostral gradient of EphAs receptors is expressed in the dorsal thalamus. These opposed gradients of ligands and receptors serve to direct TC axons to the correct topological locations within the cortex. Specifically, advancing axons from rostral regions of the dorsal thalamus are directed away from caudal regions of the VT (Dufour et al. 2003).

Finally, recent data suggest that TC guidance signals may also come from a class of tangentially migrating cells within the VT, the so-called corridor cells (Lopez-Bendito et al. 2006). Corridor cells have been shown to migrate ventrally from the lateral ganglionic eminence (LGE) along the margin of the medial ganglionic eminence (MGE) in a band that corresponds to the projection pathway of TC axons as they enter the VT. The corridor cells express *Nrg1*, producing two gene products (CRD-Nrg1 and lg-Nrd1) that serve as guidance cues for TC axons, providing a kind of bridge from the prethalamic region to the VT.

Available data on axon guidance for the TC and CT pathways suggest that multiple signaling centers may participate in the establishment of these primary pathways. Cortical cues contribute to signaling but do not appear to provide the exclusive source of guidance. The VT and the dorsal thalamus, and possibly the emerging fiber pathway itself, all provide cues for the projecting axons.

## Exuberance in the Developing Cortex

Two processes that are central to the normal development of the neocortex are the initial widespread overproduction of neural elements, followed by their principled and equally large-scale elimination. This pattern of exuberance and elimination is observed for both neurons, in the form of naturally occurring cell death or apoptosis, and for connections between neurons, in the form of synaptic and axonal exuberance and pruning. The timescales for the two sets of subtractive events are somewhat different. Most naturally occurring cell death happens prenatally and includes loss of both neurons and neural progenitor cells. Synaptic exuberance and pruning also occur prenatally but become most prominent in the postnatal period. Both cell-intrinsic and activity-dependent extrinsic factors have been shown to affect the initiation and progress of both classes of subtractive events (Innocenti and Price 2005). Both cell death and synaptic exuberance and pruning reflect the dynamic and ongoing processes of change and elaboration in cortical networks that shape the emerging organization of the developing neocortex.

## Programmed Cell Death

A critical set of events in early cortical development involves the large-scale death of neurons and neural progenitors. The rate of cell death varies greatly across cortical areas and is estimated to range from 30 to 80 percent across regions (Buss, Sun, and Oppenheim 2006; Oppenheim 1991; Rabinowicz et al. 1996). A number of different functions have been ascribed to the cell-death process, including correction of erroneous connections, elimination of abnormal cells, removal of transient cell populations with time-delimited utility, and, most important, target matching within cortical circuits (Buss, Sun, and Oppenheim 2006). For many years, the focus of investigation in the study of neural cell death was on postmitotic neurons in the period after the initiation of synapse formation. The large-scale loss of cells during this period is attributed to a competition for cell-extrinsic resources. The specific resources in question are the survival-promoting substances, referred to as neurotrophic factors, that are produced by target cells. This account of cell-death modulation is referred to as the Neurotrophic

Theory. Although the competitive loss of cells described by the Neurotrophic Theory has been well documented, more recently it has become clear that programmed cell death is a much more pervasive phenomenon in the developing brain. Large-scale cell death has been documented much earlier in development, among dividing neural progenitor cells. The scale of cell death in the proliferative population of cells is at least as large as that observed among the postmitotic cells, with estimates ranging from 50 to 70 percent (de la Rosa and de Pablo 2000; Yeo and Gautier 2004). Regardless of timing or cell type, the sequence of events in apoptosis is similar for all cells, neural and non-neural. Programmed cell death occurs via a well-defined and well-understood cell-intrinsic process that is controlled by the sequential expression of a specific set of genes. All neurons (and many other cell types) have this intrinsic "suicide" program. The activation of the program is controlled by two sets of receptors acting individually and in combination to either promote or block the apoptotic, or cell-death, cascade.

*Apoptosis*

Apoptosis is the process of cell death associated with programmed cell death. The apoptotic cell-death pathway is distinct from other forms of cell death, such as necrotic cell death, in both the sequence of physiological events that occur and the regulatory signals that control the sequence. The sequences of physiological events in apoptosis and necrosis are summarized in Table 8.1. During apoptosis, there is progressive cleavage of the chromatin (the DNA and associated proteins in the cell nucleus) into smaller and smaller fragments. The integrity of the outer membrane of cells undergoing apoptosis persists until quite late, when characteristic membrane protrusions, or blebs, form. The structural appearance of mitochondria, the small intracellular organelles responsible for energy production and cellular respiration, remains normal and there is no evidence of inflammatory change in the surrounding tissue. Cell volume gradually decreases as apoptosis proceeds. This pattern contrasts with the necrotic process, which is characterized by degradation of the nuclear material, early swelling and rupture of the cell membrane (lysis), abnormal mitochondrial appearance, and evidence of inflammation of surrounding tissue.

Table 8.1  Comparison of processes involved in apoptosis and necrosis

|  | Apoptosis | Necrosis |
|---|---|---|
| Nucleus | Internucleosomal cleavage of DNA <br> • Early stage: > 50 kb fragments <br> • Intermediate stage: 180–200 bp fragments <br> • Late stage: 1–20 bp fragments <br> • Chromatin condensation | Degradation |
| Membrane integrity | Persists until late stage | Lost early |
| Mitochondria | Normal ultrastructural appearance | Swell and take up $CA^{2+}$ |
| Inflammatory changes in surrounding tissue | No | Yes |
| Cell volume | Decreases |  |
| Cell fragmentation | Plasma membrane forms blebs; fragments of cell form characteristic apoptotic bodies | Increases early <br> Lysis occurs |

*Source:* Reprinted with permission from D. J. Price and D. J. Willshaw, *Mechanisms of cortical development* (Oxford: Oxford University Press, © 2000), p. 182.

The apoptotic cascade is signaled by genes that have been designated "proapoptotic." In mammals, two important proapoptotic genes are *Bax* and *Bad*. Expression of these genes initiates a signaling cascade involving a number of molecules, including caspase-9 (Card 9) which, in turn, signals expression of caspase-3 (Card 3) (Kuan et al. 2000). The *Card 3* expression pathway plays a central role in inducing the cell-death cascade in many but not all neuron types. This pathway can be blocked by "antiapoptotic" genes. In mammals the two important antiapoptotic genes, that is, genes that promote cell survival, are *Bcl2* and *Bclx$_L$* (Roth and D'Sa 2001). *Bcl2* is expressed in the nervous system, with highest concentrations in the peripheral motor, sensory, and sympathetic systems. *Bclx$_L$* expression is low in neural progenitors but is rapidly upregulated as new neurons begin to migrate away from the VZ; levels remain high in mature neurons. Bax and Bclx$_L$ interact to control cell death in the developing nervous system. Animals with mutation of $Bclx_L$ show a dramatic increase in cell death. However, downregulation of Bax in animals with the $Bclx_L$ mutation eliminates the increase in cell death (Shacka and Roth 2006).

### Programmed Cell-Death Neurons

The phenomenon of programmed cell death among populations of postmitotic neurons was originally documented in the classic studies of Hamburger (1975). In those studies, Hamburger excised the wing buds (including the presumptive muscle tissue) of chick embryos, thus eliminating the primary target for a population of motor neurons in the chick spinal column. The wing bud was excised on E2, before the formation of motor neurons in the spinal cord was complete. By E5, the populations of motor neurons in the spinal cord were observed to have developed normally; however, by E10, the motor neurons died. In subsequent studies, Hamburger and colleagues demonstrated that the death of cells occurred during the period when the cells would normally have established connections with their target. They speculated that the loss of cells was due to the elimination of some then-unspecified "trophic" resource from the target site. The ablation of the target eliminated the availability of both the type and amount of trophic factors necessary for neuronal survival, resulting in neuronal cell death.

In the late 1950s and early 1960s, the first neurotrophic factor, nerve growth factor (Ngf), was identified by Levi-Montalcini (1964). In a variety of in vitro and in vivo studies, she demonstrated that the survival of certain classes of neurons is critically dependent on the availability of Ngf. Specifically, she showed that modulation of the availability of neurotrophic factors systematically affects neuron survival. Overexpression or injection of neurotrophic factors reduces cell death, while ablation of the target or downregulation of available neurotrophic factors increases cell death (Figure 8.4). This phenomenon of trophic-factor-dependent survival has now been demonstrated in many systems. In addition to their role in cell survival, neurotrophic factors have also been shown to play an essential role in the regulation of neurite growth and guidance, the formation of synaptic structures, neurotransmitter release, synaptic plasticity, and perhaps, paradoxically, cell death (Chao 2003).

Since the original studies of Levi-Montalcini identifying Ngf, a number of different neurotrophins have been identified. The most important of these are brain-derived neurotrophic factor (Bdnf), neurotrophin3 (Ntf3), and neurotrophin5 (Ntf5). Each is effective in different neuronal cell populations. Further, a number of studies have demonstrated that neurotrophins are expressed in an activity-dependent manner (Chao 2003). The effects of activity on levels of neurotrophins were first observed in studies of epilepsy, where significant increases in Bdnf production were found to be associated with epileptic seizure activity (Binder et al. 2001; Gall and Isackson 1989). Subsequent experimental studies have confirmed these findings. For example, a sevenfold increase in levels of Bdnf is observed following a 25-second period of stimulation of hippocampal neurons (Isackson et al. 1991).

The availability of neurotrophic factors is essential for normal brain development. Mouse mutants that lack the genes for a variety

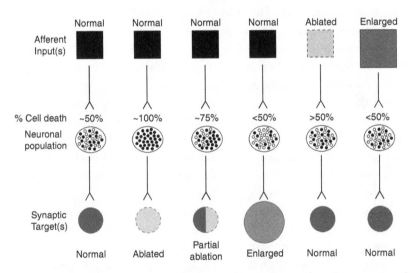

Figure 8.4. Effects of experimentally increasing or decreasing the amount of neurotrophic factor (NTF). NTFs are produced by postsynaptic cells. The amount of NTF produced is modulated by the activity of the cell; NTF production is enhanced by increases in activity. The first four examples illustrate changes in rate of neuronal cell death when the size of the available synaptic target cell population is manipulated. When the target site is ablated, neurons cannot make connections, the source of NTF is eliminated, and the neurons die; when the target site is enlarged, more synaptic space is available, the supply of NTF is increased, and fewer neurons die. Similar effects are observed with alteration of input to a neuron population.

of neurotrophic factors die very soon after birth. Mutants that under-express neurotrophins manifest a number of more subtle, factor-specific deficits. Underexpression of Ngf results in deficits of memory acquisition and retention, while mutants with underexpression of Bdnf are aggressive and hyperphagic (they eat obsessively). Injection of neu-rotrophins into the ventricles of these animals mitigates their deficits. Though subtle effects on behavior are associated with neurotrophin modulation within the neocortex, the impact on neuronal numbers in the cortex is minimal compared with the effects of neurotrophic-factor modulation in peripheral systems. These findings suggest that the reg-ulatory pathways in cortical regions may be more complex, relying on multiple factors or the interaction of factors to regulate cell numbers (Huang and Reichardt 2001; Price and Willshaw 2000).

Neurotrophins are produced and released from neurons in the target-site populations. The released neurotrophins bind receptors on the presynaptic membrane of the axons of cells that send projections to a target site (Huang and Reichardt 2001). The survival of neurons depends critically on their capacity to establish contact with target cells and to obtain the neurotrophic factors produced by the targets. When the neurotrophic factor binds with the receptor, the trophic-factor–receptor complex is internalized into membrane-coated vesi-cles in the recipient cell. The packets of neurotrophic factor are then transported in a retrograde fashion back to the cell body. When the vesicles reach the cell body, they signal the nucleus, inducing in many but not all cases a signaling cascade of survival-promoting gene tran-scription that blocks apoptosis. In the cell, many neurotrophic factors work by activating the P13k pathway, which in turn activates the Akt pathway. Akt acts both to inhibit proapoptotic genes and to directly in-hibit expression of Card9, the cell-death trigger molecule. In addition, neurotrophic factors induce the expression of $Bcl2$ and $Bclx_L$, anti-apoptotic genes.

The activity of neurotrophic factors depends on the action of two types of transmembrane cell receptors. The first is a family of tyrosine kinase receptors, TrkA, TrkB, and TrkC. The second is a receptor called p75$^{NTR}$. The three Trk receptors preferentially interact with different neurotrophic factors. TrkA binds with Ngf, TrkB with Bdnf and Ntf5, and TrkC with Ntf3. The p75$^{NTR}$ receptor binds equally to all four neurotrophic factors. Different classes of neurons require different neurotrophic factors to survive. Ngf/TrkA signaling is found in the sympathetic nervous system, the basal forebrain cholinergic system, and the nociceptor afferents. Bdnf/TrkB signaling is important in the cerebral cortex, the hippocampus, and retinal ganglion cells, and Ntf3/TrkC is found in proprioceptive afferents and the hippocampus.

It was originally thought that there was a clear distinction between the Trks and the p75$^{NTR}$ receptor signaling pathways. Specifically, Trk receptor signaling was thought to promote cell survival, while p75$^{NTR}$ signaling was thought to play a central role in regulation of cell death. More recent work suggests that although the dominant signaling patterns confirm this separation of roles for the two classes of receptors, the story is more complex. The synthesis of neurotrophic factors occurs in stages. The initial products of the synthesis process are progenitor neurotrophic factors, or proNTs, which later cleave to form mature neurotrophic factors. ProNTs have a high affinity for the p75$^{NTR}$ receptors and initiate cell-death programs, while mature neurotrophic factors bind Trk receptors and promote cell survival (Chao 2003). However, the interaction of receptor activity can modulate survival or cell death by both classes of receptors (Chao 2003; Kalb 2005; Nykjaer, Willnow, and Petersen 2005). Specifically, in addition to their independent functioning within the cell-death pathway, p75$^{NTR}$ receptors can act in concert with Trk receptors, serving as co-receptors in cell survival-promoting programs. The role of the p75$^{NTR}$ receptor in these contexts is to modulate Trk responsiveness at different points in development, thus enhancing or reducing the effectiveness of specific neurotrophic factors in different developmental contexts (Nykjaer, Willnow, and Petersen 2005).

The primary role of cell death in postmitotic cell populations is thought to concern the regulation of cell numbers and patterns of connectivity in the developing cortical system. The establishment of functioning neural circuits requires fairly precise matching between projection and target cell populations. Cell death, in conjunction with the second related subtractive process, synapse elimination, provides a mechanism for achieving an optimal balance without the need to pre-specify the billions of connections that make up the mature brain circuitry. However, other functions for the cell-death programs have also been suggested. Cell death could serve as a mechanism for eliminating transient structures that are needed for a short time in embryonic or fetal development but are not a necessary part of the mature system. The subplate of the developing neocortex is an example of such a transient structure. Similarly, cell death may serve to eliminate transient branching of fiber systems. Finally, cell death may serve to eliminate errors that might arise during the complex and dynamic process of neuronal development.

### Programmed Cell Death among Neural Progenitors

Apoptosis in the proliferating neural progenitor population is the earliest known instance of cell death in the developing brain. It is estimated that between 50 and 70 percent of neural progenitors die during proliferation (de la Rosa and de Pablo 2000; Yeo and Gautier 2004). In postmitotic cell populations, cell death is controlled by well-defined apoptotic pathways that are modulated by the availability of neurotrophic factors at connection sites in target cell populations. Cell death in the proliferative cell population occurs before the onset of synaptogenesis. Thus the triggers for apoptosis in the progenitor population are likely to be somewhat different from those in the postmitotic populations, but they are not well understood. In the mouse, the first evidence of progenitor cell death is seen during gastrulation (E6.5) within the anterior neural plate. Programmed cell death is later observed in the hindbrain at E8–9, and in the dorsal VZ and IZ on E12–15 (Yeo and Gautier 2004). Data from human studies indicate a similar profile (Chan et al. 2002; Rakic and Zecevic 2000). The first sign of apoptosis in the human neural tube is evident at GW4.5, but levels of cell death are very low. By GW6–7, the preplate begins to form, and an increase in programmed cell death is detected. By GW11, cell death is evident in all layers of the cortex and in all cortical proliferative zones, including the VZ, the SVZ, and the GEs. The overall rate of cell death in the proliferative zones increases during the peak period of neurogenesis, GW12–15, but remains low in the cortical plate through weeks GW17–21. This pattern is consistent with a predominance of progenitor cell death during periods of differentiation. By late gestation, there is significant apoptosis in the postmitotic neuron populations within all cortical layers, with loss in many areas reaching 70 percent based on estimates from sampling regions of sensorimotor and association areas (Rabinowicz et al. 1996).

As is the case for postmitotic neurons, the apoptotic cascade in neural progenitors is regulated by both antiapoptotic and proapoptotic genes. Further, the same sets of genes appear to play similar roles in both neuronal and progenitor populations; specifically, *Bcl2* and *Bclx*$_L$ serve antiapoptotic roles, *Bax* is the primary proapoptotic gene, and *Card9* provides the cell-death trigger. Regulators of cell death in progenitor populations appear to be the same classes of signaling factors that regulate other aspects of early neuronal development. These include Bmps, Wnts, and Shh, as well as a variety of growth factors. All these molecules have been implicated in either enhancement or inhibition of programmed cell death in progenitor populations (Yeo and Gautier 2004).

Programmed cell death in progenitor populations appears to be initiated as progenitors begin to differentiate and to divide asymmetrically. Apoptosis is increased when differentiation is accelerated and reduced by factors that prevent progenitors from differentiating. The functions of early cell death in progenitor populations are thought to mirror those in postmitotic cell groups. The role of error correction may be more significant among the progenitor populations. The spatial organization of many brain regions emerges from the expression of morphogenic gradients of secreted proteins. For example, the specification of cell types at different dorsal-ventral levels of the spinal column is the product of the graded expression of *Shh* in ventral regions and *Bmps* in dorsal regions. Programmed cell death may serve to eliminate cells that disrupt the patterning of cell types along these gradients. During formation of the cortical plate, progenitors must produce different cell types at different times. Programmed cell death may serve to eliminate progenitors that generate the wrong cell types. Finally, programmed cell death may serve to regulate cell numbers within the proliferative regions (de la Rosa and de Pablo 2000; Yeo and Gautier 2004).

## Exuberant Synapse Formation and Elimination

The development of neural networks requires that precise sets of connections be established between developing neurons and their targets. Within the cerebral cortex, this is an extremely complex process that involves billions of synaptic connections. The production and elimination of connections can be observed both at the level of individual neurons and at the level of neuronal populations (Innocenti and Price

2005). The original studies of synaptic exuberance and pruning took a microscopic view, examining change at the level of individual synapses within the neuromuscular junctions of the peripheral nervous system. The size and structure of the synapses in the neuromuscular junction made it possible to identify the formation and elimination of individual synapses and allowed for clear documentation of synaptic exuberance within the developing nervous system. Microscopic examination of synaptogenesis within the neocortex has been more difficult until recently. The density and complexity of connectivity within the cortex make it difficult to study the process of cortical exuberance at the level of the individual synapse. However, recent real-time imaging studies of axons and growth cones as they move toward their cortical targets suggest that very rapid formation and elimination of synapses may provide a means for cells to sample their local environments. That rapid sampling may serve to guide axons to their final target. Overproduction and elimination have also been observed within cell populations. In many cases, connections must be made over considerable distances, involving the guidance of axons over indirect and circuitous pathways. These pathways create afferent or efferent connections among remote brain regions and can involve both cortico-cortical and cortico-subcortical pathways. Exuberant production and elimination of these long-range pathways are widespread.

### Microscopic Analysis of Synaptogenesis

Ramon y Cajal was the first to note that the density of synaptic connection sites was greater in early development than in adulthood (Hua and Smith 2004). The first and most precise documentation of synaptic exuberance and elimination at the neuronal level came from studies of synaptogenesis at the neuromuscular junction (Sanes and Lichtman 1999). In adult rats, each motor neuron innervates one muscle fiber. However, in newborn rats, multiple motor neurons innervate a single muscle fiber. With development, all but one of these connections are retracted. The retraction of synapses appears to be associated both with the activity of the neuron and with the capacity of the neuron to access trophic factors at the synaptic site. Cells that fail to activate the muscle fiber lose their connection. Overexpression of nerve growth factor at the connection sites results in hyperinnervation, while blockage results in loss of connectivity (Brown, Keynes, and Lumsden 2001).

There is considerable evidence that neurons initially receive widespread input, and that input elimination serves to sharpen neural circuitry. Two models of this dynamic process are possible. A sequential formation-elimination model suggests a two-step process that includes a wave of synaptic exuberance followed by a period of synapse elimination. A concurrent model proposes a continuous process of synapse formation and elimination. Recent studies using real-time imaging methodologies support the concurrent account (Hua and Smith 2004) and suggest that synapse formation and elimination proceeds as an ongoing, rapid, and balanced process. For example, in a study of xenopus (newt) retinal ganglion cells recorded over a two-hour period, 150 percent of the initial complement of connections was generated, and 137 percent was eliminated. The postsynaptic partners of these cells (that is, cells within the target region within the tectum) added 180 percent of their original number of connections and retracted 124 percent (Hua and Smith 2004). These data suggest that the formation of connections within the cortex involves a rapid sampling process in which inappropriate contacts are quickly eliminated without further elaboration, and only functional connections are maintained. Initially, connectivity with a region is sparse and nonselective. Later projections become more target specific, and increased density and complexity are observed in the arbors of the target cells. The molecular mechanisms for these rapidly changing processes are just beginning to be understood.

### Synaptic Exuberance and Pruning in Populations of Neocortical Neurons

Rakic provided some of the first studies that examined widespread overproduction and loss of synapses in primates. His initial studies focused on developmental change in synaptic density within the motor cortex in rhesus monkeys (Zecevic, Bourgeois, and Rakic 1989). In that work, Rakic and colleagues observed that synapses first emerge in the marginal and subplate layers of the cortex on approximately E65 and through all layers of the cortical plate by E89. Rapid synapse production was reported during the last two prenatal months; numbers in all cortical layers increased eightfold during this period. By the second postnatal month, synapse density reached its maximum. The number of synapses in the brain of the two-month-old monkey plateaus at nearly twice that observed in adult animals. A slow decrease in synapse number was observed between two months and three years of age (the age of sexual maturity for the rhesus) and was followed by a period of more rapid decline. Subsequent studies by Rakic and colleagues focused on patterns of synaptic exuberance and pruning in the visual cortex (Bourgeois and Rakic 1993) and in the prefrontal cortex (Bourgeois, Goldman-Rakic, and Rakic 1994). These studies documented very similar patterns of exuberant synapse production and loss over similar timescales within these two regions.

Two studies of synaptogenesis in human brains reported a similar pattern of exuberant increase into early childhood, with maximum numbers of synapses far exceeding those of adults (Huttenlocher and Dabholkar 1997; Huttenlocher and de Courten 1987). That period of exuberance is followed by a gradual reduction in synapse numbers (Figure 8.5). Huttenlocher reported regional differences in the temporal trajectories of this basic pattern of exuberance and pruning. While all areas show the characteristic pattern of rise and fall in synapse density, the timing of peak exuberance differs across areas. Specifically, within sensory areas, peak levels are reached within the first year of life, while in frontal regions the peak is not attained until the late preschool period. The much more protracted term of human development may account for the ability to detect regional differences in the timing of synaptogenesis.

*Factors That Influence Synaptic Formation and Elimination*
The construction of neural circuits in the CNS is a dynamic process that involves the formation and elimination of synapses. There is considerable evidence that cells initially receive widespread input, and that input elimination serves to sharpen neural circuitry. Both activity-dependent and activity-independent factors appear to contribute to synapse formation.

Synapse formation can occur in the absence of neural firing. Evidence for this comes from mice with a mutation of a gene *(Munc18-1)* that prevents synaptic vesicles from fusing with the presynaptic membrane and releasing neurotransmitters. The failure of vesicle fusion eliminates synaptic transmission in these animals, yet they form synapses that are normal in appearance (Cohen-Cory 2002). In addition, the formation of postsynaptic receptors can occur when receptor activity is blocked. These two findings suggest that the formation of synapses can proceed in the absence of synaptic activity. One factor that has been shown to promote synapse formation is the neurotrophic factor Bdnf. Infusion of Bdnf increases both the number of synapses and axonal branching, while blocking Bdnf activity decreases synapse and branch numbers. It is thought that Bdnf modulates synapse formation by regulating the synthesis of synaptic proteins that are involved in vesicle fusion, thus modulating neurotransmitter release (Alsina, Vu, and Cohen-Cory 2001). Furthermore, there is evidence that synapse formation itself induces elaboration of the axonal arbors, and that synapse elimination is associated with pruning of axonal arbors. Real-time imaging studies of synapse and axonal branch formation demonstrate that a disproportionately large number of synapses are located at axon branch points. The formation of the synapses precedes and may precipitate axonal branching, and the elimination of synapses precedes and may precipitate branch pruning (Alsina, Vu, and Cohen-Cory 2001).

Although data on activity-independent effects on synapse formation are limited, activity-dependent effects on synapse formation and

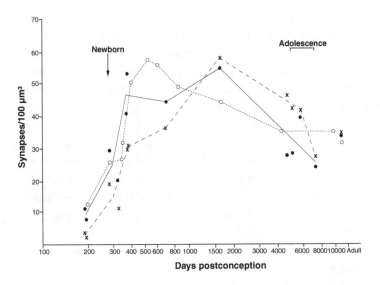

Figure 8.5. Patterns of synaptic exuberance and pruning in humans for three brain areas: visual cortex (open circles), auditory cortex (filled circles), and prefrontal cortex (x's). (From Huttenlocher and Dabholkar 1997. Adapted with the permission of John Wiley & Sons.)

elimination are better understood; indeed, a full discussion of this topic is beyond the scope of this book. The current discussion will focus on one important class of activity-dependent synaptic change, that associated with Hebbian learning. It has been suggested that one class of postsynaptic ionotropic glutamate receptors, NMDA receptors, may provide the neural basis for Hebbian learning (Berardi et al. 2003; Hua and Smith 2004). The response characteristics of the NMDA receptor optimize implementation of the Hebbian learning principle that connections between neurons that are simultaneously active are strengthened (i.e., cells that "fire together wire together"). In a typical (non-Hebbian) synaptic transmission, an action potential in the presynaptic cell induces the release of a neurotransmitter into the synaptic cleft. The neurotransmitter crosses the cleft and binds with a receptor on the postsynaptic membrane. The signal is thus transferred, and the postsynaptic neuron fires. Importantly, in this type of connection, the firing of the pre- and postsynaptic cells is temporally offset; firing of the postsynaptic neuron follows the firing of the presynaptic neuron. NMDA receptor activity differs in a critical way that serves to synchronize the timing of pre- and postsynaptic cell firing. Specifically, when the postsynaptic cell is polarized (i.e., when it is not firing), its NMDA receptor is blocked by magnesium ions. Thus under most conditions, the neurotransmitter produced by the presynaptic cell cannot bind to the NMDA receptor on the postsynaptic cell membrane and transmit a signal. However, when the postsynaptic cell is at or near depolarization (i.e., ready to fire), the magnesium ions on the NMDA receptor are displaced, allowing the neurotransmitter to bind to the NMDA receptor. The co-occurrence of neurotransmitter release, which is brought about by the activity of the presynaptic cell, and depolarization of the postsynaptic cell allows for concurrent firing of the pre- and postsynaptic cells. Thus NMDA receptor activity requires simultaneous activation of the pre- and postsynaptic cells, and that is the prerequisite for Hebbian learning. NMDA receptors bind the neurotransmitter glutamate, the most abundant excitatory neurotransmitter in the brain. They have been widely implicated in learning and memory. They are also important during development.

As suggested earlier, neurotrophins play an important role in synapse formation and elimination. The availability of neurotrophins is regulated by activity-dependent mechanisms. Specifically, there is substantial evidence that electrical activity modulates neurotrophin expression and release. Bdnf, in particular, plays an essential role in establishing connectivity by modulating branching and regulating neurotransmitter release and synapse formation. Bdnf has also been shown to play a role in regulating the elimination of synapses. Synapses that would normally be eliminated following NMDA receptor blockade can be rescued by local injection of Bdnf (Hu, Nikolakopoulou, and Cohen-Cory 2005). Bdnf has also been shown to affect the development of the inhibitory GABA-mediated system. Mice that overexpress Bdnf show initial acceleration in development of the inhibitory GABAergic system, and that is followed by accelerated stabilization of the activity-dependent connectivity within the visual system (Berardi et al. 2003). This modulation is particularly important because of recent evidence that the development of the inhibitory system plays a central role in activity-dependent modulation of neural circuitry (Hensch and Fagiolini 2005).

## Clinical Correlation: Pathological Induction of Apoptosis in the Prenatal Period

As discussed earlier, apoptosis, or programmed cell death, is a widely occurring neural event that extends over a protracted period during prenatal development. It serves a number of important functions in the developing brain, from the elimination of transient neural elements or structures to error correction and population matching. The mechanism of apoptosis is a ubiquitous and well-described cell-intrinsic signaling cascade involving specific genes that initiate and promote the cell-death cascade. Given the prevalence of cell death in early neural development, it is not surprising that a wide variety of factors have been shown to affect the cell-death program within the developing nervous system. The diversity of these factors and potential pathogenic pathways are illustrated by two types of early neural insult: early postnatal concussive head trauma and late prenatal exposure to alcohol (ethanol). Each of these events is complex in its pathology and has multiple effects on the developing nervous system. But for each, one part of the pathological profile is the abnormal acceleration of programmed cell death.

## Animal Studies of Concussive Head Trauma

Studies of concussive head trauma in neonatal rats suggest that this period may be one of unusual vulnerability to factors that trigger pathological apoptotic events (Pohl et al. 1999). In these studies, rat pups ranging in age from 3 to 30 days were experimentally injured in a localized region over the parietal lobe. Neural response to the traumatic injury occurred in two phases. In the initial, acute phase, there was immediate evidence of excitotoxic effects in the vicinity of the injury that were associated with cell damage and necrotic cell death. Necrotic cell death was observed within 30 minutes of injury and increased over a period of hours, reaching its maximum at approximately 4 hours after the injury. In young animals, a second phase of response occurred later in widespread and distal regions of the brain, and importantly, the cellular response was that of apoptotic rather than necrotic cell death. Evidence for apoptosis was first observed after 6 hours and increased progressively, reaching its maximum at about 24 hours after trauma. The effects were observed bilaterally but were more pronounced on the ipsilesional side, that is, the same side of the brain as the concussive trauma. Areas of distal apoptosis associated with the parietal lesions included the retrosplenial cortex (in the most posterior regions of the cortex), the frontal cortex, nonlesioned regions of the parietal cortex, and the dorsal thalamus, and involved the loss of 25–33 percent of neurons within a region, nearly 100 times greater than the level of cell loss observed at the site of the lesion (Olney et al. 2000, 2002). However, the developmental time window for the apoptotic cell loss in the more distal regions of the brain was very limited. Apoptosis was most pronounced among rat pups injured between 3 and 7 days, but had declined substantially in pups injured at 14 days and was not observed in pups injured at 30 days. Thus the secondary loss of neurons through apoptotic cell death was confined to a very specific period of development that corresponded to the period of maximal synaptogenesis. The authors suggest that head trauma may either activate the apoptotic mechanism or interfere with a mechanism that normally suppresses it (Pohl et al. 1999). Recent work has shown that neonatal head trauma results in the downregulation of the antiapoptotic genes $Bcl2$ and $Bclx_L$. It has been suggested that the suppression of activity brought about by the injury may lead to a decrease in the production of neurotrophic-initiated survival signals, which leads to the decrease in transcription of the antiapoptotic survival genes (Felderhoff-Mueser et al. 2002).

## Effects of Ethanol Exposure on Patterns
## of Neonatal Apoptotic Cell Death

More than 30 years ago, the effects of intrauterine exposure to ethanol, brought about by maternal ingestion of alcohol, were described and termed Fetal Alcohol Syndrome (FAS) (Jones and Smith 1973). The effects of FAS vary with degree and timing of alcohol exposure, but in serious cases problems include retarded physical growth, facial abnormalities, poor coordination, hyperactivity, learning disabilities, mental retardation, and reduction in brain size. The effects of alcohol exposure on the developing fetus are complex and are just beginning to be understood. One factor that may contribute to the poor neurocognitive outcomes observed in at least some subgroups of children with FAS is the effect of ethanol exposure on apoptosis in the late prenatal period.

Interestingly, the findings about FAS and apoptosis are related to a finding from the neonatal head trauma study. Specifically, in addition to documenting the differential effect of head trauma on the degree of pathological apoptosis in neonates, Pohl and colleagues (Pohl et al. 1999) also examined the effects of a particular pharmacological intervention. It has been shown that the degree of excitotoxic cell death following head trauma can be ameliorated in adults by the administration of an antagonist that blocks NMDA receptor activity, thus blocking the activity of the injured cells. In 3- and 7-day-old rat pups, the administration of the NMDA antagonist also reduces necrotic cell death at the site of the injury, but it has the additional effect of greatly increasing apoptotic cell death in remote regions of the brain (Ikonomidou et al. 1999; Pohl et al. 1999). The reduction in activity associated with blocking NMDA receptors has the effect of increasing the rate of apoptotic cell death within a critical neurodevelopmental window. Thus the intervention, which has an ameliorative effect in adult populations, produces far more extensive cell death in neonates.

There is evidence that ethanol acts as an NMDA antagonist, and thus, similar to the effects of NMDA antagonist administration in the study of head trauma, one avenue for ethanol's adverse effects on the developing brain could be through a mechanism that promotes pathological apoptotic cell death (Olney et al. 2000, 2002). When 7-day-old neonatal rats were administered ethanol, marked increases in apoptotic cell death were observed throughout widely dispersed regions of the brain (Figure 8.6; Olney et al. 2000). These findings are consistent with reports of reduced brain size in children with severe FAS. The degree of cell death was related to the concentration and duration of exposure to ethanol (200 mg/dl for more than four hours). Although the most pronounced effects of ethanol exposure on apoptotic neuronal cell death are in the early postnatal period for rats, an equivalent potential window of vulnerability for humans for these specific neural effects is the third trimester of pregnancy. This is a period of rapidly accelerating synaptogenesis in the human brain. It is notable that other observed effects of ethanol, for example, craniofacial abnormalities, cannot be attributable to factors occurring that late in development. Thus alcohol consumption appears to have different effects on different physical systems, each operating on a separate developmental timetable.

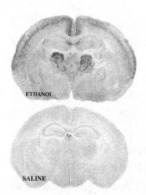

Figure 8.6. Dark staining in the upper figure indicates widespread apoptotic cell death associated with neonatal administration of ethanol. The lower figure shows dramatically lower levels of cell death in control animals administered saline. (From Olney et al. 2000. Reprinted with the permission of Springer.)

## Chapter Summary

- The surface of the mature neocortex is relatively uniform in its macroscopic appearance. However, it is composed of structurally and functionally distinct areas. Brodmann's (1909) map of the cytoarchitectonic areas of the human brain included 47 areas distinguishable from each other by cell type and patterns of connectivity.
- The protomap view of neocortical arealization argues that neural progenitor cells of the VZ provide molecular signals that specify for their neural progeny both their position in the cortex and their associated function. The protocortex view argues that the initial organization of the cortex is comparatively undifferentiated and that areal specification derives from activity within the developing neural system.
- Apoptotic cell death is a widespread phenomenon within the developing central nervous system. It serves to correct errors in connectivity, eliminate abnormal cells, and facilitate target matching within cortical circuits. The apoptotic cascade is signaled by genes that have been designated "proapoptotic." In mammals, critical proapoptotic genes are *Bax* and *Bad*. Expression of these genes initiates *Card3* expression, which plays a central role in inducing cell death. This pathway can be blocked by "antiapoptotic" genes. In mammals, the critical antiapoptotic genes, that is, genes that promote cell survival, are *Bcl2* and *Bclx*$_L$.
- The relationship between nerve growth factor and programmed cell death was first documented in the 1950s and 1960s in studies that demonstrated that overexpression of neurotrophic factors reduces cell death, while ablation of the target or downregulation of available neurotrophic factors increases cell death. The most important CNS neurotrophic factors are Ngf, Bdnf, Ntf3, and Ntf5. Each is effective in different neuronal cell populations, and each is expressed in an activity-dependent manner.
- The activity of neurotrophic factors depends on the action of two types of transmembrane cell receptors, tyrosine kinase receptors (TrkA, TrkB, and TrkC) and the receptor p75[NTR]. The three Trk receptors preferentially interact with different neurotrophic factors, while the p75[NTR] receptor binds equally with all four neurotrophic

factors. The primary role of neurotrophin/Trk receptor complexes is to promote cell survival, while the neurotrophin/p75$^{NTR}$ complexes play a central role in regulation of cell death.

- Apoptotic cell death is prominent in the dividing of the neural progenitor population, where it is estimated at 50 to 70 percent. Unlike the well-defined profiles of postmitotic cell death in the developing cortical plate, the triggers for apoptosis in the proliferating progenitor population are not well understood.

- The process of synaptogensis involves the exuberant production of many more connections than will be necessary for mature patterns of connectivity. Many of these early exuberant connections are subsequently eliminated.

- Synaptogenesis has been examined both at the level of the individual synapse and at the level of neuronal populations. Studies of individual synapse formation and elimination at the neuromuscular junction allowed for clear documentation of synaptic exuberance within the developing nervous system. Real-time imaging studies of axons and growth cones within the developing cortex show that rapid sampling of the local environment may serve to guide axons to their final target.

- Overproduction and elimination have also been observed within neuronal populations. Throughout the mammalian neocortex, synapses are produced exuberantly, reaching 200 percent of adult levels in the early postnatal period. Gradual elimination of these exuberant connections has been observed in all areas of the cortex studied.

## References

Alsina, B., T. Vu, and S. Cohen-Cory. 2001. "Visualizing synapse formation in arborizing optic axons in vivo: Dynamics and modulation by BDNF." *Nature Neuroscience,* 4: 1093–1101.

Auladell, C., P. Perez-Sust, H. Super, and E. Soriano. 2000. "The early development of thalamocortical and corticothalamic projections in the mouse." *Anatomy and Embryology,* 201: 169–179.

Berardi, N., T. Pizzorusso, G. M. Ratto, and L. Maffei. 2003. "Molecular basis of plasticity in the visual cortex." *Trends in Neurosciences,* 26: 369–378.

Binder, D. K., S. D. Croll, C. M. Gall, and H. E. Scharfman. 2001. "BDNF and epilepsy: Too much of a good thing?" *Trends in Neurosciences*, 24: 47–53.

Bishop, K. M., S. Garel, Y. Nakagawa, J. L. Rubenstein, and D. D. O'Leary. 2003. "*Emx1* and *Emx2* cooperate to regulate cortical size, lamination, neuronal differentiation, development of cortical efferents, and thalamocortical pathfinding." *Journal of Comparative Neurology*, 457: 345–360.

Bishop, K. M., G. Goudreau, and D. D. O'Leary. 2000. "Regulation of area identity in the mammalian neocortex by *Emx2* and *Pax6*." *Science*, 288: 344–349.

Bishop, K. M., J. L. Rubenstein, and D. D. O'Leary. 2002. "Distinct actions of *Emx1*, *Emx2*, and *Pax6* in regulating the specification of areas in the developing neocortex." *Journal of Neuroscience*, 22: 7627–7638.

Bourgeois, J. P., P. S. Goldman-Rakic, and P. Rakic. 1994. "Synaptogenesis in the prefrontal cortex of rhesus monkeys." *Cerebral Cortex*, 4: 78–96.

Bourgeois, J. P., and P. Rakic. 1993. "Changes of synaptic density in the primary visual cortex of the macaque monkey from fetal to adult stage." *Journal of Neuroscience*, 13: 2801–2820.

Braisted, J. E., S. M. Catalano, R. Stimac, T. E. Kennedy, M. Tessier-Lavigne, C. J. Shatz, and D. D. O'Leary. 2000. "Netrin-1 promotes thalamic axon growth and is required for proper development of the thalamocortical projection." *Journal of Neuroscience*, 20: 5792–5801.

Brodmann, K. 1909. *Vergleichende Lokalisationslehre der Grosshirnrinde in ihren Prinzipien dargestellt auf Grund des Zellenbaues*. Leipzig: J. A. Barth.

Brown, M., R. Keynes, and A. Lumsden. 2001. *The developing brain*. Oxford: Oxford University Press.

Buss, R. R., W. Sun, and R. W. Oppenheim. 2006. "Adaptive roles of programmed cell death during nervous system development." *Annual Review of Neuroscience*, 29: 1–35.

Catalano, S. M., and C. J. Shatz. 1998. "Activity-dependent cortical target selection by thalamic axons." *Science*, 281: 559–562.

Chambers, D., and G. Fishell. 2006. "Functional genomics of early cortex patterning." *Genome Biology*, 7: 202.

Chan, W. Y., D. E. Lorke, S. C. Tiu, and D. T. Yew. 2002. "Proliferation and apoptosis in the developing human neocortex." *Anatomical Record*, 267: 261–276.

Chao, M. V. 2003. "Neurotrophins and their receptors: A convergence point for many signalling pathways." *Nature Reviews Neuroscience*, 4: 299–309.

Cohen-Cory, S. 2002. "The developing synapse: Construction and modulation of synaptic structures and circuits." *Science*, 298: 770–776.

Cowan, W. M., J. W. Fawcett, D. D. O'Leary, and B. B. Stanfield. 1984. "Regressive events in neurogenesis." *Science*, 225: 1258–1265.

de la Rosa, E. J., and F. de Pablo. 2000. "Cell death in early neural development: Beyond the neurotrophic theory." *Trends in Neurosciences*, 23: 454–458.

Dufour, A., J. Seibt, L. Passante, V. Depaepe, T. Ciossek, J. Frisen, K. Kullander, J. G. Flanagan, F. Polleux, and P. Vanderhaeghen. 2003. "Area specificity and topography of thalamocortical projections are controlled by ephrin/Eph genes." *Neuron*, 39: 453–465.

Felderhoff-Mueser, U., M. Sifringer, S. Pesditschek, H. Kuckuck, A. Moysich, P. Bittigau, and C. Ikonomidou. 2002. "Pathways leading to apoptotic neurodegeneration following trauma to the developing rat brain." *Neurobiology of Disease*, 11: 231–245.

Frappe, I., M. Roger, and A. Gaillard. 1999. "Transplants of fetal frontal cortex grafted into the occipital cortex of newborn rats receive a substantial thalamic input from nuclei normally projecting to the frontal cortex." *Neuroscience*, 89: 409–421.

Gall, C. M., and P. J. Isackson. 1989. "Limbic seizures increase neuronal production of messenger RNA for nerve growth factor." *Science*, 245: 758–761.

Grove, E. A., and T. Fukuchi-Shimogori. 2003. "Generating the cerebral cortical area map." *Annual Review of Neuroscience*, 26: 355–380.

Hamasaki, T., A. Leingartner, T. Ringstedt, and D. D. O'Leary. 2004. "EMX2 regulates sizes and positioning of the primary sensory and motor areas in neocortex by direct specification of cortical progenitors." *Neuron*, 43: 359–372.

Hamburger, V. 1975. "Cell death in the development of the lateral motor column of the chick embryo." *Journal of Comparative Neurology*, 160: 535–546.

Hensch, T. K., and M. Fagiolini. 2005. "Excitatory-inhibitory balance and critical period plasticity in developing visual cortex." *Progress in Brain Research*, 147: 115–124.

Hevner, R. F., E. Miyashita-Lin, and J. L. Rubenstein. 2002. "Cortical and thalamic axon pathfinding defects in *Tbr1*, *Gbx2*, and *Pax6* mutant mice: Evidence that cortical and thalamic axons interact and guide each other." *Journal of Comparative Neurology*, 447: 8–17.

Hu, B., A. M. Nikolakopoulou, and S. Cohen-Cory. 2005. "BDNF stabilizes synapses and maintains the structural complexity of optic axons in vivo." *Development*, 132: 4285–4298.

Hua, J. Y., and S. J. Smith. 2004. "Neural activity and the dynamics of central nervous system development." *Nature Neuroscience*, 7: 327–332.

Huang, E. J., and L. F. Reichardt. 2001. "Neurotrophins: Roles in neuronal development and function." *Annual Review of Neuroscience,* 24: 677–736.

Huttenlocher, P. R., and A. S. Dabholkar. 1997. "Regional differences in synaptogenesis in human cerebral cortex." *Journal of Comparative Neurology,* 387: 167–178.

Huttenlocher, P. R., and C. de Courten. 1987. "The development of synapses in striate cortex of man." *Human Neurobiology,* 6: 1–9.

Ikonomidou, C., F. Bosch, M. Miksa, P. Bittigau, J. Vockler, K. Dikranian, T. I. Tenkova, V. Stefovska, L. Turski, and J. W. Olney. 1999. "Blockade of NMDA receptors and apoptotic neurodegeneration in the developing brain." *Science,* 283: 70–74.

Innocenti, G. M., and D. J. Price. 2005. "Exuberance in the development of cortical networks." *Nature Reviews Neuroscience,* 6: 955–965.

Isackson, P. J., M. M. Huntsman, K. D. Murray, and C. M. Gall. 1991. "BDNF mRNA expression is increased in adult rat forebrain after limbic seizures: Temporal patterns of induction distinct from NGF." *Neuron,* 6: 937–948.

Jones, K. L., and D. W. Smith. 1973. "Recognition of the fetal alcohol syndrome in early infancy." *Lancet,* 2: 999–1001.

Kalb, R. 2005. "The protean actions of neurotrophins and their receptors on the life and death of neurons." *Trends in Neurosciences,* 28: 5–11.

Kostovic, I., and N. Jovanov-Milosevic. 2006. "The development of cerebral connections during the first 20–45 weeks' gestation." *Seminars in Fetal and Neonatal Medicine,* 11: 415–422.

Kuan, C. Y., K. A. Roth, R. A. Flavell, and P. Rakic. 2000. "Mechanisms of programmed cell death in the developing brain." *Trends in Neurosciences,* 23: 291–297.

Levi-Montalcini, R. 1964. "Growth control of nerve cells by a protein factor and its antiserum: Discovery of this factor may provide new leads to understanding of some neurogenetic processes." *Science,* 143: 105–110.

Lopez-Bendito, G., A. Cautinat, J. A. Sanchez, F. Bielle, N. Flames, A. N. Garratt, D. A. Talmage, L. W. Role, P. Charnay, O. Marin, and S. Garel. 2006. "Tangential neuronal migration controls axon guidance: A role for neuregulin-1 in thalamocortical axon navigation." *Cell,* 125: 127–142.

Lopez-Bendito, G., and Z. Molnar. 2003. "Thalamocortical development: How are we going to get there?" *Nature Reviews Neuroscience,* 4: 276–289.

Miller, B., L. Chou, and B. L. Finlay. 1993. "The early development of thalamocortical and corticothalamic projections." *Journal of Comparative Neurology,* 335: 16–41.

Molnar, Z., and C. Blakemore. 1995. "How do thalamic axons find their way to the cortex?" *Trends in Neurosciences,* 18: 389–397.

Nykjaer, A., T. E. Willnow, and C. M. Petersen. 2005. "P75NTR—Live or let die." *Current Opinion in Neurobiology*, 15: 49–57.

O'Leary, D. D., and D. Borngasser. 2006. "Cortical ventricular zone progenitors and their progeny maintain spatial relationships and radial patterning during preplate development indicating an early protomap." *Cerebral Cortex*, 16 (Suppl. 1): i46–i56.

O'Leary, D. D., and Y. Nakagawa. 2002. "Patterning centers, regulatory genes and extrinsic mechanisms controlling arealization of the neocortex." *Current Opinion in Neurobiology*, 12: 14–25.

O'Leary, D. D., B. L. Schlaggar, and R. Tuttle. 1994. "Specification of neocortical areas and thalamocortical connections." *Annual Review of Neuroscience*, 17: 419–439.

Olney, J. W., M. J. Ishimaru, P. Bittigau, and C. Ikonomidou. 2000. "Ethanol-induced apoptotic neurodegeneration in the developing brain." *Apoptosis*, 5: 515–521.

Olney, J. W., D. F. Wozniak, V. Jevtovic-Todorovic, N. B. Farber, P. Bittigau, and C. Ikonomidou. 2002. "Drug-induced apoptotic neurodegeneration in the developing brain." *Brain Pathology*, 12: 488–498.

Oppenheim, R. W. 1991. "Cell death during development of the nervous system." *Annual Review of Neuroscience*, 14, 453–501.

———. 1999. "Programmed cell death." In *Fundamental neuroscience*, ed. M. J. Zigmond, F. E. Bloom, S. C. Landis, J. L. Roberts, and L. R. Squire, 581–609. San Diego, CA: Academic Press.

Pohl, D., P. Bittigau, M. J. Ishimaru, D. Stadthaus, C. Hubner, J. W. Olney, L. Turski, and C. Ikonomidou. 1999. "N-Methyl-D-aspartate antagonists and apoptotic cell death triggered by head trauma in developing rat brain." *Proceedings of the National Academy of Sciences of the United States of America*, 96: 2508–2513.

Price, D. J., and D. J. Willshaw. 2000. *Mechanisms of cortical development*. Oxford: Oxford University Press.

Rabinowicz, T., G. M. de Courten-Myers, J. M. Petetot, G. Xi, and E. de los Reyes. 1996. "Human cortex development: Estimates of neuronal numbers indicate major loss late during gestation." *Journal of Neuropathology and Experimental Neurology*, 55: 320–328.

Rakic, P. 1988. "Specification of cerebral cortical areas." *Science*, 241: 170–176.

———. 2001. "Neurobiology: Neurocreationism—making new cortical maps." *Science*, 294: 1011–1012.

Rakic, S., and N. Zecevic. 2000. "Programmed cell death in the developing human telencephalon." *European Journal of Neuroscience*, 12: 2721–2734.

Roth, K. A., and C. D'Sa. 2001. "Apoptosis and brain development." *Mental Retardation and Developmental Disabilities Research Reviews*, 7: 261–266.

Sanes, J. R., and J. W. Lichtman. 1999. "Development of the vertebrate neuromuscular junction." *Annual Review of Neuroscience,* 22: 389–442.

Shacka, J. J., and K. A. Roth. 2006. "Bcl-2 family and the central nervous system: From rheostat to real complex." *Cell Death and Differentiation,* 13: 1299–1304.

Sur, M., and J. L. Rubenstein. 2005. "Patterning and plasticity of the cerebral cortex." *Science,* 310: 805–810.

Vanderhaeghen, P., and F. Polleux. 2004. "Developmental mechanisms patterning thalamocortical projections: Intrinsic, extrinsic and in between." *Trends in Neurosciences,* 27: 384–391.

von Economo, C., and G. N. Kostinas. 1925. *Die Cytoarchitektonik der Hirnrinde des erwachsenen Menschen.* Vienna: Springer.

Yeo, W., and J. Gautier. 2004. "Early neural cell death: Dying to become neurons." *Developmental Biology,* 274: 233–244.

Zecevic, N., J. P. Bourgeois, and P. Rakic. 1989. "Changes in synaptic density in motor cortex of rhesus monkey during fetal and postnatal life." *Brain Research. Developmental Brain Research,* 50: 11–32.

Zhou, C., Y. Qiu, F. A. Pereira, M. C. Crair, S. Y. Tsai, and M. J. Tsai. 1999. "The nuclear orphan receptor COUP-TFI is required for differentiation of subplate neurons and guidance of thalamocortical axons." *Neuron,* 24: 847–859.

# NINE

# Late Prenatal and Postnatal
# Changes in Human Brain Structure

THE DYNAMIC CHANGES in brain organization that occur at the microscopic level of neurons and their connections reflect both intrinsic signaling and the response of the developing nervous system to extrinsic cues. As will be discussed in greater detail in Chapter 10, during the postnatal period, experience plays a more and more prominent role in shaping and directing the emerging patterns of neural connectivity. The macroscopic changes in cortical morphology that accompany these developments are significant and reflect the complex interplay of cortical elaboration and sculpting that converge to give rise to the mature central nervous system (CNS). This chapter will provide an overview of changes in cortical morphology in the late prenatal and postnatal periods at both a macroscopic and a microscopic level. It will begin with a discussion of the process of gyrification, that is, the macroscopic transformations that take place in the cerebral mantle during the initial period of rapid cortical expansion. Gyri and sulci emerge in an orderly sequence during the second half of gestation, beginning with the primary sulci and followed by the secondary sulci and finally the tertiary sulci. Gyral patterning reflects both species-specific regularities and individual variation. There have been a number of attempts to model the processes that underlie gyrification, and these will be discussed.

Another critical event that begins in the prenatal period is the myelination of axonal processes. In the cerebral cortex, the oligodendrocytes, a subclass of glial cells, form the myelin sheaths that envelop cortical axons, providing insulation and regulating the propagation of electrical signals. Myelination is a protracted process that, in some brain regions, extends well into adolescence. Myelin is composed of lipoproteins and thus has a white appearance that contrasts with the gray of neuronal assemblies. The segregation of gray and white matter into well-defined bands and pathways provides landmarks for defining and identifying structures in the mature brain. The changing patterns and relative densities of gray and white matter within different regions of the brain also provide a means of quantifying structural changes in the brain across development. Measures of overall regional volume, as well as separate measures gray and white matter volumes within and across regions, have proved to be useful tools for calibrating developmental change in the neural system from the early postnatal period through adolescence. Patterns of regional change in the macroscopic organization of the cortex during the periods of childhood and early adolescence will be reviewed.

## Gyrification

Until approximately GW18, the surface of the developing human brain is smooth, or lissencephalic, in appearance. By the middle of GW22, the first convolutions are clearly evident on the cortical surface, and by postnatal week 14 (PW4), the patterns of gyral and sulcal folding have reached near-adult levels (Armstrong et al. 1995; Chi, Dooling, and Gilles 1977; Garel et al. 2001). The degree of cortical folding has been quantified using a measure referred to as the gyrification index (GI) (Zilles et al. 1988). The GI is the ratio of the total length of the cortical surface contour to the length of an outer, superficially imposed, contour (both measured in two-dimensional brain sections; Figure 9.1A). A score of 1.0 on the GI indicates correspondence between the cortical and outer surfaces and thus a smooth brain. Higher values represent the expanded cortical surface area that is folded into the gyral and sulcal convolutions of the cortex. The average adult GI ratio is 2.57.

A study by Armstrong and colleagues (1995) examined developmental change in cortical folding using the GI. They computed the GI on a sample of 32 brains ranging in age from GW11 to 6 years postnatal plus an adult sample. They reported a rapid increase in the GI ratio during the last half of gestation, an overshoot of the mean adult values in the late preschool period, and a gradual return to adult levels during the school years. These findings reflect the very rapid growth of the cortical surface during the last half of gestation and the associated emergence of the typical gyrencephalic appearance of the mature human brain.

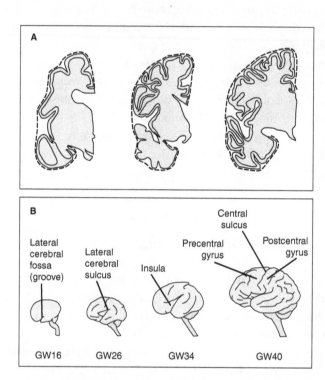

Figure 9.1. A. The gyrification index (GI) is the ratio of the difference between the total length of the cortical surface contour and the length of an outer, or superficially imposed, contour. A score of 1.0 on the GI indicates correspondence between the cortical and outer surfaces and thus a smooth brain. Higher values represent the expanded cortical surface and thus a difference between the cortical and outer surfaces. B. The progression of gyral and sulcal folding follows a regular pattern: primary, secondary, tertiary. At GW16 the brain is smooth. Primary sulci and rudimentary secondary sulci emerge at GW26. Secondary sulci are well defined by GW 34. At birth, tertiary sulci have begun to emerge. The labels provide basic landmarks within the developing brain. (A from Armstrong et al. 1995. Adapted with the permission of Oxford University Press. B from Larsen 2001. Adapted with the permission of Elsevier.)

## The Developmental Progression of Gyral Formation

The progression of gyral and sulcal folding follows a uniform trajectory, particularly in the early phases of gyrification (Figure 9.1B). The primary sulci first emerge as regularly positioned grooves or indentations on the surface of the brain. With development, the indentations become deeper, and a network of side branches begins to form. These side branches are considered the secondary sulci. These, in turn, form branches that are referred to as the tertiary sulci (Garel et al. 2001). The formation of the primary sulci and most of the secondary sulci is complete by GW34. The formation of the tertiary sulci continues until well into the postnatal period. The patterns of human gyral and sulcal formation have been well documented. Early findings were based on studies that examined fixed human tissue samples (Armstrong et al. 1995; Chi, Dooling, and Gilles 1977; Dorovini-Zis and Dolman 1977), while more recent studies have used prenatal magnetic resonance imaging (MRI) analyses (Abe et al. 2003; Garel et al. 2001, 2003). Although there is some variability in the precise estimates of when individual gyri and sulci emerge, overall, the data from the different studies provide a consistent picture of gyral and sulcal development.

The earliest fissure to develop is the interhemispheric or longitudinal fissure, which separates the two cerebral hemispheres along the anterior to posterior axis. Some studies report that it begins to emerge as early as GW8 (Chi, Dooling, and Gilles 1977) and is clearly defined by GW22 (Garel et al. 2001). The interhemispheric fissure first appears in rostral regions and proceeds to develop caudally. Other primary sulci begin to emerge between GW22 and GW25 (Chi, Dooling, and Gilles 1977; Garel et al. 2001). A representative series of images taken from an MRI study illustrating the progression of gyrification in frontal and temporal brain regions is shown in Figure 9.2 (Abe et al. 2003). Image A shows the smooth surface of the developing fetal brain at GW19. At this point, only an early hint of the emerging Sylvian fissure is evident. However, as seen in image B, by GW26, the Sylvian fissure clearly separates the frontal and temporal lobes. By GW28, shallow indentations mark the emergence of the inferior frontal sulcus and the superior temporal sulcus (image C). By GW30, the frontal lobe begins to divide into three subregions demarcated by the shallow indentations of the prospective superior and inferior frontal sulci (image D). These become well defined by GW32 (image E). By GW34, the primary division of the temporal lobe into the superior, middle, and inferior gyri is marked by the emergence of the superior and inferior temporal sulci (image F). Within frontal regions, secondary sulci are clearly apparent by GW36 (image G), and by GW39 the elaboration of secondary and tertiary gyri is evident throughout the developing brain (image H).

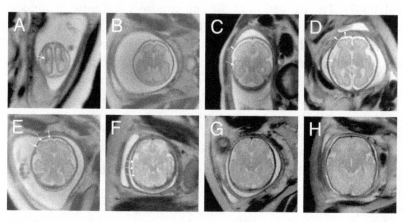

Figure 9.2. A representative series of images taken from an MRI study illustrating the progression of gyrification in frontal and temporal brain regions. In these axial images, anterior brain regions are at the top, and posterior at the bottom. A. At 19 weeks postconception, the developing fetal brain is smooth. B. By 26 weeks, the Sylvian fissure separates the frontal and temporal lobes. C. By 28 weeks, shallow indentations mark the emergence of the inferior frontal sulcus and the superior temporal sulcus. D. By 30 weeks, the frontal lobe begins to divide into three subregions. E. The subdivisions are well defined by week 32. F. The primary division of the temporal lobe into the superior, middle, and inferior regions is marked by the emergence of the superior and inferior temporal sulci at week 34. G. Within frontal regions, secondary sulci are clearly apparent by week 36. H. By 39 weeks, gyral and sulcal morphology is adultlike. (From Abe et al. 2003. Adapted with the permission of John Wiley & Sons.)

## Mechanisms of Gyral Formation

The mechanisms that underlie the process of gyrification are not well understood. Brain growth within a limited cranial volume has traditionally been cited as the primary factor that drives the development of cortical convolutions (Le Gros 1945), and indeed, across species, brain size is correlated, though not perfectly, with the degree and complexity of cortical convolutions (Toro and Burnod 2005). However, the conserved order of emergence of convolutions and the regularity of patterning cannot be accounted for by limitations imposed by cranial size alone. A number of passive, mechanical factors have been implicated in the emergence of gyral patterning. These include the constraints imposed by early sulcus formation on adjacent sulci that emerge later; differential bending of cortical cell columns in the gyral crowns and sulcal fundi; differential curvature of cortical layers; displacement by fiber tracts; changes in nonneural elements, such as the skull, ventricles, and meninges; and flexure of the neuraxis (Welker 1990). However, there is agreement that although all these factors likely contribute to the process of gyrification, these passive processes cannot by themselves account for the observed changes in gyral patterning. More active processes associated with brain development have also been implicated. Regional differences in the cytoarchitectonic organization, differences in the cortical lamina, the effect of afferent innervation and synaptogenesis, and subtractive events such as naturally occurring cell death and synapse elimination are all thought to contribute to the process of gyrification. Multifactor models of gyrification have been successful in capturing basic processes involved in the development of cortical convolutions.

Van Essen (1997) proposed a tension-based model of gyrification. He noted that the brain-size parameters most critical for understanding the phenomenon of cortical folding concern the evolutionary expansion of the cortical sheet relative to underlying cerebral volume. Across species, the horizontal surface expansion of the cortex is ten times greater than the vertical, or radial, expansion. Accompanying the horizontal expansion is a dramatic increase in the amount of neocortical gray matter expressed as a proportion of total brain size (e.g., 13 percent in insectivores versus 50 percent in humans). Both of these changes are associated with increased complexity of cortical convolutions, suggesting that enhanced gyrification may, in part, be the result of neocortical expansion outpacing increases in the size of the underlying brain volume. However, expanded cortical size alone does not explain the complex folding of the cortical sheet. Van Essen has proposed that, for a given species or individual, the specific pattern of gyrification is the product of this neocortical size differential coupled with the development of optimally efficient connectivity within and across neural systems. By this account, the emerging patterns of connectivity within the developing brain should act to maximize the efficiency of neural transmission within neural networks. Optimally efficient systems are those that are compact, with connections traversing the shortest distances possible (see also Klyachko and Stevens 2003 for discussion of the interareal optimization of connectivity). Within strongly connected networks, the tension of axons functioning together as a signaling pathway acts to pull together strongly interconnected neural regions, while weakly connected regions drift apart. This tension-based model is sensitive to the range of factors outlined earlier, including cortical thickness and curvature, differences in laminar structure, and regional cytoarchitecture. It can also account for individual differences in patterns of gyrification.

In a recent computer-based simulation, Toro and Burnod (2005) proposed a morphogenic model of gyrification that also incorporates a multifactor approach. Their model characterizes the developing cortex as a closed surface with radially connected fibers pulling nonuniformly against the surface. Their model incorporates a range of dynamic factors associated with brain growth, coupled with mechanical properties of the cortex and connecting fibers that confer both elasticity and plasticity on both the cortical sheet and the radial connections. The results of their simulation studies demonstrated that their model can generate successively more complex patterns of deformation in the cortical surface that approximate the process of gyrification. By systematically varying the parameters of their model, they demonstrated that a wide range of factors, including brain size and cortical thickness, can affect specific outcomes. Furthermore, they suggested that the initial definition of the primary sulci may arise from either architectonic inhomogeneities in the cortical surface or the initial, nonuniform geometry of the cortical sheet. Specifically, they suggest that the early "bean-shape" geometry of the cortex just before the period of rapid growth associated with gyrification (Figure 9.2A) may provide the initial template for the formation of the primary gyri within this dynamically coupled and changing system.

## Myelination

The efficient and rapid transmission of electrical signals in the CNS is facilitated by the sheaths of myelin that encase the axons of neurons. In mammals, axons larger than 1 micrometer (one millionth of a meter) are myelinated. The cells that provide the myelin sheaths within the CNS are the oligodendrocytes. Myelin in the peripheral nervous system is provided by Schwann cells.

### The Structure of Myelin

In the CNS, the myelin sheath is the cell membrane of the oligodendrocyte. It is a two-layered structure that contains several large proteins, including proteolipid protein (PLP) and myelin basic protein (MBP). Both are important for compacting of the membrane during myelination (Sampaio and Truwit 2001). The outer layer of the membrane is composed of cholesterol and glycolipids, while the inner layer is composed of phospholipids.

The process of myelination in the CNS begins with the alignment of the oligodendrocyte and the axon. As myelination proceeds, the tongue of the oligodendrocyte membrane first engulfs and then begins to wrap around the shaft of the axon. The wrapping process continues in successive spirals around the axon. Each new layer of myelin maintains contact with the axon, and earlier produced layers of myelin are pushed farther and farther away from the center of the emerging coil (Figure 9.3). An individual oligodendrocyte can myelinate up to 40 axons, depending on axon diameter (Coman et al. 2005). Further, there is a correlation between axon thickness and the thickness of the myelin sheath (Sherman and Brophy 2005).

### The Developmental Progression of Myelination

Myelination begins in the human spinal column as early as GW12 to GW14. Myelination within the cerebral cortex does not begin until the third trimester (Kinney 2005; Yakovlev and Lecours 1967). Although much of myelination is complete by the end of the second postnatal year, there is evidence that it continues into the sixth decade of life (Benes et al. 1994; Yakovlev and Lecours 1967). The progression of myelination is very systematic: it begins in caudal regions and progresses toward central cerebral regions and finally to the anterior and posterior poles. Myelination in the occipital pole is complete before

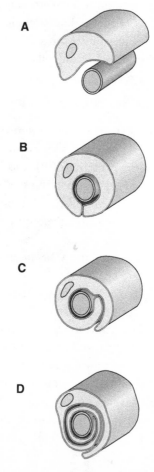

Figure 9.3. Sequence of axon myelination by an oligodendrocyte. A. The cytoplasmic tongue of the oligodendrocyte contacts the axon. B. The tongue then engulfs the axon, surrounding it. C, D. The tongue then spirals around the axon, forming the myelin sheath.

myelination in the frontal pole. Further, proximal portions of pathways myelinate earlier than distal pathways, so, for example, the optic tract myelinates before the optic radiations, which in turn myelinate before the visual association fibers.

The first detailed studies of the developmental sequence of myelination were conducted in the late 1890s and early 1900s (Flechsig 1920; Thompson 1900). Kaes (Thompson 1900) and Flechsig (1920) elucidated the principles that have been the basis for subsequent studies of the relation between myelination and function. Flechsig traced the course of myelination across development and noted that within a neural system, the completion of myelination signals the onset of full functional capacity. Further, he observed that in general, sensory and motor systems become myelinated earlier than brain systems that subserve higher-level functions, such as learning, memory, and other higher cognitive processes. With these observations, Flechsig introduced both the concept that myelination follows a highly regular temporal sequence reflecting the complexity of the underlying systems and the idea that myelination is a marker of CNS maturation. In the late 1960s, Yakovlev and Lecours (1967) provided a comprehensive and detailed study of 200 human brains ranging in age from GW4 through the first postnatal year, plus a large sample of adult brains. In that work, they traced the emergence of myelin using histological staining methods. Their study largely confirmed earlier work by Flechsig and has, in turn, been confirmed by later work using both preserved brain tissue and neuroimaging techniques (Sampaio and Truwit 2001). On the basis of their studies, Yakovlev and Lecours refined early definitions of the timing of myelination. They noted that not only do different areas begin to myelinate at different times in development, but they also have different characteristic rates of myelination. Thus within a neural system, timing of the onset of myelination does not necessarily predict the timing of completion. They described this variable temporal aspect of myelination across brain areas as the myelogenetic cycle (Figure 9.4).

Myelination begins in the midbrain, the brainstem, and some areas of the cerebellum prenatally. At birth, there is very little evidence of gray and white-matter differentiation in cortical areas. However, microscopic analyses indicate the onset of myelination by the time of birth in a range of brain areas (Kinney et al. 1988), including the

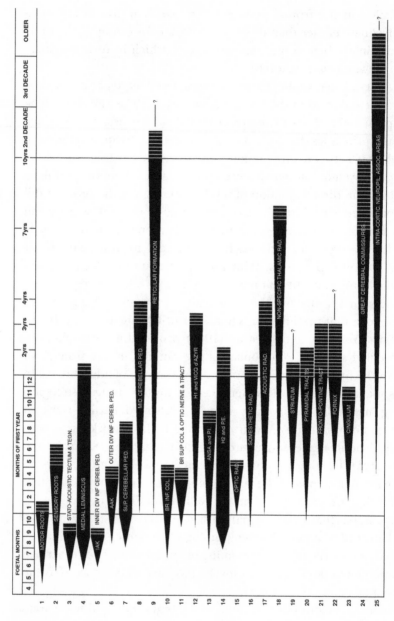

Figure 9.4. The myelogenetic cycle. (From Yakovlev and Lecours 1967. Adapted with the permission of Blackwell Publishing.)

midbrain corticospinal tract, the corona radiata, the pons, the cerebellum, portions of the anterior commissure, and the posterior limb of the internal capsule. By the sixth postnatal week (PW6), substantial myelination is observed in the posterior limb of the internal capsule, though the anterior limb does not fully myelinate until the end of the first year of life. Mature myelination is observed in the corona radiata and in the optic radiations by three months and within the auditory radiation by seven months (Kinney et al. 1988). During the second half of the first year of life, myelination advances into all the cortical lobes and is well established by the end of the second year. However, cortical myelination is a protracted process that extends throughout childhood and well into adolescence within frontal regions.

## Factors That Signal Myelination

Although the signaling pathway is not well understood, it is thought that the axon provides both secreted and surface molecules that modulate the final differentiation of the immature oligodendrocyte into the mature myelinating cell. Two growth factors secreted from axons, insulin-like growth factor (Igf) and fibroblast growth factor (Fgf), play differing roles in oligodendrocyte development. Igf has been shown to promote both oligodendrocyte differentiation and survival (Butt and Berry 2000), while Fgf2 appears to play multiple roles in oligodendrocyte development. Early in development, Fgf2 promotes differentiation in the oligodendrocyte progenitor (OLP) population and supports the differentiation of premyelinating oligodendrocytes. However, after myelination begins, Fgf2 acts to arrest the further differentiation of oligodendrocytes and has been implicated in their loss (Butt and Dinsdale 2005).

The effects of cell adhesion molecules also appear to vary at different points in development, inhibiting myelination early and promoting it later. For example, a specific isoform of N-CAM, PSA-NCAM, is expressed on the surface of axons early in development and appears to inhibit myelination (Coman et al. 2005); its disappearance coincides with the onset of myelination. A different cell adhesion molecule, L1, is also expressed on the surface of axons for a brief period that coincides with the onset of myelination. It is thought that the role of L1 may be to facilitate the initial contact of the oligodendrocyte tongue with the surface of the axon. L1 disappears as the wrapping process proceeds (Coman et al. 2005).

Finally, electrical activity of the cell plays an important role in promoting myelination, as evidenced by findings that dark-reared mice have reduced myelination, and premature eye opening in rabbits increase myelination. Blockade of activity has been shown, specifically, to reduce the progress of myelination. When activity is blocked in mice at P4, which is two days before the onset of myelination in this species, a 60 percent decrease in myelination is observed in the population of myelinated axons at P6 (Coman et al. 2005). Further, the effects of activity on myelin formation extend beyond the period of early development. A number of studies have documented the effects of environmental complexity on the density of myelin across a wide range of cortical areas for both juvenile and adult animals, supporting the association between neural activity and myelin formation (Sanchez et al. 1998; Sirevaag and Greenough 1987; Szeligo and Leblond 1977). Increases in density of myelination within localized brain regions have also been reported in response to a specific activity. Local areas of myelination were assessed in concert pianists and compared with non-musician controls (Bengtsson et al. 2005). Greater myelination was observed in musicians than controls, and within the group of musicians, density of myelination varied systematically within specific regions depending on hours of practice during childhood, adolescence, and adulthood.

Although the association between activity and myelination is well documented, the signaling mechanisms are not well understood. While most activity-dependent signaling occurs at the synapse, the signaling between the oligodendrocyte and axon occurs in the absence of a synapse. Adenosine triphosphate (ATP), a purine, has been shown to be a widespread source of nonsynaptic intercellular signaling in populations of both neurons and glial cells, and is considered to constitute an alternative form of signaling in the brain referred to as purinergic signaling (Fields and Burnstock 2006). When neurons fire, ATP is released along the extent of the axon. Oligodendrocytes and Schwann cells have receptors for ATP, though the types of receptors on the two classes of cells differ, creating varying signaling pathways for the two populations of cells. ATP signaling inhibits Schwann cell proliferation, differentiation, and subsequent myelination. In contrast, for oligodendrocytes,

ATP signaling stimulates differentiation of premyelinating cells and promotes myelination (Fields 2006).

## Clinical Correlation: Periventricular Leukomalacia and Oligodendrocyte Maturation

Periventricular leukomalacia (PVL) is a disorder of the deep, central cerebral white matter that is common among premature infants and is the major neuropathology associated with cerebral palsy (Folkerth 2005). It was first identified in 1853 by Little, who described the predominant form of cerebral palsy, spastic diplegia, and defined the association between this serious neuromotor disorder, prematurity, and prenatal asphyxia. Soon after, Virchow (1867) described a "softening" of the tissue in the vicinity of the ventricles in human brains of CP patients examined at autopsy. In 1877 Parrot noted that the brain areas most vulnerable to the disorder were also those farthest from the brain blood supply and thus postulated an association with ischemia, or deficiency in the local blood supply. Banker and Larroche (1962) were the first to use the term *PVL* to describe the disorder.

PVL is a frequent complication of prematurity, particularly among very low birth weight (500 to 1,500 gms, approximately 1 to 3 pounds) infants. Each year 55,000 children are born prematurely in the United States, and 90 percent of these children survive (Kinney 2005). Approximately 10 percent of these children are diagnosed with cerebral palsy. PVL manifests in two distinct forms, cystic and diffuse. Cystic PVL has a well-defined temporal course. In the acute phase (24 to 48 hours postinjury), there is localized necrosis reflecting the loss of all cellular elements that may be difficult to visualize using ultrasound or even slice-preparation methodologies (Folkerth 2005). The subacute phase extends from 3 to 10 days postinjury and is marked by the appearance of cavities reflecting the activity of microphages as they clear away the dying tissue. The chronic phase lasts from weeks to months, and it is during this period that the periventricular cysts can be readily visualized using ultrasound techniques. The cysts usually collapse and form scars, and in older children ventricular enlargement may be the most prominent remnant of the neural involvement (Blumenthal 2004; Kinney 2005). The diffuse form of PVL has a less obvious temporal course. There is evidence of damage to glia, including oligodendrocytes, and compromise of the blood-brain barrier can be identified. Myelination is delayed and can become a permanent marker of the disorder (Folkerth 2005). Diffuse PVL is far more common than cystic PVL, and recent imaging studies suggest that the frequency of the cystic form may be dropping and now accounts for only 5 percent of cases (Back and Rivkees 2004).

Two primary pathological conditions have been associated with PVL, hypoxic-ischemic (HI) events, which result in ischemic-reperfusion injury (brain damage caused by abnormal fluctuations in blood supply), and inflammatory events associated with maternal or fetal infection. Both conditions appear to target cells within the deep periventricular white matter of fetal brains during a specific narrow developmental window, GW23 to GW32.

The pathophysiology of PVL suggests that the immaturity of the cerebrovascular system may be implicated in periventricular ischemic-reperfusion injury observed in preterm infants (Back et al. 2001). Postmortem studies have shown that deep periventricular regions of the brain are sparsely supplied by the prenatal vascular system (Folkerth 2005). The middle cerebral artery (MCA) provides most of the blood flow to the periventricular region. The MCA vasculature extends from the pial surface through the subcortical white matter, extending what have been called short penetrations, as well as to the deep periventricular white matter, extending so-called long penetrations (Blumenthal 2004). Between GW24 and GW32, there are very few short penetrations, long penetrations have only limited branching, and there are few connections between the short and long penetration networks. The result of this sparse vascularization within the cerebral white matter is the creation of "watershed" areas, that is, brain regions at the distal extreme of the cerebral blood supply system that receive only minimal perfusion and are thus predisposed to ischemia. Furthermore, the autoregulatory mechanisms of the immature cerebrovascular system are vulnerable to stress. In adults and older children, cerebral blood flow is kept constant via autoregulatory mechanisms, regardless of changes in blood pressure. Premature infants under stressful conditions exhibit "pressure-passive circulation" (Tsuji et al. 2000). Small changes in blood pressure can result in local ischemia, particularly within watershed regions; that, in turn, triggers the cascade that results in cellular necrosis (Blumenthal 2004).

Inflammatory processes associated with maternal or fetal infection have also been implicated in PVL. Histological chorioamnionitis is an intrauterine infection caused by an infectious agent that originates in the vagina and enters the amniotic fluid. In many cases the infection is "silent" and is diagnosed only after the birth of the infant. The infection is common in preterm pregnancies, but the incidence declines with increasing gestational age. In 20- to 24-week-old preterm infants, the incidence rate is 66 percent, but the frequency drops to 16 percent among infants 34 weeks old or older (Lahra and Jeffery 2004). A small percentage of exposed infants develop PVL, suggesting that the infection contributes to a more complex pathological pathway. Infection can trigger an inflammatory response in the infant that can result in cytokine (proteins produced as part of the immune system response) release. Cytokines can cross the blood-brain barrier and activate microglia. Microglia are derived from macrophages and are part of the brain response to inflammation (Back and Rivkees 2004). Recent studies have begun to define the pathway by which both cerebral ischemia and infection can lead specifically to PVL. The key to understanding the pathophysiology of PVL appears to lie in the selective vulnerability of immature oligodendrocytes to the effects of injury.

One important feature of PVL is that it manifests within the very specific developmental window from GW23 to GW32. Interestingly, this period corresponds with an important period of change in the development of the oligodendrocytes (OLs) that constitute myelin and thus the white matter of the developing brain. Work by Back and colleagues (2001) has explored the maturation of human OLs that occurs during the critical window between GW23 to GW32. Three ordered stages of development were observed: OL progenitors, immature OLs, and mature OLs. OL progenitors were found as early as GW18 within the cerebral white matter and cortex, and they were the predominant OL cell type throughout the second half of gestation. Immature OLs were evident in small numbers between GW18 and GW27, and their numbers increased after GW30. Mature OLs increased in concert with the immature OLs and were located specifically within the periventricular white matter. This pattern of development suggests change in the maturational status of the principal component of white matter, the OL cells, during a period that corresponds to the changing pattern of susceptibility to the effects of HI injury and infection. These changes suggest that OL maturity may predict vulnerability to the effects of HI injury and infection and thus predisposition to PVL.

Both ischemia-reperfusion injury and the inflammatory events that accompany infection are associated with the release of reactive oxygen species (ROS) and reactive nitrogen species (RNS). ROS include both free radicals and nonradicals such as hydrogen peroxide (Haynes et al. 2005). Free radicals are atoms that contain one or more unpaired electrons. They exist for a short time before forming a stable molecule (Blumenthal 2004). RNS, and in particular the radical nitric oxide (NO) play an important role in regulating cell functions, including synaptic transmission. The production of both ROS and RNS must be tightly coupled with metabolism. Overproduction of either class of substance can result in conditions referred to as oxidative (associated with overproduction of ROS) and nitrative (associated with RNS) stress (Haynes et al. 2005), both of which can be toxic to vulnerable classes of cells, such as premyelinating OLs. Both ischemia and infection processes can alter the balance of ROS and RNS production. HI causes initial depletion of both oxygen and glucose, disrupting cellular energy production and homeostasis. This initiates a complex cascade that triggers the production of ROS and NO. The inflammatory response associated with infection activates astrocytes and possibly microglia, which in turn release both ROS and NO into the surrounding environment. Recent studies have suggested that OL susceptibility to the toxic effects of ROS and NO overproduction depends on the maturational state of the cell (Haynes et al. 2005). Specifically, premyelinating OLs appear to be vulnerable to the effects of ROS and NO, but, mature OLs are not. Both in vitro studies that examined directly the effects of ROS and NO on OL cells at different stages of development (Back and Rivkees 2004) and autopsy studies of the brains of fetuses with and without PVL (Kinney 2005) have demonstrated the selective vulnerability of premyelinating OLs to oxidative and nitrative stress injury.

In summary, the maturational state of the vasculature system in the 23- to 32-week developmental window makes the periventricular region particularly vulnerable to the effects of both HI and infection. Both HI and infection are associated with oxidative and nitrative stress reactions that release high levels of ROS and NO into the local environment. Immature OLs are vulnerable to the effects of ROS and NO, but mature OLs are not. The close correspondence between the timing of OL maturation and the developmental window for PVL, coupled with evidence of the selective vulnerability of immature OLs to oxidative and nitrative stress conditions, provides significant insight into the neuropathology of this prevalent neurodevelopmental disorder.

## Changes in Prenatal and Postnatal Cortical Morphology

The rate of brain growth during the late prenatal and early postnatal periods is very rapid. Imaging studies of neurologically normal preterm infants suggest that total brain volume, including the cerebral hemispheres, the brain stem, and the cerebellum, is approximately 150 ml (9 in$^3$) at GW29, but by term it increases to 400 ml (24 in$^3$), approximately 25 percent of the average adult volume (Huppi et al. 1998). Postnatal brain growth initially continues at a rapid pace, and by the time children are six years old, average brain volume has reached approximately 90 percent of adult levels (Courchesne et al. 2000; Iwasaki et al. 1997; Kennedy et al. 2002; Kennedy and Dehay 2001; Lenroot and Giedd 2006; Paus et al. 2001; Reiss et al. 1996). Subsequent development is more gradual, with total brain volume reaching adult levels in early adolescence (Courchesne et al. 2000).

Although total brain volume increases continuously from the prenatal period through early adolescence, patterns of change in the volume of the different neural constituents are more varied. Measures of white matter volume, gray matter volume, and cerebrospinal fluid (CSF) volume each reflect change across the age range, but the profiles of change differ for each of the constituents.

## Changes in White Matter

Changes in white matter reflect the elaboration of connecting fiber pathways in the developing brain. In the prenatal period, unmyelinated axons (referred to as unmyelinated white matter) constitutes the largest percentage of intracranial tissue volume. At GW30, unmyelinated white matter pathways make up 50 percent of total intracranial volume, but that percentage drops dramatically by term (GW 42) to approximately 35 percent. Overall brain growth during this period is dramatic, increasing by 250 percent, and thus, although the amount of unmyelinated white matter declines relative to other neural constituents during the last trimester of pregnancy, the absolute volume of unmyelinated white matter increases from 100 ml at GW30 to 150 ml at term.

In contrast, myelinated white matter makes up only 1 to 2 percent (less than 5 ml) of brain volume at GW30, increasing to 5 percent (20 ml) by term (Huppi et al. 1998). During the preschool and school-age periods, white matter volume continues to increase in a linear fashion (Courchesne et al. 2000; Giedd et al. 1999; Iwasaki et al. 1997; Lenroot and Giedd 2006; Pfefferbaum et al. 1994; Reiss et al. 1996). Data from a large cross-sectional study that included 50 normally developing children aged between 19 months and 12 years and 66 adults suggest that white matter volume increases by 74 percent between the early preschool period and early adolescence and then shows more modest increases into adulthood (Courchesne et al. 2000). These findings were consistent with data from a longitudinal study that included 98 participants who were scanned at least twice between 4 and 21 years of age (Giedd et al. 1999). That study reported a linear increase in white matter volume across the age period, with a total net increase in white matter of 12.4 percent. A comparison of these two studies in conjunction with earlier work suggests that a substantial portion of the change in white matter volume must occur during the preschool period.

Many studies do not report systematic regional differences in white matter increase across development (Courchesne et al. 2000; Giedd et al. 1999; Huppi et al. 1998; Iwasaki et al. 1997). However, a large cross-sectional study including 85 children between 5 and 17 years of age suggested more prominent increases within frontal regions (Reiss et al. 1996). This finding is consistent with evidence from behavioral studies suggesting that higher cognitive abilities thought to be mediated by frontal brain systems improve during the period of pronounced change in frontal white matter. Further, a recent study using diffusion tensor imaging (DTI) techniques provides additional evidence of selective changes in white matter within both anterior subcortical and frontal regions (Barnea-Goraly et al. 2005). DTI can be used to measure movement of water molecules in brain tissue. In gray matter or CSF, water disperses isotropically, that is, symmetrically, from a source (like a drop of ink in a container of water). However, in the presence of fiber pathways, water moves anisotropically, following the direction of the adjacent fibers. DTI can be used to index regional differences in the degree of anisotropy, measured as fractional anisotropy, or FA, within the brain. It thus provides an indirect measure of white matter development and maturity. In their study, Barnea-Goraly and colleagues (2005) scanned 34 children between 6 and 19 years of age. They found systematic age-related changes in their measure of anisotropy within prefrontal regions, within the internal capsule, and between pathways extending within the basal ganglia and between the basal ganglia and the thalamus. Further, a number of studies reported developmental differences in the corpus callosum, the large fiber bundle that connects the two cerebral hemispheres. Fibers passing through the corpus callosum generally connect homologous regions of the two hemispheres; thus fibers between anterior regions of the brain pass through the anterior region of the corpus callosum. The corpus callosum undergoes a protracted period of development, but patterns of change are not uniform. Anterior regions of the corpus callosum develop relatively early in childhood, while posterior regions do not mature until adolescence (Durston et al. 2001). These studies suggest that although white matter volume increases throughout the brain during infancy and childhood, there may be region-specific differences in the rate and/or duration of developmental change.

## Changes in Gray Matter

Gray matter consists of neuronal cell bodies, as well as some nerve fibers, capillaries, and glial cells. Most of the gray matter in the brain is in the cerebral and cerebellar cortices (cortical gray matter), but the subcortical nuclei make up the subcortical gray matter. During the last trimester of the prenatal period, gray matter volumes increase linearly by approximately 1.4 percent per week. At GW30, gray matter makes up 35 percent of total intracranial volume, and that percentage increases to 50 percent by term. Absolute gray matter volume goes from 60 ml at GW30 to 200 ml at term. Cortical gray matter contributes by far the most to this volume increase, making up 40 percent of intracranial volume at term (Huppi et al. 1998). The increase in absolute volume of cortical gray matter between GW30 and term is 400 percent

(40 ml to 160 ml), while subcortical gray matter doubles in volume (20 ml to 40 ml) during that time.

In contrast to the pattern of volumetric change observed across age for white matter, gray matter volumes initially increase and then decline (Courchesne et al. 2000; Giedd 2004; Giedd et al. 1999; Jernigan and Tallal 1990; Jernigan et al. 1991; Sowell et al. 2002; Sowell, Thompson, and Toga 2004; Toga, Thompson, and Sowell 2006 for review). In the early 1990s, Jernigan and colleagues used MRI to examine gray matter volumes in 8-year-old children and adults. They reported that adults had less cortical gray matter, even though their overall brain volume was greater than that of children, suggesting that the gray matter loss is a marker of brain development. In a later study, they confirmed this pattern of systematic reduction across the period from 8 years to adulthood and also noted that the timing of loss was not uniform across brain areas (Jernigan et al. 1991). Subsequent work has confirmed and elaborated upon these initial findings.

In their large cross-sectional study, Courchesne and colleagues (2000) reported that gray matter increases by 13 percent from the early preschool period through middle childhood (6 to 9 years) and then decreases linearly by approximately 5 percent per decade across the rest of the lifespan. In their longitudinal study, Giedd and colleagues (1999) reported a similar nonlinear pattern of change in gray matter volumes. Further, they reported regional differences in the developmental timing of the increase and decline. Within frontal regions, increases in gray matter volume were observed throughout preadolescence, reaching peak volume at approximately 12 years of age (11 years for females; 12.1 years for males). Parietal lobe volumes reached their peak a little earlier, at about 11 years of age (10.2 for females; 11.8 for males). Temporal regions were considerably later, peaking at approximately 16 years (16.7 for females; 16.5 for males). Occipital regions showed a continuing linear increase in gray-matter volume during the term of the study (children were not assessed beyond 20 years of age).

A number of groups have begun to examine the question of developmental change in gray matter volume by measuring the density or thickness of gray matter in different regions of the brain (Gogtay et al. 2004; Sowell et al. 2003, 2004; Sowell, Thompson, and Toga 2004). These studies have begun to provide a more detailed picture of change in the developing cortex that goes considerably beyond simple characterization of development as following a caudal-to-rostral or inferior-to-superior trajectory. Sowell and colleagues (2004) measured regional cortical thickness in a longitudinal study of 45 children ranging in age from 5 to 11 years. Each child in the study was scanned twice; the second scan was obtained at least two years after the first. Measurements of cortical thickness were taken across the surface of the brain for each data set. On the basis of evidence from earlier studies documenting a nonlinear developmental progression, areas showing evidence of maximal thinning were presumed to be developing earliest, while those areas showing thickening were presumed to be developing later. The pattern of progressive cortical thinning across development is thought to reflect the underlying subtractive processes of synapse retraction that are associated with the elimination of exuberant connections and with the stabilization of mature neural pathways. The major findings of the Sowell studies included significant thinning in dorsolateral frontal regions, particularly in the right hemisphere, and gain in cortical thickness in perisylvian regions of the ventral frontal lobe and superior temporal lobe. In addition, marked thinning was observed in parietal-occipital regions. The developmental patterns observed in these studies are largely, though not entirely, consistent with those obtained in earlier studies. Further, they provide much more detail about the patterns of change than earlier studies that used measures that averaged over whole brain lobes. For example, frontal regions contain regions that develop both early (dorsal) and late (ventral). Thus averaging over the data from those regions in a "lobar" measure can mask more intricate patterns of change.

A recent longitudinal report examined cortical density in 13 children between 4 and 20 years of age (Gogtay et al. 2004). Measures of cortical density differ from, but are very highly correlated with, measures of cortical thickness. Thus the two measures are thought to reflect very similar developmental processes. Each child in the sample was scanned a minimum of three times at minimum intervals of two years. The study measured the density of the cortex across the surface of the brain. The results of this study are again consistent with the earlier findings but provide greater detail on patterns of change in the developing cortex. There were three major findings from this study. First, the regions of the brain involved in the most basic sensory and motor functions develop earliest. These include the precentral gyrus of the frontal lobe, including the primary motor cortex, the primary sensory areas of the parietal cortex, and the occipital pole, including the primary visual cortex. The next regions to develop are those involved in spatial orientation and attention (more inferior parietal regions) and complex pattern processing (inferior, posterior temporal regions). The regions maturing latest in this study were orbitofrontal and superior temporal regions, those involved in complex planning and multimodal integration. The findings of this study are consistent with a model of development that begins with the early maturation of primary sensorimotor regions, followed by the ordered elaboration and stabilization of progressively more complex perceptual and cognitive systems.

Finally, there is very recent evidence that patterns of cortical thinning may be associated with overall intelligence levels in children. Sowell and colleagues (2004) found a modest and region-specific association in their study of cortical thinning in 7- to 11-year-old children. Specifically, they found that greater cortical thinning within dorsolateral frontal regions of the left hemisphere was associated with higher performance on the vocabulary subtest of the Wechsler IQ test. This finding hints at an association between maturation within a major brain language region and an important aspect of linguistic functioning. In a much larger study, Shaw and colleagues (2006) examined profiles of cortical thinning in a sample of 307 individuals whose ages ranged from 3.8 to 29 years. The study stratified the sample into three groups based on their performance on a Wechsler IQ test (superior, high, and average). Although an overall pattern of progressive cortical thinning was reported for all three groups, the developmental trajectories differed. Specifically, in the early childhood period (3.8 to 8.4 years), cortical thickness was negatively correlated with IQ, particularly within frontal and parietal regions. Children in the superior group initially had the thinnest cortices, but then showed a rapid and protracted increase in cortical thickness that peaked at about 11 years and was followed by a rapid decline. By contrast, cortical thickness was initially higher in the average group, peaked at age 7, and then showed a steady decline. These findings suggest that the patterns of increase and decline in regional cortical thickness may be associated with level of intellectual functioning.

## Changes in Cerebrospinal Fluid

The other main element that makes up intracranial volume is the CSF. CSF is a clear fluid that fills the ventricles and the subarachnoid spaces that surround the brain and spinal cord. The specific gravity of CSF is lower than neural tissue, thus the brain essentially floats in a bath of CSF that provides cushioning and protection from potential trauma (Bergsneider 2001). CSF is produced continuously in the lateral ventricles and exits via the venous system. In addition to its cushioning function, CSF serves to transport a variety of ions, molecules, and proteins, and acts to clear waste products. Across the last trimester of the prenatal period, CSF volume declines slightly from 10 to 15 percent of intracranial volume at GW30 to 8 to 10 percent at term (Huppi et al. 1998). Between the early preschool period and adulthood, the absolute volume of CSF more than doubles (from approximately 100 to 250 ml), increasing linearly with age (Courchesne et al. 2000). However, as a fraction of total intracranial volume, CSF volume remains constant at 7 to 9 percent from the early preschool period to adolescence and then increases again during adulthood.

## Changes in Complexity of Dendritic Branching

In addition to changes in the volume of the major tissue components during postnatal development, there is complementary evidence of change at a more microscopic level in the complexity of the dendritic arbors (Travis, Ford, and Jacobs 2005). Recall that Huttenlocher reported regional differences in the profiles of synaptic exuberance and pruning in humans. Although all areas initially generated an excess of synaptic connections indexed by density of dendrites, followed by elimination of connections, the timing of peak exuberance and decline differed across areas (Huttenlocher and Dabholkar 1997). These findings are mirrored by recent work examining regional differences in the complexity of dendritic arbors at different points in development.

Among adult monkeys and humans, differences in the complexity of the dendritic arbor, indexed by total length of dendritic segments, mean segment length, segment counts, dendritic spine number, and density, are observed in different cortical regions. In human adults

(Jacobs et al. 1997), cortical regions involved in primary sensory and motor processes (e.g., BA3, 1, 2—somatosensory, BA4—motor) have less complex dendritic arborization than areas involved in higher cognitive processing (e.g., BA10—prefrontal cortex). However, examination of these regions in the brains of neonates reveals a very different distribution of dendritic complexity (Travis, Ford and Jacobs 2005). Neonates show the most complex dendritic arborization in primary cortices, such as BA4 and BA3, 1, 2, and the least complex patterns in prefrontal regions (BA10). These findings are consistent with the data described by Huttenlocher but provide greater detail on the patterns of developmental change that underlie these larger-scale events (Travis, Ford, and Jacobs 2005).

## Chapter Summary

- The surface of the developing human brain is smooth until approximately GW18. The first convolutions are clearly evident on the cortical surface by GW22, and by PW4 the patterns of gyral and sulcal folding have reached near-adult levels.
- Gyrification follows a regular progression. The primary sulci begin as regularly positioned indentations on the surface of the brain that gradually become deeper. Side branches from the primary sulci form the secondary sulci, and these, in turn, form the branches that are the tertiary sulci. The formation of primary sulci and most of the secondary sulci is complete by GW34. Formation of tertiary sulci continues postnatally.
- The mechanisms of gyrification are not well understood. Multifactor models that include both passive mechanical and dynamic developmental factors have been most successful in capturing basic processes involved in the development of cortical convolutions.
- In the CNS, oligodendrocytes form sheaths of myelin that encase the axons of neurons. The formation of myelin facilitates efficient and rapid transmission of electrical signals between neurons.
- Myelination within the cerebral cortex begins during the third trimester and while it is largely complete by the end of the second postnatal year, there is good evidence of region-specific

change through late adolescence. The progression of myelination is very systematic. It begins in caudal regions and progresses rostrally. Proximal portions of pathways myelinate earlier than distal pathways.

- Brain growth during the late prenatal period and particularly the early postnatal period is very rapid. Total intracranial volume doubles in the last trimester of pregnancy. Patterns of change in the volume of the different neural constituents are not uniform. White matter increases in a linear fashion throughout childhood and into early adolescence. Change is fairly constant across regions, though there is some evidence of regional differences in the rate of white matter development within frontal regions. Gray matter initially increases throughout the school-age period and then begins to decline. There are significant regional differences in the patterns of gray matter change.

## References

Abe, S., K. Takagi, T. Yamamoto, Y. Okuhata, and T. Kato. 2003. "Assessment of cortical gyrus and sulcus formation using MR images in normal fetuses." *Prenatal Diagnosis*, 23: 225–231.

Armstrong, E., A. Schleicher, H. Omran, M. Curtis, and K. Zilles. 1995. "The ontogeny of human gyrification." *Cerebral Cortex*, 5: 56–63.

Back, S. A., N. L. Luo, N. S. Borenstein, J. M. Levine, J. J. Volpe, and H. C. Kinney. 2001. "Late oligodendrocyte progenitors coincide with the developmental window of vulnerability for human perinatal white matter injury." *Journal of Neuroscience*, 21: 1302–1312.

Back, S. A., and S. A. Rivkees. 2004. "Emerging concepts in periventricular white matter injury." *Seminars in Perinatology*, 28: 405–414.

Banker, B. Q., and J. C. Larroche. 1962. "Periventricular leukomalacia of infancy: A form of neonatal anoxic encephalopathy." *Archives of Neurology*, 7: 386–410.

Barnea-Goraly, N., V. Menon, M. Eckert, L. Tamm, R. Bammer, A. Karchemskiy, C. C. Dant, and A. L. Reiss. 2005. "White matter development during childhood and adolescence: A cross-sectional diffusion tensor imaging study." *Cerebral Cortex*, 15: 1848–1854.

Benes, F. M., M. Turtle, Y. Khan, and P. Farol. 1994. "Myelination of a key relay zone in the hippocampal formation occurs in the human brain during childhood, adolescence, and adulthood." *Archives of General Psychiatry*, 51: 477–484.

Bengtsson, S. L., Z. Nagy, S. Skare, L. Forsman, H. Forssberg, and F. Ullen. 2005. "Extensive piano practicing has regionally specific effects on white matter development." *Nature Neuroscience*, 8: 1148–1150.

Bergsneider, M. 2001. "Evolving concepts of cerebrospinal fluid physiology." *Neurosurgery Clinics of North America*, 12: 631–638.

Blumenthal, I. 2004. "Periventricular leucomalacia: A review." *European Journal of Pediatrics*, 163: 435–442.

Butt, A. M., and M. Berry. 2000. "Oligodendrocytes and the control of myelination in vivo: New insights from the rat anterior medullary velum." *Journal of Neuroscience Research*, 59: 477–488.

Butt, A. M., and J. Dinsdale. 2005. "Opposing actions of fibroblast growth factor-2 on early and late oligodendrocyte lineage cells in vivo." *Journal of Neuroimmunology*, 166: 75–87.

Chi, J. G., E. C. Dooling, and F. H. Gilles. 1977. "Gyral development of the human brain." *Annals of Neurology*, 1: 86–93.

Coman, I., G. Barbin, P. Charles, B. Zalc, and C. Lubetzki. 2005. "Axonal signals in central nervous system myelination, demyelination and remyelination." *Journal of the Neurological Sciences*, 233: 67–71.

Courchesne, E., H. J. Chisum, J. Townsend, A. Cowles, J. Covington, B. Egaas, M. Harwood, S. Hinds, and G. A. Press. 2000. "Normal brain development and aging: Quantitative analysis at in vivo MR imaging in healthy volunteers." *Radiology*, 216: 672–682.

Dorovini-Zis, K., and C. L. Dolman. 1977. "Gestational development of brain." *Archives of Pathology and Laboratory Medicine*, 101: 192–195.

Durston, S., H. E. Hulshoff Pol, B. J. Casey, J. N. Giedd, J. K. Buitelaar, and H. van Engeland. 2001. "Anatomical MRI of the developing human brain: What have we learned?" *Journal of the American Academy of Child and Adolescent Psychiatry*, 40: 1012–1020.

Fields, R. D. 2006. "Nerve impulses regulate myelination through purinergic signalling." *Novartis Foundation Symposium*, 276: 148–158; discussion, 158–161, 233–237, 275–281.

Fields, R. D., and G. Burnstock. 2006. "Purinergic signalling in neuron-glia interactions." *Nature Reviews Neuroscience*, 7: 423–436.

Flechsig, P. 1920. *Anatomie des menschlichen Gehirns und Rückenmarks auf myelogenetischer Grundlage*. Leipzig: G. Thieme.

Folkerth, R. D. 2005. "Neuropathologic substrate of cerebral palsy." *Journal of Child Neurology*, 20: 940–949.

Garel, C., E. Chantrel, H. Brisse, M. Elmaleh, D. Luton, J. F. Oury, G. Sebag, and M. Hassan. 2001. "Fetal cerebral cortex: Normal gestational landmarks identified using prenatal MR imaging." *AJNR: American Journal of Neuroradiology*, 22: 184–189.

Garel, C., E. Chantrel, M. Elmaleh, H. Brisse, and G. Sebag. 2003. "Fetal MRI: Normal gestational landmarks for cerebral biometry, gyration and myelination." *Child's Nervous System*, 19: 422–425.

Giedd, J. N. 2004. "Structural magnetic resonance imaging of the adolescent brain." *Annals of the New York Academy of Sciences*, 1021: 77–85.

Giedd, J. N., J. Blumenthal, N. O. Jeffries, F. X. Castellanos, H. Liu, A. Zijdenbos, T. Paus, A. C. Evans, and J. L. Rapoport. 1999. "Brain development during childhood and adolescence: A longitudinal MRI study." *Nature Neuroscience*, 2: 861–863.

Gogtay, N., J. N. Giedd, L. Lusk, K. M. Hayashi, D. Greenstein, A. C. Vaituzis, T. F. Nugent 3rd, D. H. Herman, L. S. Clasen, A. W. Toga, J. L. Rapoport, and P. M. Thompson. 2004. "Dynamic mapping of human cortical development during childhood through early adulthood." *Proceedings of the National Academy of Sciences of the United States of America*, 101: 8174–8179.

Haynes, R. L., O. Baud, J. Li, H. C. Kinney, J. J. Volpe, and D. R. Folkerth. 2005. "Oxidative and nitrative injury in periventricular leukomalacia: A review." *Brain Pathology*, 15: 225–233.

Huppi, P. S., S. Warfield, R. Kikinis, P. D. Barnes, G. P. Zientara, F. A. Jolesz, M. K. Tsuji, and J. J. Volpe. 1998. "Quantitative magnetic resonance imaging of brain development in premature and mature newborns." *Annals of Neurology*, 43: 224–235.

Huttenlocher, P. R., and A. S. Dabholkar. 1997. "Regional differences in synaptogenesis in human cerebral cortex." *Journal of Comparative Neurology*, 387: 167–178.

Iwasaki, N., K. Hamano, Y. Okada, Y. Horigome, J. Nakayama, T. Takeya, H. Takita, and T. Nose. 1997. "Volumetric quantification of brain development using MRI." *Neuroradiology*, 39: 841–846.

Jacobs, B., L. Driscoll, and M. Schall. 1997. "Life-span dendritic and spine changes in areas 10 and 18 of human cortex: A quantitative Golgi study." *Journal of Comparative Neurology*, 386: 661–680.

Jernigan, T. L., and P. Tallal. 1990. "Late childhood changes in brain morphology observable with MRI." *Developmental Medicine and Child Neurology*, 32: 379–385.

Jernigan, T. L., D. A. Trauner, J. R. Hesselink, and P. A. Tallal. 1991. "Maturation of human cerebrum observed in vivo during adolescence." *Brain*, 114 (pt. 5): 2037–2049.

Kennedy, D. N., N. Makris, M. R. Herbert, T. Takahashi, and V. S. Caviness Jr. 2002. "Basic principles of MRI and morphometry studies of human brain development." *Developmental Science*, 5: 268–278.

Kennedy, H., and C. Dehay. 2001. "Gradients and boundaries: Limits of modularity and its influence on the isocortex. [Commentary]." *Developmental Science*, 4: 147–148.

Kinney, H. C. 2005. "Human myelination and perinatal white matter disorders." *Journal of the Neurological Sciences*, 228: 190–192.

Kinney, H. C., B. A. Brody, A. S. Kloman, and F. H. Gilles. 1988. "Sequence of central nervous system myelination in human infancy. II. Patterns of myelination in autopsied infants." *Journal of Neuropathology and Experimental Neurology*, 47: 217–234.

Klyachko, V. A., and C. F. Stevens. 2003. "Connectivity optimization and the positioning of cortical areas." *Proceedings of the National Academy of Sciences of the United States of America*, 100: 7937–7941.

Lahra, M. M., and H. E. Jeffery. 2004. "A fetal response to chorioamnionitis is associated with early survival after preterm birth." *American Journal of Obstetrics and Gynecology*, 190: 147–151.

Larsen, W. J. 2001. *Human embryology*. 3rd ed. New York: Churchill Livingstone.

Le Gros, C. W. 1945. "Deformation patterns in the cerebral cortex." In *Essays on growth and form presented to D'Arcy Wentworth Thompson*, ed. W. E. Le Gros Clark and P. B. Medawar, 1–22. London: Oxford University Press.

Lenroot, R. K., and J. N. Giedd. 2006. "Brain development in children and adolescents: Insights from anatomical magnetic resonance imaging." *Neuroscience and Biobehavioral Reviews*, 30: 718–729.

Paus, T., D. L. Collins, A. C. Evans, G. Leonard, B. Pike, and A. Zijdenbos. 2001. "Maturation of white matter in the human brain: A review of magnetic resonance studies." *Brain Research Bulletin*, 54: 255–266.

Pfefferbaum, A., D. H. Mathalon, E. V. Sullivan, J. M. Rawles, R. B. Zipursky, and K. O. Lim. 1994. "A quantitative magnetic resonance imaging study of changes in brain morphology from infancy to late adulthood." *Archives of Neurology*, 51: 874–887.

Reiss, A. L., M. T. Abrams, H. S. Singer, and J. L. Ross. 1996. "Brain development, gender and IQ in children: A volumetric imaging study." *Brain*, 119: 1763–1774.

Sampaio, R. C., and C. L. Truwit. 2001. "Myelination in the developing brain." In *Handbook of developmental cognitive neuroscience*, ed. C. A. Nelson and M. Luciana, 35–44. Cambridge, MA: MIT Press.

Sanchez, M. M., E. F. Hearn, D. Do, J. K. Rilling, and J. G. Herndon. 1998. "Differential rearing affects corpus callosum size and cognitive function of rhesus monkeys." *Brain Research*, 812: 38–49.

Shaw, P., D. Greenstein, J. Lerch, L. Clasen, R. Lenroot, N. Gogtay, A. Evans, J. Rapoport, and J. Giedd. 2006. "Intellectual ability and cortical development in children and adolescents." *Nature*, 440: 676–679.

Sherman, D. L., and P. J. Brophy. 2005. "Mechanisms of axon ensheathment and myelin growth." *Nature Reviews Neuroscience*, 6: 683–690.

Sirevaag, A. M., and W. T. Greenough. 1987. "Differential rearing effects on rat visual cortex synapses. III. Neuronal and glial nuclei, boutons, dendrites, and capillaries." *Brain Research*, 424: 320–332.

Sowell, E. R., B. S. Peterson, P. M. Thompson, S. E. Welcome, A. L. Henkenius, and A. W. Toga. 2003. "Mapping cortical change across the human life span." *Nature Neuroscience*, 6: 309–315.

Sowell, E. R., P. M. Thompson, C. M. Leonard, S. E. Welcome, E. Kan, and A. W. Toga. 2004. "Longitudinal mapping of cortical thickness and brain growth in normal children." *Journal of Neuroscience*, 24: 8223–8231.

Sowell, E. R., P. M. Thompson, D. Rex, D. Kornsand, K. D. Tessner, T. L. Jernigan, and A. W. Toga. 2002. "Mapping sulcal pattern asymmetry and local cortical surface gray matter distribution in vivo: Maturation in perisylvian cortices." *Cerebral Cortex*, 12: 17–26.

Sowell, E. R., P. M. Thompson, and A. W. Toga. 2004. "Mapping changes in the human cortex throughout the span of life." *Neuroscientist*, 10: 372–392.

Szeligo, F., and C. P. Leblond. 1977. "Response of the three main types of glial cells of cortex and corpus callosum in rats handled during suckling or exposed to enriched, control and impoverished environments following weaning." *Journal of Comparative Neurology*, 172: 247–263.

Thompson, H. B. 1900. "A brief summary of the researches of Theodore Kaes on the medullation of the intra-cortical fibers of man at different ages." *Journal of Comparative Neurology*, 10: 358–374.

Toga, A. W., P. M. Thompson, and E. R. Sowell. 2006. "Mapping brain maturation." *Trends in Neurosciences*, 29: 148–159.

Toro, R., and Y. Burnod. 2005. "A morphogenetic model for the development of cortical convolutions." *Cerebral Cortex*, 15: 1900–1913.

Travis, K., K. Ford, and B. Jacobs. 2005. "Regional dendritic variation in neonatal human cortex: A quantitative Golgi study." *Developmental Neuroscience*, 27: 277–287.

Tsuji, M., J. P. Saul, A. du Plessis, E. Eichenwald, J. Sobh, R. Crocker, and J. J. Volpe. 2000. "Cerebral intravascular oxygenation correlates with mean arterial pressure in critically ill premature infants." *Pediatrics*, 106: 625–632.

Van Essen, D. C. 1997. "A tension-based theory of morphogenesis and compact wiring in the central nervous system." *Nature*, 385: 313–318.

Virchow, R. 1867. "Zur pathologischen Anatomie des Gehirns: 1. Congenitale Encephalitis und Myelitis." *Archiv für pathologische Anatomie und Physiologie und für klinische Medicin*, 38: 129–142.

Welker, W. 1990. "Why does cerebral cortex fissure and fold? A review of determinants of gyri and sulci." In *Cerebral cortex*, vol. 8, *Comparative structure and evolution of cerebral cortex,* ed. E. G. Jones and A. Peters, 3–136. New York: Plenum Press.

Yakovlev, P. I., and A. R. Lecours. 1967. "The myelogenetic cycles of regional maturation of the brain." In *Regional development of the brain in early life,* ed. A. Minkowski, 3–69. Philadelphia: Davis.

Zilles, K., E. Armstrong, A. Schleicher, and H. J. Kretschmann. 1988. "The human pattern of gyrification in the cerebral cortex." *Anatomy and Embryology,* 179: 173–179.

TEN

◆ ◆ ◆

# Plasticity and the Role of Experience
# in Neocortical Development

THE EARLY AREAL patterning of the neocortex relies on intrinsic signaling that emanates from the neuroprogenitor cells in the ventricular zone. As discussed in Chapter 8, this early intrinsic signaling involves the interaction of multiple patterning genes expressed in competing gradients and generating signaling cascades that confer initial positional value on cells in different regions of the emerging neocortex. Extrinsic factors also play a role in directing the very early patterning of the neocortex, but it is the intrinsic factors that predominate in the initial interareal specification, or areal parcellation, of the neocortex.

However, it is also clear that early patterning is malleable. Downregulation of one of the major early patterning genes such as *Pax6* or *Emx2* can shift the initial distribution of cortical areas. Further, in the late prenatal and postnatal periods, large-scale overproduction and subsequent elimination of both neurons and neural connections play an important role in directing the emerging organization of the neocortex. From very early in development, neuron production significantly outpaces the mature steady-state needs of the organism. Apoptotic processes associated with programmed cell death serve to scale back the initial overproduction of neurons. Overproduction of neural connections is also characteristic of the immature organism. Early in development, transient connections are exuberantly established between brain areas. Many of these connections have no counterpart in the mature brain. This exuberant production of connections is widespread and involves most brain areas. These pervasive early exuberant events affect patterns of both intra-areal organization and interareal connectivity, making them subject to change with development. There is substantial evidence that these patterns are significantly influenced by the experience of the developing organism. Indeed, in many cases input is necessary for the emergence of typical patterns of cortical organization. While intrinsic signaling plays an essential role at all stages of brain development, the effects of experience become particularly prominent in the late prenatal and postnatal periods (Sur and Rubenstein 2005).

This chapter focuses primarily on the role of extrinsic factors in pre- and postnatal brain development. It begins by considering a series of studies that explored the role of intrinsic and extrinsic factors in the elaboration of the features of organization within a cortical area. Early Pax6 and Emx2 signaling confers rudimentary specification of cortical areas, but mature organization of neocortical areas is considerably more complex. The elaboration of intra-areal organization involves both intrinsic and extrinsic signaling. The example of intra-areal elaboration discussed in this chapter focuses on the development of the primary visual cortex (PVC) and specifically the development of a characteristic feature of PVC organization, the ocular dominance columns (ODCs). Within the mature PVC, input from the two eyes remains segregated into eye-specific bands; these bands are the ODCs. A key question in the field has been whether the establishment of this characteristic pattern of organization is the product of intrinsic signaling or whether it is activity dependent.

The next issue considered in this chapter concerns the extent to which cells that receive early cues for positional value are restricted to that early-defined fate. The central question is whether the intrinsic or extrinsic signaling in the late prenatal and early postnatal period can fundamentally alter the function of tissue in the neocortical areas defined during the embryonic period. Put simply, the question posed here is whether, for example, early specified "visual" neurons can be signaled to assume a somatosensory fate. Two series of studies will be discussed. The first series examines studies that use "explant" methodologies in which tissue taken from one brain area in a donor animal is transplanted to a different brain area in a host animal. The central question posed by these studies is whether the transplanted tissue will retain the initially specified characteristics of the donor animal or adopt the characteristics specified by a different set of cues in the alternative brain region of the host. The second series of studies examines whether alterations in the nature of the input to a primary sensory area can alter its function. Studies examining experimental modulation of input to the primary auditory cortex (PAC) have explored whether modification of interareal connectivity can significantly alter patterns of intra-areal organization within the PAC during the early postnatal period. These studies focus on a dramatic, experimental intervention that results in the stabilization of normally transient visual system inputs to the PAC. These studies address the question of whether the function of a cortical area can be respecified by experimental manipulations that force the anatomical rewiring of cortical connections.

To address the basic issue concerning the extent of the brain's capacity for plastic adaptation, the effects of circumscribed, late prenatal or postnatal brain injury will be examined. The processes associated with synaptic exuberance and pruning extend well into the postnatal period and are influenced by the experience of the organism. The effects of extrinsic factors on postnatal brain development reflect the plasticity of the developing brain, that is, the capacity of the developing neural system to organize in response to the contingencies of specific experience. The studies of ODC development document the importance of early experience in maintenance of basic patterns of areal organization, as well as the capacity of the developing neural system to adapt to significant alterations of input. Studies of animals and children with early localized brain injury provide an opportunity to further explore the range and limits of early brain plasticity and the role of experience in shaping the organization of the developing brain.

Finally, the general effects of postnatal experience on brain development will be explored by examination of studies in which the experimental manipulations are confined to the rearing environment. In these studies, there is no direct manipulation of the neural system. Rather, animals and, in some unfortunate "natural experiments," human children are exposed to either impoverished or experientially complex living environments. These studies demonstrate that rearing conditions can have a dramatic effect on brain development, altering the number and kinds of neural elements and connections. They provide important evidence of the role of experience in postnatal brain development.

## Elaboration and Modification of Areal Organization in the Cortex

As discussed in Chapter 5, graded expression of Pax6 and Emx2 provided the initial, very primitive specification of brain areas in the presumptive embryonic neocortex. That early patterning provided a rudimentary definition of sensory and motor cortical areas. However, within each of these primitive areas, organization is poorly defined. As development proceeds, both intrinsic and extrinsic factors will contribute to the ongoing elaboration of these cortical areas. Central questions about the ongoing process of specifying areal organization concern the extent to which intrinsic or extrinsic factors direct the elaboration and maintenance of areal fate.

This section will first examine the issue of how patterns of intra-areal organization emerge, using the emergence of ODCs in the PVC as an example. It begins with a summary of the classic work by Hubel and Wiesel on the effects of postnatal monocular deprivation on ODC organization, and introduces a widely accepted model of activity-dependent modulation of PVC organization to account for the observed changes. However, while this classic work documents an important role for extrinsic input in the modulation or maintenance of early postnatal PVC organization, it does not address the origins of this organization. A second question considered in this section asks whether the initial establishment, as opposed to maintenance, of ODCs is intrinsically controlled or dependent on extrinsically generated neural activity.

### Areal Organization of the Primary Visual Cortex

In a seminal series of studies, Hubel and Wiesel explored the role of experience in the emerging organization of the PVC. Their studies focused on a particular aspect of PVC organization, the ocular dominance columns. In the normal adult mammal, the PVC is organized into eye-specific columns referred to as ocular dominance columns (ODCs). Input projections from each eye remain segregated as the fibers of the optic nerve project from the retina to the primary subcortical visual relay nucleus, the lateral geniculate nucleus (LGN) of the thalamus. The segregation of eye-specific information is preserved at the level of the LGN, where visual inputs are partitioned into eye-specific layers (Figure 10.1). This segregation of information from the two eyes is maintained in projections from the LGN to layer 4, the principal input layer of the PVC (Figure 10.2A). The experiments by Hubel and Wiesel involved depriving young animals (cats and monkeys) of patterned visual input by suturing their eyelids closed. In some cases, deprivation was binocular, while in others only one eye was deprived. These manipulations had very different effects on the emerging organization of the PVC. The two key findings from that initial series of studies concerned the early emergence of cortical organization and its susceptibility to change depending on visual input.

Binocularly deprived animals showed very little effect of input loss. Three weeks of binocular deprivation had no effect on brain organization. By four weeks, visual selectivity began to deteriorate. By seven weeks, neural responses to patterned information were weak; however, basic ODC organization remained. This first finding suggests that the basic ODC organization of the PVC must be present at birth or within a few days of it, and that the development of this pattern of connectivity occurs even in the absence of patterned visual experience. Once the basic organization is established, complete deprivation can degrade the responsivity of cells to visual input, but basic organization into ODCs is preserved.

The experiments involving monocular deprivation produced a very different pattern of results. Animals that were deprived of input to one eye had profoundly defective vision in that eye. Their ability to visually follow a target or to use visual cues to direct motor activity was absent, and there was no hint of any ability to perceive form. Examination of the anatomical organization of emerging visual structures in the deprived animals was consistent with these data. For the anatomical studies, a retrograde, transneuronal tracer was injected into one of the animal's eyes. The tracer is taken up into the axons of the cells projecting from the retina to the LGN and is transported to the LGN cell bodies. From the LGN, the tracer is transported to cells within the PVC. Cells infused with the tracer appear dark on examination, while cells lacking tracer appear light. In normal, nondeprived animals, the tracer marks evenly spaced bands in both the LGN (Figure 10.1) and the PVC representing the inputs from the two eyes (Figure 10.2A). Examination of the organization of the LGN from monocularly deprived animals using the tracer methodology showed that although there was some change in size of LGN cells receiving input from the deprived eye, the differences were small, and the cells were functionally normal. By contrast, in the PVC, the patterns of innervation were dramatically altered by monocular deprivation (Figure 10.2B). The proportion of

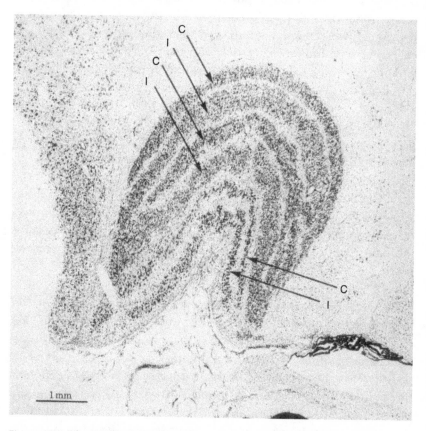

Figure 10.1. The LGN of the thalamus relays visual information from the retina to the PVC. The LGN is partitioned into eye-specific layers. The order of inputs in the dorsal (parvocellular) division of the LGN is contralateral (C), ipsilateral (I), contralteral, ipsilateral. The order of inputs to the ventral (magnocellular) layers is ipsilateral, contralateral. (From Hubel and Wiesel 1977. Reprinted with the permission of The Royal Society.)

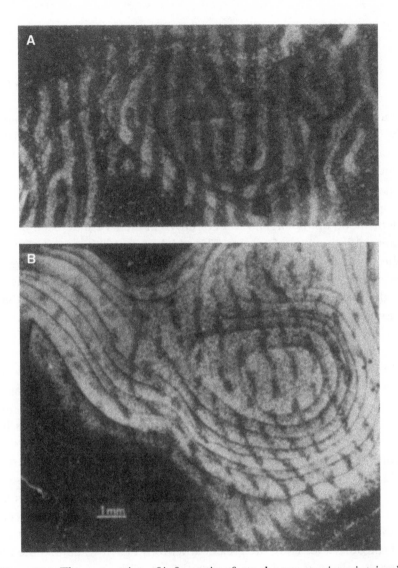

Figure 10.2. The segregation of information from the two eyes is maintained in projections from the LGN to layer 4 of the primary visual cortex. A. Ocular dominance column organization of a normal monkey. Cells receiving input from one eye are stained dark; inputs from the other eye are unstained. B. When young animals are deprived of patterned visual input via experimental eyelid suturing, the pattern of ocular dominance organization is altered. Inputs from the deprived eye (dark bands) have shrunk, while inputs from the nondeprived eye have expanded (light bands). (From Hubel, Wiesel, and LeVay 1977. Reprinted with the permission of The Royal Society.)

cells receiving input from the nondeprived eye (light bands) expanded relative to normal controls, while the proportion of cells receiving input from the deprived eye (dark bands) was dramatically reduced. Further, the effects of monocular deprivation were modulated by both the timing of the onset and the duration of the period of deprivation. Later onset and shorter periods of monocular deprivation mitigated the effects. These findings suggested an important role for input in the emerging organization of the cortical visual system.

Since the original studies of Hubel and Wiesel, the effects of early deprivation on the organization of ODCs in the PVC have been documented in a range of species. The widely accepted interpretation of the findings from these studies stresses the importance of extrinsic input in establishing the basic ODC organization of the PVC. That is, it is the specific pattern of visual input impinging on the two eyes that modulates patterns of neural activity along the visual pathway and ultimately determines the organization of ODC in the PVC. The concept most commonly associated with activity-dependent organization is Hebbian learning, in which a high correlation between pre- and post-synaptic firing is associated with increases in the strength of a connection, while a low correlation is associated with a reduction in connection strength. Thus the activity of a cell and its effectiveness in activating other cells are key to establishing connections within the brain. Furthermore, networks of cells firing synchronously will establish common pathways. Within the visual system, extrinsic visual input to each eye induces synchronous firing of the receptor cells in each retina, but the firing of cells in the retina of one eye is not necessarily correlated nor synchronous with the firing of cells in the retina of the other eye. Thus, the greater synchrony of activity among the receptor cells in a single eye directs the establishment of eye-specific pathways.

In the normal course of development the extrinsic inputs to the two eyes are comparable, and the two eyes compete in a balanced fashion for synaptic space within the PVC. These typical patterns of activation produce eye-specific bands within layer 4 of the PVC that are equal. When input is altered, as in the case of monocular deprivation, a disparity in input to the two eyes is introduced, thus creating a disparity in activity that results in the dominance of the more active, nondeprived eye. The mechanism underlying the change in PVC organization under conditions of monocular deprivation involves the processes of synaptic exuberance and elimination. The reduction of activity in the deprived eye makes that eye less able to compete for synaptic space; and in the absence of competition the active, nondeprived eye creates exuberant connections, resulting in the dramatic shifts in patterns of ODC banding observed within the PVC.

There is considerable evidence supporting this model of activity-dependent modulation of PVC organization during the postnatal period. That is, for a period beginning at approximately PW3 and extending for several months (in cats), experience has significant effects on the organization of the ODCs. It is during this period that the dramatic effects on ODC organization reported by Hubel and Weisel, and others, are observed. However, there is ongoing controversy over the role of activity in the initial specification of the ODC organization of the PVC. The key question revolves around whether neural activity is required for the initial ODC organization to emerge, or whether early ODC patterning is driven by intrinsic factors. The next sections consider the question of the origins of ODCs.

### The Origins of Ocular Dominance Columns

Activity-dependent models of cortical organization assume that the initial cortical projections are comparatively heterogeneous, lacking clear structure and organization. Early models of activity-dependent ODC development predicted that connections from the two eyes would initially be overlapping and interspersed, lacking the clear segregation of the mature eye-specific columns. Supporting this idea, the initial tracer studies of cats younger than three postnatal weeks (P22) exhibited a lack of eye-specific segregation. The evidence from this methodology was that ODCs begin to emerge at approximately P22 and reach adult levels of specification within approximately one month (LeVay, Stryker, and Shatz 1978).

However, studies using newer fiber-tracing methodologies suggest that ODC organization in the PVC may emerge earlier than predicted from the tracer studies. In ferrets, for example, sharp boundaries and clear segregation of the eye-specific inputs are reported at P16 to P21, three weeks earlier than reported for this species with tracer methods. Further, the ODCs form bands that are comparable in width and definition with those of adults (Crowley and Katz 2000, 2002). Even in monocularly deprived animals, column spacing is comparable with that in nondeprived animals (Schmidt et al. 2002). All these findings point to limitations on the role of activity in the initial phases of ODC formation.

Studies examining ODC organization over a more extended developmental period show that ODC organization emerges gradually along the extent of the visual pathway. Studies by Crair and colleagues (2001) reported that ODC development in cats extends from P7, which is two weeks earlier than previous estimates, through P21. These studies reported no evidence of eye-specific segregation in PVC at P7. However, at the time, they found clear eye-specific segregation within the LGN, suggesting that organization along the primary visual pathway had begun to emerge. By P14, they found initial evidence for eye-specific segregation in PVC, one week earlier than had previously been reported. The ODCs observed at P14 were spatially similar to, although somewhat less distinctive than, those of adult animals (Crair et al. 2001; Hua and Smith 2004). However, functional differences provided an index of immaturity at P14. Specifically, that data showed that functional input from the two eyes was imbalanced at this point in development, such that, within each cerebral hemisphere, inputs from the contralateral eye dominated those of the ipsilateral eye. By P21, clear evidence of eye-specific separation within the ODC and comparable responsiveness from the cells driven by the two eyes were observed. A similar profile of ODC development has been documented in ferrets (Crowley and Katz 2002).

These studies of early visual pathway development suggest that the emergence of mature patterns of ODC organization begins very early and proceeds gradually. However, they provide only suggestive evidence about the factors that influence the earliest stages of development. A number of studies have examined the possible contributions of various intrinsic and extrinsic factors in the initial formation of ODCs. First, it has been argued that spontaneous retinal firing occurring during early visual system development may provide the activity-dependent input required for the initial establishment of ODCs. It is well documented that from early in development, waves of retinal activity occur spontaneously and are typically confined to one eye (Meister et al. 1991; Wong et al. 1993), thus providing a possible basis for very early activity-driven, eye-specific organization within the visual pathway. However, enucleation studies have raised questions as to whether this spontaneous retinal activity is necessary for the formation of ODCs (Crowley and Katz 1999; Katz and Crowley 2002). In a typical enucleation study the presumed source of spontaneous retinal firing, the eye, is removed before the formation of ODCs in PVC begins. These studies report that ODCs develop normally in the absence of retinal activity in the enucleated animals, suggesting that some other, intrinsically based factor must underlie development of the ODC. However, more recent data have reasserted the possible importance of spontaneous retinal firing in the establishment of ODCs (Huberman, Speer, and Chapman 2006). Specifically, new techniques for silencing retinal neuron firing during the normal period of ODC formation resulted in degradation of the normal ODC patterning and an increase in the number of neurons exhibiting binocular responsivity. Thus the role of spontaneous retinal activity in early ODC development remains unclear.

A second line of evidence that has challenged the priority of activity-driven factors in ODC development comes from the data documenting an imbalance of eye-specific inputs during early visual system development. A number of investigators (e.g., Crair et al. 1998, 2001; Katz and Crowley 2002) have reported an imbalance of functional input to the PVC of each cerebral hemisphere during early stages of ODC formation. As discussed earlier, within each hemisphere, although a balanced anatomical distribution of inputs from the two eyes is observed, the contralateral inputs initially dominate ipsilateral inputs. These findings are not consistent with a simple activity-dependent account of ODC formation, because if activity determines ODC organization, the dominant inputs should take over the available cortical area and eliminate the weaker ipsilateral inputs. Studies of monocular deprivation in older animals clearly document that imbalanced input from the two eyes has precisely this effect on the organization of ODCs later in development. However, anatomical studies show that, early in development, the dominant activity from the contralateral eye does not drive the redistribution of neural resources within PVC (e.g., Crair et al. 2001); the spatial distribution of the ODCs is not affected by the early imbalanced input. These findings argue against a simple Hebbian account in which activity-dependent factors determine the initial organization of ODCs.

Finally, although there is clear evidence that ODCs begin to form by P14 in cats, in the period from P14 through P21, the organization of the eye-specific columns is not susceptible to the effects of monocular deprivation (Crowley and Katz 2002). Deprivation appears to have little effect on the emerging ocular dominance organization until after P21. These findings are consistent with the data on the effects of imbalanced input on early ODC development. Taken together, these data suggest that while activity may well contribute to the establishment of ODCs, intrinsic factors must also play a significant role. These findings have led to the suggestion that there may be two phases or stages in visual cortical development, an early precritical period and a later critical period.

### Two Stages in ODC Formation: A Precritical Period and a Critical Period

The distinction between what has been termed a precritical period of ODC formation and a critical period has been suggested as a way of unifying the data on ODC development (Feller and Scanziani 2005). There is considerable agreement that the critical period is dominated by activity-dependent reorganization and refinement of cortical networks. The hallmark of this period, which begins at P21 in cats (P38 in ferrets), is the overproduction and elimination of synaptic connections in response to input. In typical development, the activity-dependent modulation of synaptic connectivity gives rise to the mature patterns of organization within the cortex. Under conditions of early neural pathology, the plasticity exhibited by cells in response to input provides the opportunity to establish alternative patterns of brain organization that may in some cases serve to compensate for the early pathology.

Although the events of the critical period are well defined, there is less agreement about the characterization of the earlier precritical period. In some accounts, the precritical period is an activity-independent phase in which molecular cues and signaling serve to establish the basic adult profile of cortical organization (Crowley and Katz 2002; Ruthazer 2005). In other accounts, it is a period during which a rudimentary pattern of cortical organization is established, and that pattern is elaborated and refined during subsequent developmental periods to achieve the adult state. The early developmental mechanisms in these latter accounts include both activity-dependent and activity-independent factors (Feller and Scanziani 2005; Grubb and Thompson 2004; Kantor and Kolodkin 2003).

The onset of the critical period in the development of the visual system is closely linked to the development of the GABAergic system (Hensch 2005). For example, brain derived nerve growth factor (BDNF) accelerates GABA system development and leads to early onset of the critical period in studies of the effects of monocular deprivation (Hensch 2004). As discussed in the last section, before the onset of the critical period, activity appears to have little effect on the development of excitatory neural systems that define ODC functioning. However, early, precritical period activity has been shown to be essential for the early development of the inhibitory systems, and thus necessary for the transition to the critical period (Bence and Levelt 2005). Dark rearing has been shown to interfere with the development of GABAergic neurons, resulting in more spontaneous activity and longer responses to visual stimuli. Under conditions of early monocular deprivation, arbors of the GABAergic neurons of the deprived eye show less branching and reduced total length, while the nondeprived eye shows the opposite effect. These findings define a role for input in the early development of this system. The inhibitory system appears to play a critical modulatory role in the initiation of the critical period, in which activity-dependent modification and refinement of the excitatory system are essential for normal cortical development. Further, activity appears to play a critical role in the development of the inhibitory GABAergic system.

Finally, the defining characteristic of the critical period is the capacity of activity to shape and direct cortical organization. A primary mechanism of activity-dependent change during the critical period has been associated with Hebbian learning and more particularly with NMDA receptor activity. NMDA receptor activity has been specifically implicated in ODC formation during the critical period. When NMDA receptor activity is experimentally blocked in monocularly deprived animals, critical-period effects on column formation are eliminated. Specifically, no shift in the organization of columns is observed. NMDA receptors also play an important role in dendritic spine growth in that the activity of NMDA receptors induces spine formation (Hua and Smith 2004). Blocking the activity of NMDA receptors inhibits dendritic arbor growth

(Cohen-Cory 2002). In addition, NMDA receptors induce the movement of a second type of ionotropic glutamate receptor, the AMPA receptor, to the synaptic sites (Cohen-Cory 2002). AMPA receptors play a complementary role to NMDA receptors in dendritic spine development. While NMDA receptors act in an activity-dependent fashion to induce spine formation, AMPA receptors act later to induce changes that serve to stabilize and regularize the shape and thus the functionality of the spines (Fischer et al. 2000). NMDA receptor activation also induces the synthesis and release of neurotrophins, specifically BDNF (Hua and Smith 2004).

## Clinical Correlation: Effects of Congenital Cataracts on Human Visual Development

Studies of visual development in children with congenital cataracts parallel the experimental animal studies in their investigation of the role of activity-dependent and activity-independent factors in affecting outcome. Cataracts are any clouding or opacity of the lens of the eye (Levin 2003). When the cataract is dense, it can block patterned vision, allowing only diffuse light to reach the retina (Maurer, Lewis, and Mondloch 2005). Congenital cataracts occur in approximately 2.2 to 2.5 of 10,000 live births and can be either unilateral or bilateral (Francis and Moore 2004). Maurer and colleagues have studied a large group of children with binocular or monocular congenital cataracts and compared their visual development with that of typical controls. Typically developing newborn children have very poor acuity, approximately 40 times worse than that of adults. Acuity improves quickly. By six months acuity is only 8 times worse than normal adult acuity, and by age four to six years it reaches adult levels. Other aspects of visual functioning develop on different timetables, with some maturing as early as three months and others as late as early adolescence (Lewis and Maurer 2005).

Examination of the initial effects of deprivation on visual development (Maurer et al. 1999) came from a study of infants less than one year of age. The children were tested following surgery to remove cataracts and immediately after they were fitted with corrective lenses. The children's visual acuity was tested within 10 minutes of fitting with the corrective lens and again after 1 hour, 1 week, and 1 month

(Figure 10.3). At the 10-minute test, acuity in the deprived eyes was very poor, approximating that of a typical newborn. Acuity improved from immediate test to 1 hour and continued to improve at 1 week and 1 month. Data from children obtained in the first year of life indicated that improvement did not differ by age at receipt of contact lenses, and improvement was the same for both monocular and binocular cases. However, by the end of the first year, both the long-term effects of early deprivation and the effects of competition induced by

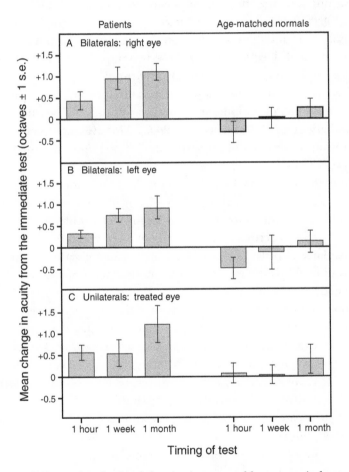

Figure 10.3. Effects of early visual deprivation caused by congenital cataracts in children less than one year of age. After surgery for removal of cataracts and provision of corrective lenses, changes in acuity were observed over time. (From Maurer et al. 1999. Adapted with the permission of AAAS.)

monocular deprivation became more evident, and factors such as onset and duration of deprivation became more prominent.

Among children with binocular cataracts operated on early, subtle and permanent deficits in visual acuity were evident when they were tested in later childhood and adolescence. When tested between 5 and 18 years, most had reduced acuity. Contrast sensitivity (the measure of the amount of contrast needed to detect a pattern) and peripheral vision were also reduced (Lewis and Maurer 2005). Importantly, two visual functions that develop very early, perception of global motion and global form, showed consistently greater compromise following bilateral than unilateral deprivation. It appears that input is essential for the normal development of these two important visual functions, but the input need not be typical. Any input early in development, such as that available when deprivation is monocular, is enough to support the normal development of these early-established visual abilities (Ellemberg et al. 2002; Lewis et al. 2002). However, complete deprivation results in permanent impairment of these important aspects of visual processing.

Although the initial effects of monocular and binocular deprivation follow a similar pattern, competitive effects of early monocular deprivation become more apparent after the first year of life. Without treatment, outcomes across a range of measures of visual function for the monocularly deprived eye can be worse than for cases of binocular deprivation. Thus the effects of intervention are a particularly important factor in determining outcome in this group of children. The typical therapeutic intervention for monocular deprivation is patching of the nondeprived eye. Maximum effects of this intervention are achieved when it is initiated early (before six to eight weeks) and there is good compliance with the daily patching regimen (six to eight hours per day). Early intensive intervention results in good final acuity and contrast sensitivity, with outcomes comparable to or better than those of binocular cases. Without compliance and early treatment, outcomes for these children are much worse than for children with bilateral cataracts on measures of visual acuity, contrast sensitivity, and peripheral vision.

The data from these studies suggest that, as is seen in other mammalian species, initial development of visual function appears to be driven by visual activity in a noncompetitive fashion. Competition emerges as an important factor only later in development. In humans, its effects begin at approximately two months and become prominent after one year of life. The effects of competitive imbalance continue until at least six years of age and for some functions continue until late childhood (Lewis and Maurer 2005).

## Respecifying Functional Identity within a Neocortical Area

A number of studies have explored questions about the extent to which early patterning within the cortical plate fixes the fate of neurons within the newly emerging cortical areas. Specifically, can the fate of cells initially induced by cortical progenitors to take on the characteristics of the visual, auditory, or somatosensory cortex be altered by subsequent exposure to a different set of signaling cues? These questions have been addressed by cortical explant studies in which, for example, tissue from the visual cortex of a donor animal is transplanted to the somatosensory area of a host animal, and by studies in which the major sensory input pathways to a cortical area are redirected, for example by directing retinal input to primary auditory cortex. The next sections will examine the effects of these kinds of manipulations on the emerging functional organization of cortical areas.

### Early Patterning and Fate Restriction of Neural Tissue

Cortical explant studies have been used to examine whether local signaling cues within a cortical region can influence the fate of transplanted cells. The findings of these studies suggest that, at least early in development, specific local signaling is necessary to maintain a cell's functional fate.

O'Leary and Stanfield (1989) transplanted sections of the sensorimotor cortex and the occipital cortex from the brain of a late fetal rat into the complementary regions of the brain of a newborn rat. Thus sensorimotor tissue of the fetal donor animal was transplanted to the visual occipital region of the newborn host, and occipital tissue was transplanted to the sensorimotor region. For both sections of explanted tissue, the cells survived and began to take on characteristics of cells in the host environment. Specifically, cells from the visual cortex transplanted into the host sensorimotor areas extended projections and established permanent axonal connections to the spinal cord, a subcortical target for sensorimotor neurons. Sensorimotor tissue transplanted into the visual cortex initially extended axons to the spinal cord, but these connections were subsequently lost. However, these cells also extended axons to the superior colliculus, a subcortical visual target, and these were retained. Transplanted tissues in both areas established callosal and thalamic projections typical of their host environment.

Other studies examined intra-areal organization of the transplanted tissues and also found evidence of adaptation of cells to the host environment. Somatosensory regions of the rat cortex typically form well-demarcated anatomical features, called "barrels," that form a "barrel-field" organization that corresponds to the input from facial vibrissae (whiskers). In this experiment, visual area tissue from a fetal donor was transplanted to the somatosensory area of a host animal. The transplanted visual tissue developed the characteristic barrel-field patterning. This result further supports the idea that neural tissue has the capacity to adapt to the local signaling cues (Schlaggar and O'Leary 1991).

These studies suggest that although cortical neurons initially receive cues that signal their differentiation and direct their development in ways appropriate to their positional value, this early specification is not fixed. Exposure to cues arising from different brain areas can induce further differentiation of the young neurons, directing an alternative developmental pathway that is appropriate for establishing connectivity within the experimentally respecified brain region.

## The Effects of Input on Brain Organization and Function

One important series of studies examining the role of input in establishing the organization of the PAC involved what have become known as "cortical rewiring" procedures. In the cortical-rewiring studies, normal connection pathways and target regions are systematically altered to eliminate either a cortical target region or the normal dominant input to a target. The key question in these studies is whether systematic alteration in competitive inputs will redirect the anatomical and functional organization of the remaining cortical targets and input pathways. The first demonstration that lesions of subcortical structures could alter the projection patterns of major sensory pathways came from Schneider's work with hamsters (Schneider 1973). Subsequent studies have elaborated upon that early work, documenting changes in the anatomical organization at the level of both the thalamus and the neocortex and demonstrating that the "rewired" cortex is able to support alternative functions.

### Rerouting Visual Input to the PAC

Cortical rewiring studies introduce experimental manipulations that are designed to alter the basic patterns of connectivity in the cortex. The normal visual pathway projects from the sensory receptors in the retina both to eye-specific layers in the LGN of the thalamus and to the superior colliculus. The LGN then projects to the PVC, establishing the primary cortical visual pathway. The normal auditory pathway projects from the sensory receptors in the cochlea to the inferior colliculus to the medial geniculate nucleus (MGN) of the thalamus and finally to the PAC. In a series of early studies, Sur and his colleagues (Pallas, Roe, and Sur 1990; Sur, Garraghty, and Roe 1988) removed the visual cortex and the superior colliculus of one-day-old ferrets, thus eliminating two major visual-system target areas. They also eliminated the major input pathways from the inferior colliculi to the MGN of the thalamus, thus greatly reducing auditory pathway input to the PAC. The lesions induced retinal axons to project to the MGN and the MGN to carry the resulting visual information to the PAC. A visual input pathway to the PAC was thus established. Later studies showed that a visual pathway from the MGN to the PAC could be established by simply destroying the auditory inputs to the MGN; elimination of the primary visual cortical target is neither necessary nor sufficient to induce rewiring of the auditory cortex (Angelucci et al. 1997).

### Anatomical Consequences of Rewiring

More detailed examination documented significant change in anatomical organization at the level of both the thalamus and the cortex. As discussed earlier, the normal LGN is organized into distinct layers that reflect the separation of inputs from the two eyes, and that separation is reflected in the eye-specific bands within the input layer of the PVC. Further, the topographical organization of visual input is projected onto the retina, and that retinotopic organization provides a two-dimensional map of visual space that is maintained at the level of the thalamus and the PVC. In the normal MGN, terminal clusters of axons that provide input from the inferior colliculus are aligned in a linear sequence within the ventral division of the MGN. Each terminal cluster transmits information about a small range of sound frequencies. Input to the clusters then projects to the PAC, establishing its characteristic one-dimensional tonotopic organization.

In rewired animals, retinal inputs to the MGN initially overlap, but by the third postnatal week, they segregate into eye-specific clusters, thus approximating the organization of the LGN. Furthermore, MGN projections to PAC establish a two-dimensional, retinotopic pattern of connectivity, thus establishing a cortical region very similar in organization to the PVC. Other features of visual cortex organization, including orientation and direction-specific mapping, also emerge in the rewired PAC. Thus much of the effect of altering the sensory input is to transform the function of PAC from auditory to visual. However, some features of normal auditory cortex are maintained, including lamination, cell density, and thalamocortical arborization. In addition, the visual maps are somewhat less refined than those observed in the normal visual cortex (Sur and Leamey 2001).

*Does the Rewired Primary Auditory Cortex Function as a Visual Area?*
A number of studies have examined the functional integrity of the rewired cortex. One approach is to introduce the rewiring procedure in one hemisphere, leaving the other hemisphere intact. At the outset of these experiments, within the rewired hemisphere, both the normal retina-LGN-PVC and the rewired retina-MGN-PAC pathways were functional. Animals were then trained to respond to either an auditory cue or a visual cue. The visual cue was presented to either the intact or the rewired visual system. Visual performance in response to cues presented to both the intact and rewired hemispheres was high and comparable, documenting both the efficacy of training and the visual proficiency of the rewired animals. Next, the normal visual pathway was lesioned in the rewired hemisphere, leaving only the rewired "visual" pathway to the PAC. After recovery from surgery, the animals were again tested, and again their performance was high and comparable in the intact and rewired hemispheres. As a final control, the rewired

pathway was lesioned, and when visual performance was then measured, performance fell to chance for stimuli presented to the rewired hemisphere. This experiment provided strong evidence that the rewired auditory cortex was responsive to visual input. It also confirmed that the rewiring procedure altered the functional, as well as the structural, organization of the PAC, creating a second visual cortical area in these animals.

However, there was evidence that the rewired visual system may be less effective than the normal system. In a second experiment, the animals that had undergone the second surgical procedure and thus had only the rewired retina-MGN-PAC pathway intact within the rewired hemisphere were tested on measures of visual acuity. Acuity was tested by presenting spatial frequency gratings at different levels of contrast to either the rewired or the intact hemisphere. The animals were able to distinguish spatial frequency gratings presented to both the intact and rewired hemispheres. However, visual acuity mediated by the rewired visual system was substantially reduced (von Melchner, Pallas, and Sur 2000). This experiment again confirmed the capacity of neural systems to adapt to unconventional input and establish alternative patterns of connectivity and functionality. However, it also points out that although the adapted system may be functional, it may not be as optimal or as efficient in mediating the acquired function.

### Analogous Findings in Humans

A variety of functional neuroimaging techniques have been used to explore the possibility of similar patterns of functional cortical reallocation in humans. Studies of individuals with early-onset auditory or visual sensory loss have provided a means of examining functional reorganization in humans. A number of studies report findings consistent with the animal studies that use cortical-rewiring techniques. For example, Fine, Finney, and Dobkins (Fine et al. 2005; Finney, Fine, and Dobkins 2001) used functional magnetic resonance imaging (FMRI) to look at patterns of brain activation in both hearing and congenitally deaf individuals. FMRI is a rapid imaging technique that can be used to detect subtle changes in local magnetic-field signal strength associated with increases in blood flow and changes in oxygen extraction that are triggered by neural activity. Fine and colleagues imaged hearing individuals performing both auditory and visual motion-detection tasks and deaf individuals performing only the visual motion-detection task. Not surprisingly, on auditory tasks, activation was found within an extended region of the superior temporal cortex, including the PAC, in hearing individuals. These areas were used as regions of interest (ROIs) in the examination of patterns of activation on the visual task. The most critical finding from the analysis of the visual task data was that deaf individuals activated a subregion of the ROI, defined as auditory areas in hearing individuals. Specifically, regions of the right superior temporal lobe, including secondary and associative auditory areas, as well as portions of the PAC activated in deaf, but not hearing individuals on the visual task. The findings of activation within the PAC are consistent with the cortical-rewiring studies, and the more extensive activation within secondary and associative auditory areas by visual stimuli supports a larger body of work showing that effects of altered early experience may extend beyond primary sensory areas into multimodal cortical areas. For example, a number of studies have reported activation in secondary and associative auditory cortices of congenitally deaf individuals to visual presentation of sign language (MacSweeney et al. 2002; Nishimura et al. 2000). However, the findings concerning the primary sensory cortex should be interpreted with some caution. Other studies have reported that not all deaf individuals show activation in the PAC to visual stimulation (Bavelier and Neville 2002; Hickok, Bellugi, and Klima 1997; Nishimura et al. 1999), and some have reported activation by visual input among hearing individuals (Bavelier and Neville 2002). Still other reports suggest that both age at onset and degree of sensory deprivation may influence the degree to which the cortical system will reorganize (Bavelier and Neville 2002; Lambertz et al. 2005; Sadato et al. 2004).

## The Effects of Localized Postnatal Brain Injury on Neocortical Organization

Early intrinsic signaling and afferent input work in concert to define the initial organization of the developing neocortex (Sur and Rubenstein 2005) such that by the early postnatal period, cortical networks are in place that can support basic sensory and motor functions, rudimentary learning, and simple social interaction. But cortical organization in the newborn is far from complete, and over the next two decades, extrinsic factors play an essential, though not exclusive, role in shaping and defining the cortical circuits. Animal and human studies of the effects of localized cortical and subcortical injury on the developing brain have provided insight into the capacity of the developing brain to respond flexibly to perturbations of normal postnatal patterning. They have helped define the dynamic nature of early brain development and the capacity of the emerging neural system to adapt to both early insult and experience. But the capacity for adaptation also has limits that reflect both the temporal and the emerging structural constraints that underlie and define the process of brain development. The pace of development is not uniform across brain regions. Myelination, an index of pathway maturity and stabilization, proceeds in a well-defined progression from subcortical to cortical and then caudal to rostral. Within that general progression, cortical sensory areas mature earlier than association areas. Just as early intrinsic signaling defined the essential organization of the brain, progressive stabilization of the developing neural system gradually constrains the capacity for adaptation. Three examples of the effects of early localized brain injury will illustrate both the extent and the limits of early brain plasticity.

### Effects of Neonatal Lesions on the Visual Recognition Pathway

The neural pathway that underpins visual recognition memory involves ventral regions of occipital and temporal cortex, as well as medial temporal lobe (MTL) structures. In rhesus monkeys, the pathway begins in the PVC and projects to multiple prestriate areas in the occipital cortex, to the posterior inferior temporal cortex (TEO) to the anterior inferior temporal cortex (TE), and then to limbic structures in the MTL (amygdala, hippocampus, rhinal cortex; Figure 10.4). The interaction of area TE with the limbic system structures is critical for visual recognition memory (Mishkin, Ungerleider, and Macko 1983; Webster, Bachevalier, and Ungerleider 1995b; Webster, Ungerleider, and Bachevalier 1991b). In adult monkeys, lesions to cortical area TE impair performance on a variety of visual recognition memory tasks (Bachevalier and Mishkin 1994). However, the effects of lesions introduced in the neonatal period are much milder.

One task that has been widely used to test visuospatial memory performance is the delayed nonmatch to sample (DNMS) task. In the standard DNMS task, a sample object is placed over a well containing a reward, and then the animal or child is allowed to move the object and retrieve the reward. After a 10-second delay, the sample object and a novel object are placed over two separate, adjacent wells, but only the well under the novel object contains a reward. Thus the task is to select the novel object. Bachevalier and Mishkin (1994) tested normal infant and adult monkeys and infant and adult monkeys with lesions to area TE on the DNMS task (Figure 10.5A). Normal adult and infant monkeys learned to perform at above 90 percent on this task. For monkeys lesioned in adulthood, performance dropped to 71 percent, while the performance of lesioned infants (surgery at 2 weeks and tested at 10 months) was near normal at 84 percent. Furthermore, when the monkeys lesioned early were tested at age 4, their performance remained high at 85 percent (Malkova, Mishkin, and Bachevalier 1995). These

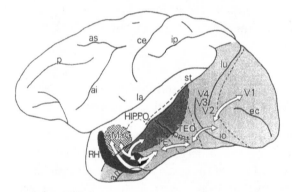

Figure 10.4. The visual recognition pathway in rhesus monkeys begins in the primary visual cortex (VI), projects to multiple prestriate areas in the occipital cortex, to area TEO in the posterior inferior temporal lobe, to area TE in the anterior inferior temporal lobe, and then to limbic structures in the medial temporal lobe (rhinal cortex [RH], amygdala [AMYG], and hippocampus [HIPPO]). Sulcal abbreviations: ai, inferior arcuate; amt, anterior middle temporal; as, superior arcuate; ce, central; ec, external calcarine; io, inferior occipital; ip, intraparietal; la, lateral; lu, lunate; p, principal; pmt, posterior middle temporal; st, superior temporal. (From Ungerleider and Murray 1992. Reprinted with the permission of Gale, a division of Thomson Learning.)

data suggest that early in development the neural substrate may be capable of compensatory reorganization. Indeed, other work by this group of investigators has suggested a possible profile of reorganization.

Webster, Ungerleider, and Bachevalier (1991a) have shown that early in development, both area TE and area TEO establish direct connections with structures in the limbic system. In the normal course of development, the connections between TE and the limbic system stabilize and become part of the primary pathway for visual recognition memory, while the connections between TEO and the limbic system are lost. However, when area TE is lesioned early in development, the normally transient connections between TEO and limbic structures are retained, thus providing a possible alternative pathway for visual memory processing. In addition, these investigators have demonstrated that a number of visual association areas, including the superior temporal polysensory area (STP), the caudal inferior parietal cortex (PG), and a region of the posterior parahippocampal gyrus (TF), which are not typically involved in visual recognition memory, become important links after early TE lesions. In separate studies, adult monkeys that had been lesioned in area TE as infants were given second lesions as adults (Figure 10.5B). In one group, the second lesion involved area TEO only, resulting in a group with an early TE and a late TEO lesion. In a second group, only areas STP, PG, and TF were involved (early TE and late SPT, PG, and TF), and in a third group areas TEO plus STP, PG, and TF were lesioned (early TE and late TEO, SPT, PG, and TF). Only the third group of monkeys, that is, the ones that had lesions of all target brain areas, showed evidence of impairment on the DNMS task. Ablation of TEO or the visual association areas alone was not sufficient to impair performance on this task. Thus, in the context of early TE lesions, it was only when both TEO and the visual association areas were removed that performance was affected (Webster, Bachevalier, and Ungerleider 1995b). These results suggest considerable reorganization and plasticity within this temporal-lobe system.

In a subsequent series of studies, these investigators examined the role of MTL structures in performance on the DNMS task and obtained results that contrasted sharply with the findings of the neocortical lesion studies. Recall that TE projects to the MTL. One particularly

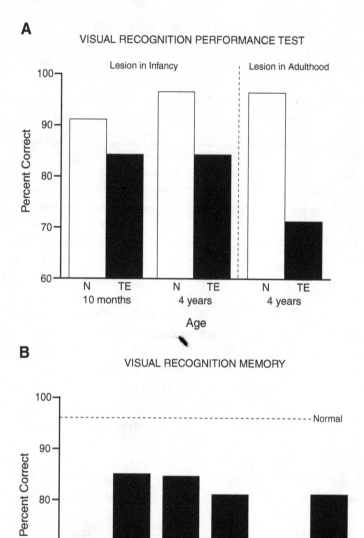

A

VISUAL RECOGNITION PERFORMANCE TEST

Lesion in Infancy          Lesion in Adulthood

Percent Correct

N    TE        N    TE        N    TE
10 months      4 years        4 years

Age

B

VISUAL RECOGNITION MEMORY

Percent Correct

- - - - - - - - - - - - - - - - - - - - - - - Normal

Adult TE    Infant TE    Infant TE    Infant TE    Infant TE    Adult STP
N=3         N=13         Adult TEO    Adult STP    Adult STP    PG, TF, TEO
                         N=4          PG, TF       PG, TF, TEO  N=4
                                      N=3          N=3

important MTL structure is the hippocampus, which in adults mediates explicit memory. In humans, neurogenesis in the hippocampus extends throughout the first year of postnatal life, and synapse formation continues until approximately age five (Seress 2001); in rhesus monkeys, the comparable period of development is approximately one year. However, although hippocampal development continues until well into early childhood, early damage to this structure does not appear to be something that can be easily compensated for. Neonatal lesions of the hippocampus have a significant and lasting effect on specific aspects of memory. Performance on a visuospatial version of the DNMS task among monkeys lesioned in the neonatal period was as compromised as the performance of monkeys lesioned as adults (Alvarado, Wright, and Bachevalier 2002). These findings provide a clear example of the limits of plasticity in the developing brain. Although the neocortical circuit involved in mediation of visual recognition exhibits considerable capacity for reorganization, the plasticity of the hippocampus is much more restricted. As the authors suggest, "Despite the special neural plasticity present early in life, no other structures or circuits can serve as a hippocampal substitute in enabling these forms of memory" (Bachevalier and Vargha-Khadem 2005, p. 170). It is important to note that a similar pattern of memory deficit has been reported among children with isolated bilateral hippocampal lesions (Isaacs et al. 2003).

## Effects of Cortical and Subcortical Lesions of the Frontal Lobe

In adult monkeys, lesions to the dorsolateral prefrontal cortex profoundly affect performance on spatial working memory tasks (Goldman 1971; Goldman, Rosvold, and Mishkin 1970). Goldman-Rakic demon-

---

Figure 10.5. *(Opposite Page)* The effects of early and late lesions on DNMS task performance. A Monkeys lesioned in adulthood are impaired in the DNMS task, while monkeys lesioned in infancy initially show considerable sparing that is retained at 4 years of age (adulthood). B. Monkeys lesioned as infants were lesioned a second time in adulthood. Only monkeys with a second lesion involving TEO, PG, STP, and TF showed significant impairment. (From Webster, Bachevalier, and Ungerleider 1995a. Adapted with the permission of Addision-Wesley.)

strated that the timing of cortical lesions has a marked effect on performance. She compared the performance of monkeys lesioned as neonates with that of monkeys lesioned at one year using a delayed-response task. On a simple spatial delayed-response task, she found that monkeys with early lesions performed significantly better than monkeys with later lesions; performance on more difficult delayed alternation was somewhat impaired in the group with early lesions, but to a lesser degree than animals with later lesions. Longitudinal examination of these same monkeys a year later revealed that the monkeys with early lesions had lost ground relative to normally developing monkeys on the delayed-alternation task. Rather than the normal profile of developmental improvement with age, no change in performance was observed.

Goldman and Rosvold (1972) also examined the effects of lesions to a critical subcortical structure, the caudate nucleus, which normally has extensive connections to the dorsolateral prefrontal cortex. Caudate nucleus lesions produce deficits on both the delayed-response and the delayed alteration tasks in adult monkeys. In contrast to the studies of the effects of early neocortical lesions on working memory tasks, Goldman-Rakic reported that neonatal lesions to subcortical structures within the frontal working memory circuit lead to levels of impairment comparable with those observed among monkeys lesioned as adults (Goldman 1974). These data suggest that the neural systems responsible for processing information at different points in development may not be identical. One account of the data reported here is that early in development, the subcortical system may play a larger role in performance on the delayed-response and delayed alteration tasks than it does later in development, thus producing the initial sparing of function with early cortical lesions on this task. However, the subcortical system is not optimal for this task, and in the normal course of development the prefrontal cortical system takes over this function. The animal lesioned early continues to rely on the subcortical system and thus appears to lose ground with development relative to its normally developing, cortically intact peers. Early subcortical lesions deprive the animal of the early primary processing, which interferes with subsequent development of the neural system. Animals with early subcortical lesions exhibit serious impairments during infancy that do not resolve with development.

## Site and Timing of Brain Lesions

Kolb and his colleagues have reported differential effects of lesions depending on the age at lesion, lesion location, and environmental input following early injury (Kolb and Whishaw 1989). They compared the effects of removing one hemisphere of the brain to those of removing either the frontal lobes or the posterior parietal lobes bilaterally, and they varied the timing of the lesion to include four groups: the 1st day (D1), 5 days (D5), and 10 days (D10) after birth, plus an adult lesion control group (DA). The Morris water-maze task was used to assess the effects of lesion on spatial problem solving (Morris 1984). In this task, which normal animals solve in a few trials, rats are placed in a tank filled with opaque liquid and trained to find a submerged platform. Kolb and his colleagues found that the effects of bilateral frontal (Kolb and Elliott 1987) or parietal lobe lesions (Kolb, Holmes, and Whishaw 1987) differed from those of hemidecortication, but the timing of lesions also affected outcome (Kolb and Tomie 1988). Overall, outcomes for animals with unilateral lesions were significantly better than for those with bilateral lesions. Regardless of the timing of lesions, hemidecorticated animals performed better than animals that had been given bilateral lesions. However, among the early unilateral-lesion groups, performance was better for the animals with earlier lesions than those with later lesions.

The effects of bilateral lesions provided a very different profile in that the most serious impairments were observed among animals with earliest lesions. For both the bilateral frontal and parietal cases, animals lesioned on D1 performed significantly worse than DA animals, while the performance of animals lesioned on D5 was comparable with that of DA animals. Critically, performance of animals with D10 lesions was significantly better than that of the DA animals. Although there was compromise of performance relative to nonlesioned or hemidecorticated animals, the later bilateral lesions allowed for greater recovery of function than earlier bilateral lesions.

A comparison of findings from these two studies suggests that unilateral lesions allow for greater neural compensation than bilateral lesions, and that the earlier the onset of a unilateral lesion, the greater the capacity for reorganization. By contrast, recovery is more limited with bilateral injury, and the effect of timing differs greatly. Early bilateral lesions are the most devastating, and although later lesions are serious, they are accompanied by some degree of compensation. These findings, like those that suggest differences in outcome with subcortical versus cortical prefrontal lesions and those that indicate limited recovery from hippocampal lesions, raise important questions about the limits on the capacity of the developing brain to respond to early injury.

In a separate study, which combined the lesion methodology with an enriched-environment technique, Kolb has shown that even the detrimental effects of lesions can be mitigated with input from the environment (Kolb and Elliott 1987; Kolb and Whishaw 1989). Animals with bilateral frontal-lobe lesions administered at D1, D5, and D10 were raised either in an enriched environment or in isolated laboratory cages. After three months, the performance of the D1 and D5 rats raised in the enriched environment was indistinguishable from that of the D10 rats, indicating a dramatic enhancement in the performance of the D1 and D5 rats (Kolb and Elliott 1987). These studies suggest that early brain development is dynamic and subject to both endogenous and external effects. Early brain damage has detrimental effects that are specific to the timing and location of the lesion, but the effects of early injury can, at least in some cases, be mitigated by the organism's interaction with the environment.

## The Effects of Rearing Environment on Brain Development

A more general case for the impact of the environment on brain development comes from studies in which the rearing conditions of young and older animals are systematically altered. These types of studies show quite dramatically that rearing conditions can affect behavioral outcome. A classic early observation by Hebb (1949) suggested superior maze learning in "home"-reared versus laboratory-reared rats. In the 1960s, studies by Rosenzweig and the Berkeley Group (e.g., Bennett, Rosenzweig, and Diamond 1969; Rosenzweig and Bennett 1972; Rosenzweig et al. 1962a, 1962b; Rosenzweig, Love, and Bennett 1968) were among the first to demonstrate explicit effects of environmental enrichment on brain anatomy and chemistry. Uylings and colleagues (1978) documented that the effects of the environment are not confined to young animals, but are also observed among adults. Adults reared in a complex environment showed significant thickening of frontal and occipital cortices that reflected lengthening of terminal dendritic segments and increased branching. More recently, Greenough and colleagues (Greenough and Chang 1988; Grossman et al. 2002; Markham and Greenough 2004), in an extensive series of studies with rats, have demonstrated that variation in environmental conditions can affect patterns of synaptic connectivity in the developing brain.

Consistent with earlier studies, Greenough and colleagues looked specifically at changes in brain morphology associated with rearing condition. Identical strains of rats were reared under three conditions: individual cage (IC), social cage (SC), and environmental complexity (EC). The individual and social cages were standard laboratory cages containing only food and water. In the IC condition, rats were reared in isolation, while in the SC condition, they were reared in small groups. In the EC condition, animals were housed in groups of 12 or more in large cages filled with a variety of objects. Animals were free to explore, and the objects in the cage were changed frequently. Different groups of rats were reared from birth to adolescence in the three conditions. Examination of the brains of animals in the three groups revealed significant differences in the number of dendrites per neuron, that is, in the amount of synaptic space available for each neuron. Animals reared in the EC condition had 20 to 25 percent more dendrites than animals reared in the other two conditions (see also Jones et al. 1997 for discussion of selective increases in multiple versus single synapse contacts). These effects were not associated with any specific feature of the enriched-environment condition, nor were they accounted for by general metabolic differences in animals reared in the enriched condition. Animals fitted with a monocular occluder and reared in the EC environment showed evidence of unilateral exuberance of dendrites in visual areas. This result linked the changes in dendritic branching specifically to the experience of the animal (Chang and Greenough 1982).

Greenough has also used cortical lesion techniques to examine the effects of experience on brain organization (Jones, Kleim, and Greenough 1996) The forelimb region of the somatosensory cortex was lesioned in a group of adult rats. Different subgroups of lesioned animals were then sacrificed at 10, 18, or 30 days after surgery. Systematic changes were observed in layer 5 of the remaining contralateral somatosensory cortex. Specifically, compared with sham operated rats, the lesioned rats showed increases both in the number of synapses per neuron and in the surface area of the dendritic membrane that were statistically significant by 30 days after surgery. These changes coincided with observed increased use of the surgically unaffected limb during the postoperative period. The authors suggest that these increases in neural elements are, at least in part, the product of lesion-induced increases in the use of the unaffected limb. Thus, once again, these data provide an example of experience-based (in this case activity-based) changes in the neural substrate.

Experience has also been shown to affect nonneural brain elements. Exposure to the EC environment increases both the number and the complexity of astrocytes in the developing brain (Jones and Greenough 1996). This result suggests that the effects of environmental complexity extend to neuronal support cells. As reported in Chapter 9, myelination is affected by rearing condition. Szeligo and Leblond (1977) were the first to report an association between experience and the amount of subcortical white matter. Later studies confirmed increases in the number of oligodendrocytes in EC-reared animals (Sirevaag and Greenough 1987). Finally, experience induces change in the cerebrovascular system. Animals reared in EC environments have larger and more complex capillary systems (Black, Sirevaag, and Greenough 1987).

The patterns of synaptic exuberance follow different developmental trajectories depending on the age of the animals in Greenough's studies. In young animals, the enhanced synaptic production is superimposed on the typical profile of synaptic exuberance and pruning. Recall that Huttenlocher (Huttenlocher and Dabholkar 1997; Huttenlocher and de Courten 1987) showed that synapse production in the postnatal period follows an inverted U-shaped function. There is an initial exuberant production of synapses that far exceeds the numbers observed for adults, which is followed by a systematic pruning back of synapses until the typical adult numbers are achieved. In Greenough's studies, the groups reared in both the isolated and complex environments exhibited an early postnatal increase in synaptogenesis followed by a pruning back of synapse numbers. However, the effect of experience was reflected in the enhanced magnitude of synapse numbers across the period. Greenough has suggested that this profile reflects the normal "experience-expectant" patterns of change that are characteristic of early development. The later enhancement of synaptogenesis found among adult animals reflects a different set of underlying processes. The acceleration of synapse production in mature animals is thought to be explicitly dependent upon the experience of the organism. The "experience-dependent" processes associated with increased synaptogenesis in adult animals are not confined to the early period of development. Rather, experience-dependent processes, such as the enhanced synapse production associated with exposure to complex environments, extend across the lifespan and are considered to be the neural basis of learning.

## Gene-Environment Interactions

As observed in the preceding sections of this chapter, a significant body of evidence documents the role of experience in brain development. In immature organisms, both central and peripheral alterations of neural systems induce the emergence of alternative patterns of brain organization, resulting in the formation of functional but atypical neural networks. Natural or experimental manipulation of sensory input can also redirect neural pathway organization and redefine stable patterns of mature connectivity. Even variations that arise entirely from conditions in the external world can have dramatic effects on the complexity of a wide range of neural elements and systems. However, although evidence for the effects of experience on the development of the neural system is substantial, specific data verifying the interaction between genes and the environment has been much more difficult to obtain. A gene-environment interaction has been defined as "a situation where risk from an environmental exposure varies according to genotype or where genotype effect varies according to environment" (Zammit and Owen 2006, p. 199). Documenting gene-environment interactions requires (1) identifying an appropriate target gene with specific and well-defined allelic variation within the population, (2) defining the specific function of the gene, and then (3) identifying an environmental factor that both selectively modulates a particular phenotypic outcome and can be associated with a specific genotype. Although many studies have looked indirectly at the relative contributions of inherited and experiential factors by exploring questions of heritability, data that directly document the interaction of genes and environment are rare. Marshalling such a complex combination of factors to support a specific gene-environment interaction is challenging, and few convincing examples are available in the literature. However, a recent study of population variations in a specific gene involved in serotonin transport has presented one possible example, and thus represents a potentially important demonstration of the feasibility of detecting gene-environment interactions.

Caspi and colleagues (2003) reported the results of a study that examined variations in the serotonin transporter gene, environmental stressors, and depression. The study was conducted as part of the Dunedin Multidisciplinary Health and Development Study (New Zealand), a longitudinal birth-cohort study that followed a sample of over 1,000 individuals with data collected at two-year intervals between ages 3 and 22 years. Data on a wide variety of topics were collected over the term of the study, including prospective assessments of stressful life circumstances. The Caspi study was conducted when the cohort was 26 years of age and included assessment of recent life stressors based on life-history calendars for the preceding four years, childhood maltreatment based on longitudinally obtained data, and self and clinician reports of incidents of major depression, as well as genotyping to determine serotonin transporter gene variants.

Serotonin (5-hydroxytryptamine, 5HT) is a neurotransmitter that is produced in a neural pathway that ascends from the raphe nuclei in the brain stem through the basal ganglia and hypothalamus to limbic-system structures (including the hippocampus and the amygdala) and to the olfactory cortex and frontal regions of the neocortex. The pathway contributes to aspects of sleep, appetite, some cognitive functions, and, importantly for these studies, expression of anxiety and depression. The serotonin transporter, 5HTT, regulates the reuptake of 5HT in the synaptic cleft after neuronal firing. The human $5HTT$ gene ($SLC6A4$) is polymorphic; that is, it has two different forms, or alleles, that are differentiated by the length of a segment of repeating nucleotides in the promoter region of the gene. Thus the two alleles are referred to as the long (l) and the short (s) variants. The genotype frequencies in the European population are well established: s/s=.36, l/s=.48, and l/l=.16. Animal studies indicate that individuals that carry the s allele are more likely to have abnormal anxiety levels and more readily acquire a conditioned fear response. In human functional neuroimaging studies, s-allele carriers show greater amygdala activation to fearful and angry faces (Hariri et al. 2002).

The Caspi study examined the association between genotype, life history, and depression. Importantly, for this current study, the incidences of both stressful life events and childhood maltreatment did not differ across the three genotype groups. All three groups were equally likely to have experienced earlier negative events at the same frequencies, thus ruling out the possible confound that members of a particular genotype group might create the negative life circumstances that then lead to their depression. There were two major findings from this study. First, the number of stressors in the four-year period immediately preceding assessment at age 26 predicted incidences of major depression in groups carrying the s allele (s/s or s/l), but not among the l/l group. Specifically, there were no group differences among individuals reporting zero or one major stressful event, but as the number of stressors increased, the probability of a major depressive event increased significantly for both the s/s and s/l groups, but not for the l/l group. These data suggest an interaction between genotype, life experience, and depressive outcome, that is, a gene-environment interaction. Further, when early life experience was examined, robust associations were obtained between childhood maltreatment and likelihood of depression for the s/s and s/l groups, but not for the l/l group. That is, a history of maltreatment during childhood predicted adulthood depression, but only among individuals with the s/s or s/l genotype for *5HTT*. For individuals with the l/l genotype, a history of childhood maltreatment did not predict later depression.

The surprising and dramatic findings in support of a gene-environment interaction reported in the Caspi study stirred considerable interest and controversy precisely because these kinds of interactions are difficult to obtain. Caspi and colleagues acknowledged the difficulty in detecting such interactions and stressed the need for replication of their findings. Thus far, there have been eight attempts to replicate the original findings (Eley et al. 2004; Gillespie et al. 2005; Grabe et al. 2005; Kaufman et al. 2004; Kendler et al. 2005; Sjoberg et al. 2006; Surtees et al. 2006; Wilhelm et al. 2006). Of these, six reported at least partial replication; in some cases, replication was

reported for the s/s group data but not the s/l group, and in one replication it was reported for females but not males. Importantly, the two
studies that failed to replicate the original findings used a broader, and
largely older, sample (Gillespie et al. 2005, ages 14 to 78; Surtees et al.
2006, ages 40 to 70). Gillespie suggested that one factor that could
account for the failure to observe the gene-environment interaction
among older adults is a phenomenon referred to as "kindling." The
onset of major depression typically occurs in the late teens or 20s, and
during that early period, depressive episodes can be linked to specific
stressors. With age, the association between specific life events and depression becomes less well defined; "as the number of previous
episodes increases, individuals require less provocation; they become
increasingly desensitized to stressful events . . . This might also suggest
that early onsets of depression are more likely to be influenced by
G×E interactions." (Gillespie et al. 2005, p. 107). In summary, although the data from the *5HTT* allele variation studies need to be considered with some caution, the growing body of evidence suggests that
it may reflect a true example of a gene-environment interaction.

## Chapter Summary

- A model for exploring the role of experience in the developing
  cortex has been the formation of ODCs. Early work suggested a
  primary role for activity-dependent, competitive interaction
  among neurons for synaptic connections. Studies of the effects of
  binocular and monocular deprivation provided evidence for two
  phases in early visual cortical development, the precritical and
  critical periods, which are thought to be distinct phases in cortical development. There is agreement that the critical period is
  dominated by activity-dependent reorganization and refinement
  of cortical networks.
- The role of the precritical period for ODC formation is less clear.
  In some accounts, the precritical period is an activity-independent phase in which molecular cues and signaling serve to establish the basic adult profile of cortical organization. In other accounts, it is a period during which a rudimentary pattern of
  cortical organization is established via both activity-dependent
  and activity-independent factors.

- The beginning of the critical period for ODC formation is associated with the development of the inhibitory GABAergic system. Precritical-period activity is important for the development of the inhibitory systems. The inhibitory system plays an important role in the initiation and maintenance of the critical period.
- Cortical transplantation studies test whether intrinsic cues can be altered by exposure to signaling from a different cortical area. For example, sensorimotor tissue transplanted into visual regions of the cortex has been shown to adopt the fate of the host regions. These kinds of studies suggest that early in development, cell fate specified by initial intrinsic signaling can be overridden and that cells retain their capacity to adapt to alternative local signaling cues.
- Cortical rewiring studies examine whether alteration of connectivity can change areal fate. In these studies, major sensory input pathways are destroyed, and the subsequent functional specification of the target sensory areas is examined. When the auditory pathway is lesioned, retinal axons project to the auditory thalamic nucleus, the MGN, and then to the PAC, thus establishing a visual input pathway to the PAC. The projections in the PAC reflect the typical pattern of visual retinotopic organization, although the patterning is somewhat less refined than that observed in the PVC. The rewired PAC responds to visual input; however, as was the case with the structural organization, the functional capacity is reduced.
- Studies of the effects of early cortical brain injury suggest that the developing brain is considerably more adaptive than the mature brain. Early patterns of cortical connectivity are more distributed than later patterns. When cortical injury occurs, the developing brain can exploit the more extensive structural connectivity, stabilizing connections that would normally be pruned back and preserving functions that are lost with comparable injury in the mature organism.
- Subcortical structures do not necessarily exhibit the same degree of plasticity in response to early injuries. Subcortical lesions of the caudate nucleus result in persistent deficits that are comparable with deficits observed in adult animals. Both animal and human

studies have shown that injury to the hippocampus can result in memory deficits that are evident early and extend into adulthood.
- Unilateral injury is generally less detrimental than bilateral injury, even when the amount of tissue lost is comparable. Further, with unilateral injury, early injury is less detrimental than later injury. Bilateral injury has a significant impact on later development, but the effects of the timing of the injury differ from those observed with unilateral injury. Early injury has a more negative impact on development than does later injury. However, enriched rearing conditions can improve outcome even under conditions of early bilateral injury.
- The role of environmental complexity has been examined in studies that manipulate the rearing environment. Animals reared in isolated cages show significant attenuation of dendritic branching throughout the brain compared with littermates reared in complex, social environments. The experience of the complex environment promotes connectivity in both younger and older animals. In young animals, enhancement of synaptic exuberance and pruning is thought to reflect the modulation of experience-expectant neural events. Importantly, environmental complexity can also induce synaptogenesis in adult animals, reflecting the kinds of experience-dependent neural processes that are associated with later learning.
- Gene-environment interactions are very difficult to detect in populations. They require a complex and diverse set of data, including an appropriate target gene with specific and well-defined allelic variation, functional specification of the gene, and identification of an environmental factor that affects phenotypic outcome and is associated with a specific genotype. Recent work suggests that allelic variation in the 5HT transporter gene and stressful life experiences may interact to determine the likelihood of depression in adulthood.

### References

Alvarado, M. C., A. A. Wright, and J. Bachevalier. 2002. "Object and spatial relational memory in adult rhesus monkeys is impaired by neonatal lesions of the hippocampal formation but not the amygdaloid complex." *Hippocampus*, 12: 421–433.

Angelucci, A., F. Clasca, E. Bricolo, K. S. Cramer, and M. Sur. 1997. "Experimentally induced retinal projections to the ferret auditory thalamus: Development of clustered eye-specific patterns in a novel target." *Journal of Neuroscience*, 17: 2040–2055.

Bachevalier, J., and M. Mishkin. 1994. "Effects of selective neonatal temporal lobe lesions on visual recognition memory in rhesus monkeys." *Journal of Neuroscience*, 14: 2128–2139.

Bachevalier, J., and F. Vargha-Khadem. 2005. "The primate hippocampus: Ontogeny, early insult and memory." *Current Opinion in Neurobiology*, 15: 168–174.

Bavelier, D., and H. J. Neville. 2002. "Cross-modal plasticity: Where and how?" *Nature Reviews Neuroscience*, 3: 443–452.

Bence, M., and C. N. Levelt. 2005. "Structural plasticity in the developing visual system." *Progress in Brain Research*, 147: 125–139.

Bennett, E. L., M. R. Rosenzweig, and M. C. Diamond. 1969. "Rat brain: Effects of environmental enrichment on wet and dry weights." *Science*, 163: 825–826.

Black, J. E., A. M. Sirevaag, and W. T. Greenough. 1987. "Complex experience promotes capillary formation in young rat visual cortex." *Neuroscience Letters*, 83: 351–355.

Caspi, A., K. Sugden, T. E. Moffitt, A. Taylor, I. W. Craig, H. Harrington, J. McClay, J. Mill, J. Martin, A. Braithwaite, and R. Poulton. 2003. "Influence of life stress on depression: Moderation by a polymorphism in the 5-HTT gene." *Science*, 301: 386–389.

Chang, F. L., and W. T. Greenough. 1982. "Lateralized effects of monocular training on dendritic branching in adult split-brain rats." *Brain Research*, 232: 283–292.

Cohen-Cory, S. 2002. "The developing synapse: Construction and modulation of synaptic structures and circuits." *Science*, 298: 770–776.

Crair, M. C., D. C. Gillespie, and M. P. Stryker. 1998. "The role of visual experience in the development of columns in cat visual cortex." *Science*, 279: 566–570.

Crair, M. C., J. C. Horton, A. Antonini, and M. P. Stryker. 2001. "Emergence of ocular dominance columns in cat visual cortex by 2 weeks of age." *Journal of Comparative Neurology*, 430: 235–249.

Crowley, J. C., and L. C. Katz. 1999. "Development of ocular dominance columns in the absence of retinal input." *Nature Neuroscience*, 2: 1125–1130.

———. 2000. "Early development of ocular dominance columns." *Science*, 290: 1321–1324.

———. 2002. "Ocular dominance development revisited." *Current Opinion in Neurobiology*, 12: 104–109.

Eley, T. C., K. Sugden, A. Corsico, A. M. Gregory, P. Sham, P. McGuffin, R. Plomin, and I. W. Craig. 2004. "Gene-environment interaction analysis of serotonin system markers with adolescent depression." *Molecular Psychiatry*, 9: 908–915.

Ellemberg, D., T. L. Lewis, D. Maurer, S. Brar, and H. P. Brent. 2002. "Better perception of global motion after monocular than after binocular deprivation." *Vision Research*, 42: 169–179.

Feller, M. B., and M. Scanziani. 2005. "A precritical period for plasticity in visual cortex." *Current Opinion in Neurobiology*, 15: 94–100.

Fine, I., E. M. Finney, G. M. Boynton, and K. R. Dobkins. 2005. "Comparing the effects of auditory deprivation and sign language within the auditory and visual cortex." *Journal of Cognitive Neuroscience*, 17: 1621–1637.

Finney, E. M., I. Fine, and K. R. Dobkins. 2001. "Visual stimuli activate auditory cortex in the deaf." *Nature Neuroscience*, 4: 1171–1173.

Fischer, M., S. Kaech, U. Wagner, H. Brinkhaus, and A. Matus. 2000. "Glutamate receptors regulate actin-based plasticity in dendritic spines." *Nature Neuroscience*, 3: 887–894.

Francis, P. J., and A. T. Moore. 2004. "Genetics of childhood cataract." *Current Opinion in Ophthalmology*, 15: 10–15.

Gillespie, N. A., J. B. Whitfield, B. Williams, A. C. Heath, and N. G. Martin. 2005. "The relationship between stressful life events, the serotonin transporter (5-HTTLPR) genotype and major depression." *Psychological Medicine*, 35: 101–111.

Goldman, P. S. 1971. "Functional development of the prefrontal cortex in early life and the problem of neuronal plasticity." *Experimental Neurology*, 32: 366–387.

———. 1974. "Functional recovery after lesions of the nervous systems. 3. Developmental processes in neural plasticity: Recovery of function after CNS lesions in infant monkeys." *Neurosciences Research Program Bulletin*, 12: 217–222.

Goldman, P. S., and H. E. Rosvold. 1972. "The effects of selective caudate lesions in infant and juvenile Rhesus monkeys." *Brain Research*, 43: 53–66.

Goldman, P. S., H. E. Rosvold, and M. Mishkin. 1970. "Selective sparing of function following prefrontal lobectomy in infant monkeys." *Experimental Neurology*, 29: 221–226.

Grabe, H. J., M. Lange, B. Wolff, H. Volzke, M. Lucht, H. J. Freyberger, U. John, and I. Cascorbi. 2005. "Mental and physical distress is modulated by a polymorphism in the 5-HT transporter gene interacting with social stressors and chronic disease burden." *Molecular Psychiatry*, 10: 220–224.

Greenough, W. T., and F. F. Chang. 1988. "Plasticity of synapse structure and pattern in the cerebral cortex." In *Cerebral Cortex*, vol. 7, ed. A. Peters and E. G. Jones, 391–440. New York: Plenum Press.

Grossman, A. W., J. D. Churchill, K. E. Bates, J. A. Kleim, and W. T. Greenough. 2002. "A brain adaptation view of plasticity: Is synaptic plasticity an overly limited concept?" *Progress in Brain Research*, 138: 91–108.

Grubb, M. S., and I. D. Thompson. 2004. "The influence of early experience on the development of sensory systems." *Current Opinion in Neurobiology*, 14: 503–512.

Hariri, A. R., V. S. Mattay, A. Tessitore, B. Kolachana, F. Fera, D. Goldman, M. F. Egan, and D. R. Weinberger. 2002. "Serotonin transporter genetic variation and the response of the human amygdala." *Science*, 297: 400–403.

Hebb, D. O. 1949. *The organization of behavior: A neuropsychological theory*. New York: Wiley.

Hensch, T. K. 2004. "Critical period regulation." *Annual Review of Neuroscience*, 27: 549–579.

———. 2005. "Critical period plasticity in local cortical circuits." *Nature Reviews Neuroscience*, 6: 877–888.

Hickok, G., U. Bellugi, and E. S. Klima. 1997. "The basis of the neural organization for language: Evidence from sign language aphasia." *Reviews in the Neurosciences*, 8: 205–222.

Hua, J. Y., and S. J. Smith. 2004. "Neural activity and the dynamics of central nervous system development." *Nature Neuroscience*, 7: 327–332.

Hubel, D. H., and T. N. Wiesel. 1977. "Ferrier Lecture: Functional architecture of macaque monkey visual cortex." *Proceedings of the Royal Society of London*, ser. B, 198: 1–59.

Hubel, D. H., T. N. Wiesel, and S. LeVay. 1977. "Plasticity of ocular dominance columns in monkey striate cortex." *Philosophical Transactions of the Royal Society of London*, ser. B, *Biological Sciences*, 278: 377–409.

Huberman, A. D., C. M. Speer, and B. Chapman. 2006. "Spontaneous retinal activity mediates development of ocular dominance columns and binocular receptive fields in v1." *Neuron*, 52: 247–254.

Huttenlocher, P. R., and A. S. Dabholkar. 1997. "Regional differences in synaptogenesis in human cerebral cortex." *Journal of Comparative Neurology*, 387: 167–178.

Huttenlocher, P. R., and C. de Courten. 1987. "The development of synapses in striate cortex of man." *Human Neurobiology*, 6: 1–9.

Isaacs, E. B., F. Vargha-Khadem, K. E. Watkins, A. Lucas, M. Mishkin, and D. G. Gadian. 2003. "Developmental amnesia and its relationship to degree of hippocampal atrophy." *Proceedings of the National Academy of Sciences of the United States of America*, 100: 13060–13063.

Jones, T. A., and W. T. Greenough. 1996. "Ultrastructural evidence for increased contact between astrocytes and synapses in rats reared in a complex environment." *Neurobiology of Learning and Memory*, 65: 48–56.

Jones, T. A., J. A. Kleim, and W. T. Greenough. 1996. "Synaptogenesis and dendritic growth in the cortex opposite unilateral sensorimotor cortex damage in adult rats: A quantitative electron microscopic examination." *Brain Research*, 733: 142–148.

Jones, T. A., A. Y. Klintsova, V. L. Kilman, A. M. Sirevaag, and W. T. Greenough. 1997. "Induction of multiple synapses by experience in the visual cortex of adult rats." *Neurobiology of Learning and Memory*, 68: 13–20.

Kantor, D. B., and A. L. Kolodkin. 2003. "Curbing the excesses of youth: Molecular insights into axonal pruning." *Neuron*, 38: 849–852.

Katz, L. C., and J. C. Crowley. 2002. "Development of cortical circuits: Lessons from ocular dominance columns." *Nature Reviews Neuroscience*, 3: 34–42.

Kaufman, J., B. Z. Yang, H. Douglas-Palumberi, S. Houshyar, D. Lipschitz, J. H. Krystal, and J. Gelernter. 2004. "Social supports and serotonin transporter gene moderate depression in maltreated children." *Proceedings of the National Academy of Sciences of the United States of America*, 101: 17316–17321.

Kendler, K. S., J. W. Kuhn, J. Vittum, C. A. Prescott, and B. Riley. 2005. "The interaction of stressful life events and a serotonin transporter polymorphism in the prediction of episodes of major depression: A replication." *Archives of General Psychiatry*, 62: 529–535.

Kolb, B., and W. Elliott. 1987. "Recovery from early cortical damage in rats. II. Effects of experience on anatomy and behavior following frontal lesions at 1 or 5 days of age." *Behavioural Brain Research*, 26: 47–56.

Kolb, B., C. Holmes, and I. Q. Whishaw. 1987. "Recovery from early cortical lesions in rats. III. Neonatal removal of posterior parietal cortex has greater behavioral and anatomical effects than similar removals in adulthood." *Behavioural Brain Research*, 26: 119–137.

Kolb, B., and J. A. Tomie. 1988. "Recovery from early cortical damage in rats. IV. Effects of hemidecortication at 1, 5 or 10 days of age on cerebral anatomy and behavior." *Behavioural Brain Research*, 28: 259–274.

Kolb, B., and I. Q. Whishaw. 1989. "Plasticity in the neocortex: Mechanisms underlying recovery from early brain damage." *Progress in Neurobiology*, 32: 235–276.

Lambertz, N., E. R. Gizewski, A. de Greiff, and M. Forsting. 2005. "Cross-modal plasticity in deaf subjects dependent on the extent of hearing loss." *Brain Research. Cognitive Brain Research*, 25: 884–890.

LeVay, S., M. P. Stryker, and C. J. Shatz. 1978. "Ocular dominance columns and their development in layer IV of the cat's visual cortex: A quantitative study." *Journal of Comparative Neurology*, 179: 223–244.

Levin, A. V. 2003. "Congenital eye anomalies." *Pediatric Clinics of North America*, 50: 55–76.

Lewis, T. L., D. Ellemberg, D. Maurer, F. Wilkinson, H. R. Wilson, M. Dirks, and H. P. Brent. 2002. "Sensitivity to global form in glass patterns after early visual deprivation in humans." *Vision Research*, 42: 939–948.

Lewis, T. L., and D. Maurer. 2005. "Multiple sensitive periods in human visual development: Evidence from visually deprived children." *Developmental Psychobiology*, 46: 163–183.

MacSweeney, M., B. Woll, R. Campbell, P. K. McGuire, A. S. David, S. C. Williams, J. Suckling, G. A. Calvert, and M. J. Brammer. 2002. "Neural systems underlying British Sign Language and audio-visual English processing in native users." *Brain*, 125: 1583–1593.

Malkova, L., M. Mishkin, and J. Bachevalier. 1995. "Long-term effects of selective neonatal temporal lobe lesions on learning and memory in monkeys." *Behavioral Neuroscience*, 109: 212–226.

Markham, J. A., and W. T. Greenough. 2004. "Experience-driven brain plasticity: Beyond the synapse." *Neuron Glia Biology*, 1: 351–363.

Maurer, D., T. L. Lewis, H. P. Brent, and A. V. Levin. 1999. "Rapid improvement in the acuity of infants after visual input." *Science*, 286: 108–110.

Maurer, D., T. L. Lewis, and C. J. Mondloch. 2005. "Missing sights: Consequences for visual cognitive development." *Trends in Cognitive Sciences*, 9: 144–151.

Meister, M., R. O. Wong, D. A. Baylor, and C. J. Shatz. 1991. "Synchronous bursts of action potentials in ganglion cells of the developing mammalian retina." *Science*, 252: 939–943.

Mishkin, M., L. G. Ungerleider, and K. A. Macko. 1983. "Object vision and spatial vision: Two cortical pathways." *Trends in Neurosciences*, 6: 414–417.

Morris, R. 1984. "Development of a water-maze procedure for studying spatial learning in the rat." *Journal of Neuroscience Methods*, 11: 47–60.

Nishimura, H., K. Doi, T. Iwaki, K. Hashikawa, T. Nishimura, and T. Kubo. 2000. "Sign language activated the auditory cortex of a congenitally deaf subject: Revealed by positron emission tomography." *Advances in Oto-rhino-laryngology*, 57: 60–62.

Nishimura, H., K. Hashikawa, K. Doi, T. Iwaki, Y. Watanabe, H. Kusuoka, T. Nishimura, and T. Kubo. 1999. "Sign language 'heard' in the auditory cortex." *Nature*, 397: 116.

O'Leary, D. D., and B. B. Stanfield. 1989. "Selective elimination of axons extended by developing cortical neurons is dependent on regional locale: Experiments utilizing fetal cortical transplants." *Journal of Neuroscience*, 9: 2230–2246.

Pallas, S. L., A. W. Roe, and M. Sur. 1990. "Visual projections induced into the auditory pathway of ferrets. I. Novel inputs to primary auditory cortex (AI) from the LP/pulvinar complex and the topography of the MGN-AI projection." *Journal of Comparative Neurology*, 298: 50–68.

Rosenzweig, M. R., and E. L. Bennett. 1972. "Cerebral changes in rats exposed individually to an enriched environment." *Journal of Comparative and Physiological Psychology*, 80: 304–313.

Rosenzweig, M. R., D. Krech, E. L. Bennett, and M. C. Diamond. 1962a. "Effects of environmental complexity and training on brain chemistry and anatomy: A replication and extension." *Journal of Comparative and Physiological Psychology*, 55: 429–437.

Rosenzweig, M. R., D. Krech, E. L. Bennett, and J. F. Zolman. 1962b. "Variation in environmental complexity and brain measures." *Journal of Comparative and Physiological Psychology*, 55: 1092–1095.

Rosenzweig, M. R., W. Love, and E. L. Bennett. 1968. "Effects of a few hours a day of enriched experience on brain chemistry and brain weights." *Physiology and Behavior*, 3: 819–825.

Ruthazer, E. S. 2005. "You're perfect, now change—Redefining the role of developmental plasticity." *Neuron*, 45: 825–828.

Sadato, N., H. Yamada, T. Okada, M. Yoshida, T. Hasegawa, K. Matsuki, Y. Yonekura, and H. Itoh. 2004. "Age-dependent plasticity in the superior temporal sulcus in deaf humans: A functional MRI study." *BMC Neuroscience*, 5: 56.

Schlaggar, B. L., and D. D. O'Leary. 1991. "Potential of visual cortex to develop an array of functional units unique to somatosensory cortex." *Science*, 252: 1556–1560.

Schmidt, K. E., M. Stephan, W. Singer, and S. Lowel. 2002. "Spatial analysis of ocular dominance patterns in monocularly deprived cats." *Cerebral Cortex*, 12: 783–796.

Schneider, G. E. 1973. "Early lesions of superior colliculus: Factors affecting the formation of abnormal retinal projections." *Brain, Behavior and Evolution*, 8: 73–109.

Seress, L. 2001. "Morphological changes of the human hippocampal formation from midgestation to early childhood." In *Handbook of developmental cognitive neuroscience*, ed. C. A. Nelson and M. Luciana, 45–58. Cambridge, MA: MIT Press.

Sirevaag, A. M., and W. T. Greenough. 1987. "Differential rearing effects on rat visual cortex synapses. III. Neuronal and glial nuclei, boutons, dendrites, and capillaries." *Brain Research*, 424: 320–332.

Sjoberg, R. L., K. W. Nilsson, N. Nordquist, J. Ohrvik, J. Leppert, L. Lindstrom, and L. Oreland. 2006. "Development of depression: Sex and the interaction between environment and a promoter polymorphism of the serotonin transporter gene." *International Journal of Neuropsychopharma-cology*, 9: 443–449.

Sur, M., P. E. Garraghty, and A. W. Roe. 1988. "Experimentally induced vi-sual projections into auditory thalamus and cortex." *Science*, 242: 1437–1441.

Sur, M., and C. A. Leamey. 2001. "Development and plasticity of cortical areas and networks." *Nature Reviews Neuroscience*, 2: 251–262.

Sur, M., and J. L. Rubenstein. 2005. "Patterning and plasticity of the cere-bral cortex." *Science*, 310: 805–810.

Surtees, P. G., N. W. Wainwright, S. A. Willis-Owen, R. Luben, N. E. Day, and J. Flint. 2006. "Social adversity, the serotonin transporter (5-HTTLPR) polymorphism and major depressive disorder." *Biological Psy-chiatry*, 59: 224–229.

Szeligo, F., and C. P. Leblond. 1977. "Response of the three main types of glial cells of cortex and corpus callosum in rats handled during suckling or exposed to enriched, control and impoverished environments fol-lowing weaning." *Journal of Comparative Neurology*, 172: 247–263.

Ungerleider, L. G., and E. A. Murray. 1992. "Primates, visual perception and memory in nonhuman." In *Encyclopedia of learning and memory*, ed. L. R. Squire, 537–541. New York: Macmillan.

Uylings, H. B., K. Kuypers, M. C. Diamond, and W. A. Veltman. 1978. "Ef-fects of differential environments on plasticity of dendrites of cortical pyramidal neurons in adult rats." *Experimental Neurology*, 62: 658–677.

von Melchner, L., S. L. Pallas, and M. Sur. 2000. "Visual behaviour medi-ated by retinal projections directed to the auditory pathway." *Nature*, 404: 871–876.

Webster, M. J., J. Bachevalier, and L. G. Ungerleider. 1995a. "Development of plasticity and visual memory circuits." In *Maturational windows and adult cortical plasticity*, ed. B. Julesz and I. Kovács, 73–86. Reading, MA: Addison-Wesley.

———. 1995b. "Transient subcortical connections of inferior temporal areas TE and TEO in infant macaque monkeys." *Journal of Comparative Neurology*, 352: 213–226.

Webster, M. J., L. G. Ungerleider, and J. Bachevalier. 1991a. "Connections of inferior temporal areas TE and TEO with medial temporal-lobe structures in infant and adult monkeys." *Journal of Neuroscience*, 11: 1095–1116.

———. 1991b. "Lesions of inferior temporal area TE in infant monkeys alter cortico-amygdalar projections." *Neuroreport*, 2: 769–772.

Wilhelm, K., P. B. Mitchell, H. Niven, A. Finch, L. Wedgwood, A. Scimone, I. P. Blair, G. Parker, and P. R. Schofield. 2006. "Life events, first depression onset and the serotonin transporter gene." *British Journal of Psychiatry*, 188: 210–215.

Wong, R. O., M. Meister, and C. J. Shatz. 1993. "Transient period of correlated bursting activity during development of mammalian retina." *Neuron*, 11: 923–938.

Zammit, S., and M. J. Owen. 2006. "Stressful life events, 5-HTT genotype and risk of depression." *British Journal of Psychiatry*, 188: 199–201.

# ELEVEN

# The Importance of Brain Development
# for Psychology

THIS BOOK BEGAN with a discussion of the psychological debate over the origins of knowledge. Central to that debate is the definition of the concept of innateness. Nativists define innate concepts as those that are acquired or available in the absence of learning. Recent constructivist accounts have attempted to define a level of innate representation that might plausibly emerge in the absence of input and rely entirely on organism-intrinsic factors. The difficulty with both of these accounts lies in the failure to provide a biologically feasible account of precisely what it means for something to be innate. One argument that has been voiced by some psychologists is that defining biological feasibility of an innate factor is the job of the biologist. Psychological models provide characterizations of sensory, motor, perceptual, cognitive, and social abilities, and although they assume that biological systems underpin behavior, the job of the psychologist is ultimately to explain behavior, not biology. It is true that the proper focus of the psychologist is psychology. However, the essential link between all behaviors and the biological systems that mediate and support them demands a more rigorous definition of the concept that is both central to psychological thought and inextricably rooted in biology. Psychology does not benefit from an impoverished or under-specified definition of what it means for something to be innate. The psychological concept of innateness might plausibly benefit from stronger and more fully articulated links to the biological systems that support it.

A central question raised in this book is, how do biologists think about the question of innateness, and can those ideas inform the psychological debate? The biological concept of innateness is focused on questions of inheritance and on explaining both intergenerational constancy and variation. What is inherited is genetic material and the cellular mechanisms for making use of the information contained in the genes. Thus, from the beginning, the biological concept of inheritance, of innateness, involves a process, specifically, a process for translating and making use of the information contained in the genes. It is that process that drives all the subsequent development and functioning of the organism. The biological view of innateness also stresses the inseparability of inherited factors and experience acting in concert to direct the development of the organism. Thus it is ultimately a concept about the process of development itself.

This chapter will explore the biological perspective on innateness and development and will consider how these ideas may be important for psychologists. It will begin with a discussion of the historical roots of the biological concept of innateness, drawing largely from topics considered in Chapter 2 in the discussion of the emergence of the concept of the gene. Next, the chapter will attempt to place the recent, dramatic advances in our understanding of brain development—the content of much of this book—into the perspective of the biological view of innateness. From the early embryonic period through the postnatal period, development entails the complex interaction of intrinsic signaling cascades coupled with extrinsic signaling. In this chapter, examples taken from earlier chapters of the book will be used to elaborate specifically on the interactive nature of neural development and to illustrate how the basic processes that drive brain development exemplify the biological view of innateness.

Development can also be construed as a series of events and processes that unfold over time. The next sections of the chapter will consider the multiple ways in which the timing of the biological events that constitute brain development serves to constrain and direct development. Over time, the influence of any particular factor is variable such that, for example, a factor that has little effect on early development may play a critical role in shaping neural organization later in life, and vice versa. Thus a complete account of the factors that influence and contribute to brain development must consider the effects of both the timing and the sequence of developmental events. In the postnatal period, the concept of the "critical period" has played an important role in thinking about the development of the sensory, perceptual, and conceptual systems. Critical or sensitive periods are temporally defined periods during which input from the environment is required to establish a particular behavior. Changing ideas about the nature and functions of critical or sensitive periods will be considered. The chapter concludes with a discussion of constancy and variability in brain development and how the model of brain development presented in this chapter can accommodate the essential demands of constancy during typical development and still allow for the degree of flexibility observed when the experience of the organism demands adaptation.

## Biological Perspectives on the Concept of Innateness

As discussed in Chapter 2, the biological concept of innateness has historically been linked to questions about the intergenerational transmission of information, that is, inheritance. How is the intergenerational transfer of information explained, what is the source of variation, and how is the competition between the opposing pulls of constancy and variability reconciled in a single account of inheritance? The history of change in these central ideas is captured in the search for the material nature of inheritance, in the quest for what became known as the gene. That history contains the press to define a source of constancy by specifying the nature and location of particulate matter that carries intergenerational information, combined with the puzzle of variation. How is constancy ensured when variation is allowed? The key to the conundrum posed by these seemingly opposing forces lies in the modern ideas about gene expression.

Genes provide the material code for the development and functioning of all biological structures and processes, but the code is neither prescriptive nor singular. Gene expression is a process, and the triggers for expression of any given gene are external to the nucleotide sequences that make up the coded genetic material. Gene expression requires the interaction of multiple factors within the environment of the cell, and cellular environments are, in turn, influenced by factors external to the cell. The layers of environments extend from the molecular to the world outside the organism. Further, the interactive influences are multidirectional. The expression of a gene initiates a cascade of events that influence and direct other processes that alter the organization or functions of the organism. Each change in the system influences other processes. In addition, the developmental and functional state of the organism at any given time constrains which factors can exert an influence. Thus sound originating in the external environment is unlikely to affect the migration of neurons, but maternal ingestion of particular drugs or alcohol during precise moments in development can interfere with migration and disrupt the laminar organization of the cortex. Similarly, a defective gene may impair development, but its effects are specific to those developmental processes that depend on the normal production of the particular proteins coded by the gene. In short, a first principle of the biological concept of inheritance is the inseparability of inherited and environmental factors. It is the orchestrated and constrained interaction of intrinsic and extrinsic factors—broadly construed—that defines and drives development.

The view of biological development as the product of the inseparable influences of inherited and environmental factors has been bolstered by recent work suggesting that environmental factors can be transmitted across generations. Work on epigenetic marking suggests that regional modification of the nuclear chromatin (via DNA methylation or histone acetylation) influences the level of specific gene expression. Modifications in the chromatin can be induced by dietary or other external environmental factors. Importantly, those externally induced modifications are transmissible to the offspring. Thus it is not just the DNA that is inherited, but also changes in the state of chromatin originating in the parent that are transmitted to the offspring. At an even more basic level, it is critical to remember that DNA is never transmitted in isolation. As Keller (2001) has emphasized, transmission of genetic material is always accompanied by transmission of the cellular machinery necessary for gene expression. What is inherited are both the genetic material and the cellular environment that gives the organism the capacity to transform the information in the coded nucleotide sequences into the active agents of biological development and function. Thus for every organism, the inseparability of inherited and environmental factors begins at conception.

## Inseparability of Inherited and Environmental Factors

The processes that underlie and guide brain development provide a particularly rich example of the interplay of inherited and environmental factors. At each period of neural development, organism-intrinsic factors interact with environmental cues to shape the increasingly complex and elaborate structures and functions of the brain. During the embryonic period, the interactive processes play out largely at the level of cell-cell interactions where one population of cells generates molecular signals that alter the developmental course of another population of cells. However, even during this earliest period, interactions involving factors in the external environment also play essential roles in the development of the embryonic brain. During the fetal and postnatal periods, organism-intrinsic factors continue to play a critical role in development, but during this extended period a wide array of factors in the external world play increasingly prominent roles in shaping and directing the course of brain development.

### *Embryonic Brain Development*

The embryonic period is a time of rapid and dramatic change. In a matter of a few weeks, the embryo acquires the cell lines necessary to generate all the organ systems of the body; it undergoes rapid growth and develops its characteristic shape. Even during this very early period, interactive processes are essential for directing the developmental course of the organism. Within the developing nervous system, the neural progenitor cell line is specified during gastrulation. As discussed in Chapter 3, the fate of particular progenitor cells is the product of complex molecular signaling cascades that occur along well-defined spatial and temporal trajectories. Many of the cues that signal the fate of particular cells are organism intrinsic, but they reflect interactive processes occurring both within cells and, most important, among cells. The migrating cells of the organizer, for example, send out molecular signals that block the production of a specific protein (BMP4) as they pass through particular regions of the developing embryo. Those signals are critical for the normal differentiation of the ectodermal cells that overlie the migratory pathway of the organizer cells. Absent the signaling from the organizer cells, the particular small population of ectodermal cells located along the midline of the embryo would fail to differentiate into neural progenitor cells, and the entire process of neural development would be interrupted. Thus it is the interaction among cells that directs the early development of this critical cell population. But the early development of the neural progenitor cell line is even more complex in that the particular fate of an individual neural progenitor cell reflects its spatial position within the embryonic nervous system. For example, some neural progenitors produce cells specific to anterior brain regions, while others produce cells that will form the hindbrain and the spinal column. The cues for anterior-posterior neural-fate specification come from regionally specific signaling cascades arising from the mesendodermal organizer cells that underlie the newly specified neural progenitor cell population. Thus whether a particular neural progenitor produces cells appropriate for the forebrain or the hindbrain is determined by the signals it receives from other nonneural cells in the local embryonic environment.

The role of interactive cell-cell signaling in early brain development is further illustrated by the morphogenic signaling cascades that give rise to different cell types. During morphogenic signaling, concentration gradients of one or more secreted molecules determine the fate of particular cells within the gradient distribution. Within the developing spinal column, for example (see Chapter 5), the genes *SHH* and members of the *TGFB* superfamily (e.g., *BMP4, BMP7*) are expressed in opposing ventral-dorsal and dorsal-ventral gradients, respectively. SHH is produced by cells of the notochord and the floor plate that are located in the most ventral region of the spinal cord, while TGFBs are produced by roof-plate cells in the most dorsal regions. The interaction of these two diffusing gradients induces the expression of different transcription factors in cells at different levels of the neural tube. The specific transcription factor expressed at a given level, in turn, activates cell-intrinsic programs that cause the local neuron populations to adopt specific cell fates. Within ventral regions, different concentration gradients give rise to a range of different motor-neuron populations, and within dorsal regions, specific classes of interneurons arise. Morphogenic signaling provides a dramatic example of the importance of the interaction among cells in the development of the central nervous system (CNS). Here the cell populations of the roof and floor plates produce opposing gradients of secreted molecules that systematically alter the fate of a large number of spinal column neurons, thus creating the layered subpopulations of cells that define the dorsal-ventral organization of the spinal column.

Factors external to the organism also play an important role in the development of the embryonic brain. In some cases, the effects of environmental factors can be damaging to the developing embryo. For example, a wide range of substances that can be introduced into the embryo from the external world are known to have teratogenic effects on the developing brain. Alcohol, drugs, lead, and radiation are just a few of the many factors that have documented pathological effects on brain development. But the developing embryo also relies on factors derived from the external world for its development. The maternal system provides many factors that are essential for the normal development of the embryo. One clear example of the importance of an externally derived factor for typical brain development is retinoic acid (RA; see Chapter 5). RA is a substance that is critical for the normal development of the hindbrain, but it cannot be produced in animal cells. Rather, it is typically derived from vitamin A available from environmental sources. For the embryo, the availability of RA depends on maternal ingestion of vitamin A. The role of RA in hindbrain development involves control of HOX gene expression. HOX genes are an important and highly conserved family of genes that control the segmental organization of the hindbrain and the spinal column. They are expressed in a nested sequence along the rostral-caudal extent of the hindbrain and the spinal column. The expression of different subsets of HOX genes is confined to specific and highly localized regions (i.e., rhombomeres or spinal-cord segments), and this specific targeting of gene expression produces the characteristic segmental organization of the hindbrain and the spinal cord. Importantly, HOX gene expression is regulated by RA in a dose-dependent manner. Either too much or too little RA can disrupt the segmental organization of the posterior nervous system and compromise the viability of the embryo. The example of RA illustrates the range of interactive processes that are essential for embryonic development. Although organism-intrinsic factors are crucial, factors in the external environment are also essential for the normal development of the embryo.

*Fetal Brain Development*

Both the increasing complexity of interactions among cell populations and the influence of environmental factors in shaping and directing brain organization and function become more prominent during the later stages of development. Molecular signaling continues to play an important role, but the range of signaling within the developing nervous system expands to include a wider range of functions, such as those involved in mediation of neuronal migration, myelination, cell adhesion, and axonal guidance. Furthermore, neuronal activity becomes an important factor influencing processes such as apoptosis and synaptic stabilization that are essential for the establishment of the neural pathways and networks. The dynamic and interactive nature of later brain development is observed in a wide array of developmental processes. This section considers examples that illustrate both the increasing complexity in the range of cellular interaction and the growing prominence of environmental input.

During the embryonic period, interactions among cell populations played an important role in the differentiation of cell types. Furthermore, the specific patterns of regional interactions defined cell types that served to establish the initial spatial organization of the embryo along the anterior-posterior, dorsal-ventral, and right-left axes. Later in development, the range of cellular interactions becomes more varied. Although cellular differentiation continues to play a role (for example, in defining the different cell types that compose the different cortical layers), interactions among cell populations also serve other functions. The two examples that follow, illustrate the role of interactions between neurons and specific classes of cells whose signaling serves to regulate the organization of neuron populations.

First, Cajal-Retzius (C-R) cells are class of cells produced early that are involved in establishing the laminar organization of the neocortex (see Chapter 7). They are among the first cells to migrate to the newly developing cortical preplate, and they remain in the marginal zone (MZ) after the cortical plate splits the preplate into the separate MZ and subplate layers. C-R cells produce the protein reelin that provides a critical signal for neurons to stop migrating and take up their positions within the developing cortical plate.

The second example involves subplate neurons that play a critical early role in establishing the major sensory pathways, the thalamocortical (TC) and corticothalamic (CT) pathways (see Chapter 8). In the mature brain, neurons from the thalamus project axons to the sensory input layer (layer 4) of the neocortex, forming the TC pathway; and cortical neurons project to the thalamus, forming the CT pathway. Early in development, before the arrival of thalamic axons to the cortex or cortical projections to the thalamus, subplate neurons establish connections with both layer 4 neurons and the thalamus. The role of these early, transient subplate connections appears to be to prepare the developing input layers of the cortex for future connections with the thalamus (Kostovic et al. 2002). Both C-R and subplate cells engage in neuronal signaling, but rather than inducing cellular differentiation in the target neuronal population, the signals produced by each of these cell populations affect aspects of the organization of neuronal populations.

C-R cells are critical for the laminar organization of the cortex, while subplate neurons act as pioneers in setting up the major sensory relay pathways. Importantly, both the C-R and the subplate cell populations are transient. Each is present early, plays an important and specific role in the development of the brain, and then dies off via apoptosis when the particular aspects of neural organization it directs are complete (Kostovic and Rakic 1990; Soriano and Del Rio 2005). The functions of both cell populations provide striking examples of the kinds of interactive processes that are essential for establishing fundamental aspects of neural organization.

### Postnatal Brain Development

In the postnatal period, the role of experience in defining patterns of brain organization and connectivity becomes more pronounced (see Chapter 9). Indeed, Greenough has described the early postnatal period as a time of experience-expectant learning, suggesting that the neurobehavioral system "expects" or depends upon certain kinds of input from the world to develop normally. These kinds of effects are clearly demonstrated in the seminal work of Hubel and Wiesel on the developing visual system (Hubel, Wiesel, and LeVay 1977; Wiesel and Hubel 1963a, 1963b, 1965). The mature primary visual cortex (PVC) is organized into ocular dominance columns that reflect the segregation of input from the two eyes. Monocular deprivation early in postnatal development alters this typical pattern of organization. PVC neurons responsive to the nondeprived eye increase in number, while neurons responsive to the deprived eye decrease. The magnitude, duration, and permanence of these effects depend on the timing of deprivation onset, the duration of deprivation, and the postdeprivation interventions that are imposed. These findings suggest that during a period after birth, the specific visual experience of the organism significantly affects the emerging organization of the neural system that supports vision.

Studies examining the effects of early brain injury also support the idea that experience can affect brain organization. Goldman-Rakic's (Goldman 1974; Goldman and Galkin 1978; Goldman and Rosvold 1972; Goldman, Rosvold, and Mishkin 1970), Bachevalier and Mishkin's (1994), and Kolb's (Kolb 1987; Kolb and Elliott 1987; Kolb, Holmes, and Whishaw 1987; Kolb and Tomie 1988) studies of the effects of early circumscribed cortical injury on the development of memory and problem-solving abilities clearly demonstrate that, unlike the mature brain, the developing brain has the capacity to organize differently to support functions that would normally have been supported by injured brain areas (see Chapter 9). For example, Bachevalier examined the effects of specific temporal-lobe lesions experimentally introduced in either adult or infant monkeys. In the adult monkeys, the lesions compromised performance on a simple memory task. However, the performance of infant monkeys was nearly comparable with that of normal controls. Furthermore, follow-up suggested that the abilities acquired early were retained into adulthood. The studies suggest that when injury occurs early in life, the initially exuberant connectivity within the temporal lobe can be exploited to preserve function. In the young animal, normally transient connections within the temporal lobe stabilize, providing an alternative neural network that supports memory function. Kolb's work provides evidence of the limits of plasticity by demonstrating that bilateral injury results in more pronounced impairment than injury confined to a single cerebral hemisphere. That work also illustrates that the effects of the timing of the injury depend on the nature of the injury. In unilateral cases, outcomes following early injury are better than outcomes following later injury, while in cases of bilateral injury, the opposite pattern is observed. Importantly, Kolb has also demonstrated that environmental enrichment following early injury can significantly reduce the level of impairment even in cases of early bilateral injury.

Findings such as those from the work on the effects of deprivation on early visual system development or the effects of early lesions on the development of memory and problem solving document both the responsiveness of the neural system to such factors as variation in input or injury and the limits on the capacity of the neural system for adaptation. These examples, which reflect a much larger body of work, illustrate what has been described as the plasticity of the developing brain. Plasticity here refers to the capacity of the developing brain to respond adaptively and to adjust patterns of neural organization and connectivity to meet the demands of the specific experience of the organism. When input is altered or diminished, the neural system adjusts to maximize remaining input. When portions of the neural system are damaged, the remaining system organizes differently to support functions that would normally have been mediated by injured brain areas. The mechanisms thought to support neural plasticity in the postnatal period are principally those associated with the exuberant production of neural connections and their subsequent elimination (see Chapter 9). The studies of deprivation or experimental injury suggest that the capacity for plastic adaptation early in development is considerable, but it is important to emphasize that although the developing system exhibits considerable plasticity, there are also limits. For example, in Bachevalier's study, it is notable that although performance in the early lesioned monkeys was good, it never fully reached the level of controls either during infancy or in the adult follow-up study. Further, there is ample evidence that not all neural systems exhibit the level of plasticity observed in the cortical-lesion studies. For example, in Goldman-Rakic's studies, while monkeys with early cortical lesions performed nearly as well as controls, performance was compromised in infant monkeys with lesions to subcortical pathways. Kolb's studies of bilateral versus unilateral injury also document variation in the capacity to compensate for injury.

Finally, the effects of experience are temporally constrained. In the visual deprivation studies, one important moderating factor was the timing of the onset of deprivation. The greatest effects were associated with very early alteration of input. When deprivation onset was delayed by even a few weeks, the effects on cortical organization were diminished. These kinds of findings are important because they place the construct of plasticity within the developmental context. The developing brain does appear to be responsive to input and to retain the capacity to organize adaptively. In that sense, plasticity of the developing brain in the postnatal period provides a very good example of the interaction between intrinsic factors and experience. However, the limits on plasticity highlight the fact that the developmental process is one of continuing change within the context of increasing specification. Development happens over time, and the timing of events and experience matters. The next section will consider some of the multiple levels at which time affects and constrains the development of the emerging organization of the CNS.

## Time as an Organizing Factor in Brain Development

Development is a complex, multilevel process that unfolds over time. At the macro level, brain development appears to be a simple, additive process, and in some respects it is. Cells differentiate, multiply, and congregate in appropriate regions of the brain in increasing numbers. Connections among cells are formed both locally and over long distances. Thus at a global level, the neural system becomes more complex over time because more and more elements are incorporated into the system. But this simple additive model fails to take account of both the dependencies among the accumulating neural elements and the effects of experience, and thus masks much of the complexity of brain development.

A more nuanced view reveals multiple levels of change that, over time, are all driven by the interactions among the emerging and constantly changing complement of elements that compose the developing neural system. Across the entire period of brain development, the neural system depends upon the availability of the right neural elements appearing at the appropriate moment in developmental time for its integrity, stability, and growth. Often the emergence of a new element depends upon developmental events that immediately precede its appearance. All of this may seem a formula for chaos, but developmental changes appear to be orderly and follow regular patterns over time. At all levels of the neural system, from the cell to the neural pathways, progressive differentiation of specific elements and structures, coupled with progressive commitment of those elements to functional systems, appear to be the governing principles of brain development.

The timescales for differentiation and commitment vary both at different levels of the system and across subsystems within a neural level. The coordination and integration of these multiple levels of change happening on multiple timescales are essential elements of brain development. The sections that follow will examine the complementary processes of progressive differentiation and commitment for different levels of the neural system. The importance of the timing of interactive processes for the orchestrated development of the neural system is illustrated with examples drawn from the morphological, cellular, and neural pathway levels.

## Progressive Differentiation

Progressive differentiation of neural elements is observed at all levels of the neural system, from basic morphology to cells to neural pathways. Differentiation is probably most obvious at the level of basic morphology, particularly during the embryonic period, when the shape of the primitive nervous system changes dramatically over a relatively short period of time (see Chapter 4). At the onset of neurulation, the embryonic disc elongates as the neural tube begins to form. By the end of neurulation (E28), three primary subdivisions of the embryo can be discerned, and by E50 the embryo has differentiated into five distinct subregions, each of which will give rise to a different part of the developing CNS. Further, rates of growth across the subregions are not uniform. During this early period, the rate of growth in the most rostral regions of the embryonic nervous system far outpaces that in more caudal regions, setting the stage for the emergence of the critical structures of the telencephalon. Within more caudal regions, the compartments that define the segmented organization of the hindbrain and the spinal cord begin to emerge. The formation of rhombencephalic compartments is achieved by a simple but elegant difference in the timing of cellular element production within alternating rhombomeres. During the embryonic period, failure of differentiation of any of the major morphological divisions results in serious deformation or death of the embryo. Later in development, telencephalic development continues to be the most prominent morphological feature of the mammalian, and particularly the primate, brain. The size of the brain increases dramatically, and as size outpaces cranial capacity, the characteristic patterns of gyral and sulcal folding begin to appear. Sulci appear in a regular sequence, beginning with the primary sulci, which mark the major divisions of the developing neocortex, followed by the secondary and finally the tertiary sulci. Differences in gray- and white-matter compartments become increasingly evident.

Progressive differentiation at the cellular level begins within the CNS with the differentiation of the neural progenitor cells (see Chapter 6). As discussed earlier, differentiation depends upon signaling from migrating organizer cells. The additional differentiation of neural progenitor cells into those that produce cells appropriate to anterior or posterior neural regions is also signaled by nonneural mesendodermal cells. By the end of neurulation, neural progenitors begin to divide. Initially, the cells divide symmetrically, producing clones of themselves and thus increasing the pool of neural progenitor cells. By about E42, a subset of progenitor cells begins to divide asymmetrically, producing a new type of daughter cell, a neuron. Across the period of cortical development, the type of neuron produced by the neural progenitors changes repeatedly, and the timing of those changes is critical for the laminar organization of the neocortex. Specifically, signals thought to arise in part from neurons generated earlier induce the progenitor cells in the ventricular zone to produce neurons appropriate for the cortical layer currently being generated. Thus at the level of cellular differentiation, signaling between neural and nonneural cell populations initially defines the progenitor cell lines that will give rise to the brain and the CNS. Later those cells receive other signals that instruct them to produce a variety of neuronal subtypes. Further, the timing of the neuronal subtype production is carefully orchestrated to ensure that the correct cell types are generated and migrate to the appropriate cortical layers. Finally, at the end of neurogenesis, progenitors begin to produce the support cells of the brain, specifically, the astrocytes and myelin-producing oligodendrocytes and Schwann cells.

There are many examples of progressive differentiation of cortical pathways, which often take the form of increasing specification of the patterns of input and output. Some of the original work documenting the progressive specialization of connectivity within the primate neocortex came from Rakic and colleagues (Zecevic, Bourgeois, and Rakic 1989). In that work, they documented the early exuberance and later pruning of synapses within motor, visual, and frontal cortices in rhesus monkeys (see Chapter 8). For all three systems, they reported initial widespread and distributed patterns of connectivity that were replaced over time with more selective patterns of connectivity. Huttenlocher (1990; Huttenlocher and Dabholkar 1997) reported similar patterns of synaptic exuberance and pruning for humans. Unlike the monkey studies, however, Huttenlocher reported different timescales for over-production and loss within different brain areas. Specifically, the temporal course within primary sensory areas was earlier than that in frontal regions in both the timing of peak production and the rates of both initial exuberance and later pruning. The refinement and stabilization of cortical pathways during the postnatal period are thought to be influenced by the experience of the organism.

## Progressive Commitment

As differentiation proceeds, the complementary processes involved in progressive commitment unfold to produce the orderly emergence of neural structures and functions. The functional commitment of neural elements to specific networks and pathways serves to organize and constrain the developing neural system. Morphological differentiation of the embryo establishes the structural basis for regional differences in function. For example, the segmental differentiation of the hindbrain and the spinal cord is morphologically suited to the functional organization of the peripheral nervous system, while the early rapid expansion of the telencephalon provides a mechanism for generating the complex and intricate neocortex. Progressive commitment is also observed at the cellular level (see Chapter 6). For example, the neural stem cells that will form the principal neocortical progenitor population are initially multipotent neurepithelial cells that transform into radial glial cells (Merkle and Alvarez-Buylla 2006). At the onset of neurogenesis, radial glial cells are capable of producing the full range of cortical neurons. However, with development their production range becomes progressively more constrained (Desai and McConnell 2000; Frantz and McConnell 1996; McConnell and Kaznowski 1991). Once production of the neurons appropriate for the first cortical layers is complete and the progenitor has begun to generate a different type of neuron for a subsequent layer, the progenitor is no longer capable of generating the initial neuron type. Later in corticogenesis, radial glial cells produce oligodendrocytes and astrocytes. Finally, there is evidence that radial glial cells eventually exit the mitotic cycle and transform into astrocytes (Merkle and Alvarez-Buylla 2006).

The progressive commitment of neural resources is probably most evident in the formation of neural pathways. In early postnatal development, pathway formation is both exuberant and flexible. As the studies of visual deprivation and early injury suggest, brain organization adapts to meet the contingencies of experience. However, as pathways stabilize and exuberant connections are eliminated, the neural system becomes increasingly committed and the capacity for flexible reorganization becomes limited. The commitment of resources is gradual and progressive and, as Huttenlocher and Dabholkar's (1997) data suggest, operates on different timescales for different neural systems. Sensory and motor pathways stabilize earliest, while pathways that mediate higher cognitive and social functions show different and more protracted patterns of commitment. Finally, the capacity for change and reorganization, while increasingly constrained over development, is never completely lost. Work documenting at least limited plasticity in the adult brain (Buonomano and Merzenich 1998; Kaas 1991; Kaas, Merzenich, and Killackey 1983) demonstrates the continuing capability for neural pathway modification. Further, the capacity for lifelong learning must be mediated by the formation of new neural circuits and pathways.

## Changing Influences across Development

As the structural and functional organization of the emerging system changes over time, the factors that are most central to the ongoing process of development also change. As discussed previously, early in development, organism-intrinsic signaling dominates the developmental process, inducing cellular differentiation and establishing the primitive spatial organization of the embryo. Organism-extrinsic factors influence early development, but play a less central role than later in development. As the neural system becomes more complex, the range of factors that direct and influence development also expands. The increasing variety of structural elements (some permanent, some transient) creates diversity in the kinds of interactions that can be engaged in the complex signaling cascades that structure the developing brain. For example, by midgestation, populations of cells have emerged that direct the movement of neurons into organized structures. In this same period, other groups of cells act to guide the advance of neuronal processes to appropriate locations within the brain where they can establish functional connections with other cells. The activity of the emerging neural circuits creates another kind of signaling that has a significant impact on brain organization. For example, in the prenatal period, a cell's survival can depend on whether it becomes integrated within active neural circuits (see Chapter 8). Cells that make connections with other cells survive, while those that fail to make connections are subject to apoptotic cell death. The establishment of sensory input systems and motor circuits creates yet another avenue for neural signaling and expands the influence of the external world on the development of the neural system.

Developmental periods are often characterized by the particular "superordinate" event that is most prominent and defines the major structural change of the period. Embryonic events include such processes as gastrulation or neurulation; later events include corticogenesis or thalamocortical pathway formation. But each of these major developmental events is composed of many smaller epochs of change, each with its own unique and well-defined spatial distribution and temporal window. It is the combination of these many smaller developmental processes unfolding over time and interacting with other temporally convergent events that constitutes the larger "superordinate" processes. Thus, although the most obvious changes may appear to be the superordinate events, they are really the product of many smaller developmental processes, each of which contributes an essential element to the larger developmental event. An example from the embryonic period illustrates this point.

Early in development, this kind of temporally convergent network of changes serves to organize the embryonic proliferative zone. Initially, spatially specific expression of BMP4 and the BMP4 antagonists noggin, chordin, and follistatin define the neural progenitor population (Chapter 3). Soon after, posteriorizing agents such as WNTs are expressed. They induce cells in posterior regions of the embryonic brain to a posterior fate but are blocked by the concurrent expression of WNT antagonists, such as Cerberus and Dickkopf, in more anterior regions. Still later in embryonic development, the regionally specific expression of the transcription factors EMX2 and PAX6 plays an important role in establishing anterior-posterior patterning within the developing neocortex, while the temporally and spatially specific expression of *HOX* family genes defines the anterior-posterior axis in the hindbrain and the spinal cord (see Chapter 5). All the signals described for these early embryonic events are single, organism-intrinsic events; they are the products of specific gene expression. But no single gene product can independently define spatial organization of the embryonic nervous system. Rather, each constitutes a small developmental event that contributes an essential element to the larger, more complex signaling cascade. Each contribution is unique in terms of the signal content, its spatial distribution, and its temporal onset and duration. But it is the combination of many small developmental events interacting in larger signaling cascades that serves to establish the structural and functional organization of the embryonic nervous system.

## "Critical Periods" in Postnatal Development

The term *critical period* has been used to describe the temporally circumscribed periods of postnatal development when specific input is required to establish a particular behavior, presumably because the input plays a central role in the establishment of the neural system that supports the behavior (Knudsen 2004). The early definitions of the critical period came from ethologists studying animal behavior. Lorenz's (1957) early work with chicks and goslings examined imprinting behaviors in which young birds establish filial relations with a moving object encountered early. Contingencies in the natural environment make it likely that the mother will be the first object encountered, but Lorenz's work suggested that the young birds would imprint on any moving visual stimulus available in a critical period after hatching. The early definitions of the critical period made very strong claims about intrinsic control of the time window during which experience could affect development. Later work on the role of early experience in the emergence of birdsong (Marler 1970) and maternal attachment (Harlow and Harlow 1965) provided support for a strong version of a critical period. The concept was also applied to studies of humans. Bowlby (1969) introduced the concept of the critical period to the study of human attachment behaviors, and Lenneberg (1967) extended the idea to explain observations of declining capacities in language learning with age.

Despite the prevalence of the critical period concept as an explanatory construct for a wide range of early-learned behaviors, subsequent work suggested that revision of the original definition of the term was necessary. A substantial body of evidence demonstrated that there was greater flexibility in both the onset and the termination of the critical period for many behaviors. Other data suggested that critical period effects could be modified or in some cases even reversed by variations in experimental conditions (Michel and Tyler 2005). These kinds of findings led to a revision of the initial concept and the introduction of the term *sensitive period* as a more moderate alternative (Johnson 2005; Knudsen 2004; Michel and Tyler 2005). The sensitive period terminology acknowledges the well-documented findings based on data from a range of behavioral domains that experience has a greater effect on particular behaviors during specific developmental windows. But the sensitive period account does not require the narrowly conceived ideas about either developmental timing or maturational mechanism that are often associated with the critical period. Indeed, the conceptual shift appears to reflect a change in basic questions that were being asked about these important early developmental events. While critical period studies focused on documenting the existence of behavior-specific developmental windows and the timing of their onset and offset, studies of sensitive period events focus more on identifying the underlying mechanism for a particular event, as well as the complement of factors that might affect the timing and plasticity of learning for the event. As Michel and Tyler (2005) noted, "Replacing 'critical' with 'sensitive' marked the recognition that once the 'what' of development was discovered, timing alone would not be critical for manipulating the developmental outcome" (p. 160).

The construct of the postnatal sensitive period fits well with the dynamic, interactive model of brain development presented here. Throughout the prenatal period, both organism-intrinsic and extrinsic factors play important roles in brain development. With development, as the range of both structural elements and neural circuits expands, extrinsic factors play an increasingly prominent role. By the early postnatal period, the importance of input in developing brain and behavioral systems is well documented and indeed is the substance of the critical-period then sensitive-period debates. The importance of experience on a wide range of systems from sensory and motor to social, affective, cognitive, and linguistic is well established. Greenough used the term *experience-expectant* to refer to those aspects of early postnatal development that appear to expect or require particular input. But not all behaviors manifest this developmental pattern. For many aspects of learning, the timing of a particular input is not critical to acquisition. Greenough referred to this kind of learning as "experience-dependent." The challenge is to define more specifically why some aspects of learning appear to manifest a sensitive period while others do not.

Johnson (2001, 2005) has offered three competing accounts of sensitive period effects: maturational, skill learning, and interactive specialization. By the maturational view, sensitive periods are defined by the physical development of the brain. As brain regions mature, they assume specific, well-defined functions but require specific input to achieve full functionality. Thus physical maturation sets the limits on the sensitive period. The skill learning view presents a very different perspective on sensitive period effects, suggesting that the apparent insensitivity to new learning after the close of the "sensitive period" actually reflects the stabilization of a particular neural system as specific expertise in a skill area is acquired. Thus stabilization constrains plasticity within the system and indirectly limits sensitivity to novel input. Interactive specialization focuses on processes involved in organizing and integrating interactions among brain regions and suggests that the response properties of a region are dependent on its connections with other brain regions. As learning proceeds, patterns of connectivity sharpen and functions within a region become more specifically defined. Thus the end of the sensitive period is associated with the learning process itself.

The maturational view most closely approximates a strong critical period view in that it emphasizes the temporal constraints of brain maturation as central to the opening and closing of the development window. For both skill learning and interactive specialization, the sensitive period appears to be an epiphenomenon of the underlying developmental processes associated with learning. Learning-associated input shapes the patterns of connectivity and refines the neural systems. It is quite possible that, depending on the specific system, maturational factors also contribute significantly to the stabilization of the neural system. The models offered by the skill learning and interactive specialization views differ in the scope of learning they define and in their account of the interactions among neural systems. However, both take a dynamic view of the effects of learning (i.e., input and its effects) on the developing neural system, suggesting that multiple factors interacting in a dynamic fashion direct the course of brain and behavioral development. Thus in these views, the principles that appear to drive prenatal brain development continue during the postnatal period. The postnatal brain is a significantly more complex structure than the prenatal brain, and the range of inputs and outputs far exceeds that of the prenatal period. But the principles of progressive differentiation and, in particular, of progressive commitment of neural resources to functional systems continue into the postnatal period. Learning itself appears to become an important factor in the postnatal commitment of neural systems to particular patterns of organization.

## Temporal Constraints on Brain Development

The view of brain development presented here is dynamic, interactive, and adaptive. Complex signaling cascades direct the formation and fate of cell populations, specify the migratory pathways and final destinations of new neurons, direct the formation of connections, and even signal cell death in targeted populations. The developmental process can adjust to contingencies and even to direct insult to brain structure. Yet there does not appear to be a blueprint, an executive, or even a homunculus directing the continuous changes in the complex array of elements, systems, and processes that emerge, expand, change, and sometimes just disappear across the period of development. How can a process with apparently so many degrees of freedom succeed so regularly in the real world of pre- and postnatal brain development?

Part of the answer lies in the fact that biological development is a process that unfolds over time. Thus at any point in time, there are limitations on how development can proceed. Therefore, at any point in time, the developing organism has both a state and a history. The history is the sum of all the events that contributed to the current state of the organism. The state represents both the current structure and the functional capacity of the organism, as well as its potential for further change. In short, development does not happen all at once; rather, it builds upon itself, often creating as it goes the tools necessary for each successive step in the developmental process.

In addition to time, there are other constraints on the process of development. It is first constrained by inheritance, that is, by the species- and parent-specific genetic material passed on at conception, coupled with the cellular machinery necessary to make use of the information in the genes. The information in the genes is very specific; it provides the coded nucleotide sequence information necessary for producing the protein products that are the active agents in development. Many genes, particularly developmental genes, have a long evolutionary history that shaped their functional role both historically and within the developing individual organism. Environment, broadly construed, also constrains development. Cells reside in a nested set of environments, and each environment has the potential to influence change in the cell either directly or through signaling cascades. Some aspects of the environment are the product of the developmental process, as in the case of newly generated cell populations whose function is to direct some other aspect of development. But many environmental factors are external to the organism. Nutrients provided by the maternal system, teratogens introduced into the fetus via ingestion by or infection of the mother, gravity, light, temperature, and sensory input are all factors that affect and constrain the development of the organism. The developmental state of the organism in turn influences whether or not it can be affected by environmental factors. For example, teratogens that have a specific effect on neuronal migration can affect development only during a very specific temporal window, and even within that window, early versus late exposure affects cells migrating to different cortical layers, thus inducing very different kinds of disorders in the developing organism.

An important part of the account of why brain development is so consistently successful lies in the process of development itself. Neural system development is constrained by both inherited and environmental factors, but the process of development also introduces its own temporal and structural constraints. Early in development, the set of available structures and the range of possible processes are comparatively limited. Interactions are governed by intrinsic signaling cascades that function to define primary cell lines and the primitive spatial organization of the embryo. Later in development, the system is structurally more complex, but the developmental process has produced greater compartmentalization and regionalization of systems, as well as increasing commitment of neural elements to specific structures with particular functions. Thus the process of development introduces levels of structure and function that constrain the range of possible developmental trajectories for the organism. In that sense, development is, in part, a self-organizing process. The idea of development as a self-organizing process is not new. It has a long and varied history in disciplines as diverse as evolutionary biology, psychology, anthropology, and computational modeling. The principle as applied to brain development is important and consonant with the growing body of evidence on the basics of brain development emerging from developmental neurobiology. There are constraints on brain development that derive from both genetics and the environment, but neither genes nor the environment can specify the complex set of events that must occur for a brain to develop normally. The particular temporal dynamics of the developmental process introduce the additional constraints necessary to account for the continuity and robustness of brain development.

The idea that brain development is a process is also important for understanding what happens when things go wrong. Some early pathological events are devastating and lethal to the organism. More often, specific factors, such as a genetic anomaly, introduction of a pathogen, hypoxia, or frank brain injury, affect the course of brain development but are not fatal to the child. One important and basic set of questions raised by such early events is how they will affect the cognitive and social abilities of the affected children (Uylings 2006). Considerable work in developmental neuropsychology has over many years attempted to address these kinds of questions for a range of disorders. The models used for studying these questions draw from studies of adult-onset disorders in that they attempt to link a specific pathology with a particular behavioral outcome. However, more recently this model has been challenged as inadequate for the study of child populations because it fails to take account of the fact that the neuropathological event occurred within a developmental context (Karmiloff-Smith et al. 1998; Thomas and Karmiloff-Smith 2002). If brain development is a dynamic and progressive event, any nonlethal neuropathological event will become one of the many factors that affect brain development because it is part of the biological experience of the individual child. It will become part of the developmental history of the child and thus part of the developmental process itself.

The effects of neural insult on the developing brain and cognitive system are illustrated by a rare condition that affects approximately 1 in 4,000 children, perinatal stroke (Nelson and Lynch 2004). Perinatal strokes typically happen during the last trimester of pregnancy and are often associated with motor-system weakness on the contralesional side of the body. Studies of the effects of these early strokes on linguistic and cognitive development suggest that although children have deficits in a range of areas, they are typically mild compared with deficits observed among adults with comparable injury (Bates et al. 1997, 2001; de Schonen et al. 2005; Levine 1993; Levine et al. 1987, 2005; Reilly et al. 2004, in press; Reilly, Bates, and Marchman 1998; Reilly and Wulfeck 2004; Stiles et al. 2005, in press; Stiles, Paul, and Hesselink 2006). Further, there appear to be differences in the magnitude of deficit across behavioral domains (de Schonen et al. 2005; Stiles et al. 2005, in press). Children usually develop normal language skills but have persistent subtle deficits in visuospatial and affect processing. Recent functional imaging data suggest that the brain systems that mediate both language and visuospatial function in these children differ from those observed in typically developing children, suggesting that alternative patterns of brain organization emerged in the wake of early injury, and these alternative patterns of neural connectivity are capable of supporting a range of cognitive and linguistic functions at normal or near-normal levels (Raja et al. 2006; Saccuman et al. 2006; Stiles et al. 2003; Stiles, Paul, and Hesselink 2006). Data of these kind suggest that although neural insult is never a good thing, when it occurs in a child, it is, by definition, part of a developmental profile and thus part of a larger developmental process. In the case of children with perinatal stroke, the process of brain development supports the emergence of an alternative pattern of neural organization that in turn supports relatively high levels of behavioral functioning. Because developing systems emerge over time, the final functional organization of the brain in a child with early brain injury reflects an alternative developmental pathway, a variant of the typical pathway, which is itself developmentally constructed. From the moment of the stroke, both the state of the neural system and the developmental history of the child diverge from those of a typically developing child. Subsequent steps in brain development must incorporate both the neuropathology and the cognitive and neural consequences of that pathology into an ongoing developmental process that is unique to that individual. Nonetheless, the developmental pathway has much in common with that of a typical child—the genetics have not changed, mechanisms for neuronal differentiation and axon guidance are the same, and the laminar organization of the cortex and the organization of major pathways within unaffected areas are intact. But the injury affects both the state of the neural system at the moment of injury and the subsequent developmental trajectory. This perturbation of the developmental process has specific effects that give rise to the patterns of deficit, adaptation, and compensation that are the hallmark of development in this population of children.

## Brain Development as a Dynamic Process

The model of brain development presented here is dynamic and adaptive. It is a temporally defined process that is constrained by both inherited factors and experience, as well as by the process of development itself. It is a model that allows for adaptation, that is, for divergence from the "typical" pathway, but adaptation is also limited and must fit within the constraints of the developmental process. Development involves production of new elements and functions via processes of progressive differentiation but also imposes limits in the form of commitment of elements to particular structures and functions. Timing is critical both for the moment-to-moment process of development and for the longer-term emergence of stable structures and functions, as well as for any influence external factors might have on development trajectories. The model of brain development presented here differs significantly from older maturational models in which systems emerge in a linear fashion. But this more dynamic model fits the growing body of data on brain development from the early embryonic period through postnatal development.

The concept of brain development as a constrained and temporally bound but flexible and adaptive process has significant implications for psychologists. First, on the question of innateness, within this model of biological brain development, innate factors, that is, inherited factors, are inextricably linked to experience, and together inheritance and experience define and direct the developmental process. This presents a very different view of what it means for something to be innate than is typically presented in psychological models. In this view, everything that develops has an innate aspect. It must because all developmental processes rely, fundamentally, on the information encoded in the genes and on the cellular mechanisms that provide access to that information. Genes themselves do not participate in developmental processes; rather, it is the products of gene expression, the proteins, that are the active agents in development. But gene products do not by themselves create neural structures or functions. Rather, they participate in complex signaling cascades that over time serve to direct the fate of cells, the organization of systems, and the establishment of signaling pathways. Indeed, the same gene product can have markedly different effects depending on the developmental context in which it is expressed. When *BMP4* is expressed during gastrulation, its gene product directs the epidermal fate of ectodermal cells (Chapter 3). However, later in development, *BMP4* expression within the spinal column contributes to defining the dorsal-ventral axis of organization within the neural tube by directing the induction of specific types of interneurons (Chapter 5). Thus development depends equally on processes that decode the information in the genes and on the ever-expanding levels of environments that arise, in part, as the product of development itself.

This is a very different way of thinking about what it means for something to be innate. It renders any attempt to classify things as innate or learned moot. By this model, the neural structures and functions are the products of developmental processes that rely upon, but are distinct from, the inherited and contextual factors that interact to create them. Innate factors and environmental context act in concert to direct the processes that generate the developing neural system. The question, by this model, becomes, what is the nature of the developmental process that gives rise to a particular biological structure, neural function, learning mechanism, or concept? It is the understanding of development, both biological and psychological, that becomes central in this model of brain and behavioral development.

This approach to thinking about brain and behavioral development raises interesting and important questions for psychologists who study the typical development of children. Specifically, to what extent can our growing understanding of the basic processes of brain development be used to inform our understanding of social and cognitive development in typical populations of children? Ideas about neural flexibility and adaptation within developmentally constrained systems should inform the way we think about how children learn or interact socially. The very old questions about whether there are "optimal" ways for children to learn new material may be informed by data that allow us to capitalize on information about the state of the neural system at particular points in development. It may also help address questions about individual differences and the extent to which performance differences among children reflect different states of readiness or flexibility at a neural level. Evidence for the effects of experience or for progressive commitment of neural systems should be reflected in how children learn. Will learning in some domains "stabilize" and become less adaptable earlier than others? What is the effect of "enriching" a child's environment? Do we know enough about the relationship between input and brain development to define, beyond cases of extreme deprivation, what it means to enrich a child's world? These are precisely the kinds of questions that motivated this book. They are questions that suggest that knowledge of the developing neural system is important for understanding cognitive and social development more generally. The goal of this book is to make accessible this important body of information to nonbiological investigators whose work might be informed by it.

## Chapter Summary

- The biological concept of inheritance stresses the inseparability of inherited and environmental factors. It is the interaction of intrinsic and extrinsic factors that defines and drives development.

- During the embryonic period, the interactive processes are principally observed at the level of cell-cell interactions where one population of cells generates molecular signals that alter the developmental course of another population of cells, but external factors also play an important role. Later in development, intrinsic factors continue to play a critical role, but extrinsic factors play increasingly prominent roles in shaping and directing the course of brain development.

- Development is a process that unfolds over time. Thus the timing of developmental events is critical. There are multiple levels of timing, and each plays an important role in shaping the developing brain.

- At all levels of the neural system, progressive differentiation of specific elements and structures, coupled with progressive commitment of those elements to functional systems, are governing principles of brain development.

- A critical period is a time in postnatal development when specific input is required to establish a particular behavior. The onset and offset of the critical period are thought to be sharp and controlled by intrinsic factors. A more moderate conceptualization of the critical period is the sensitive period. The construct of a sensitive period focuses on the importance of experience during specific developmental windows but does not require the narrowly conceived ideas about either developmental timing or maturational mechanism.

- Brain development is constrained by both inherited and environmental factors, but the process of development also introduces its own temporal and structural constraints.

- Everything that develops has an innate aspect because developmental processes rely on the information encoded in the genes and the cellular machinery that allows access to that information. Brain structure and function are the products of developmental processes that rely upon, but are distinct from, the inherited and environmental factors that interact to create them.

### References

Bachevalier, J., and M. Mishkin. 1994. "Effects of selective neonatal temporal lobe lesions on visual recognition memory in rhesus monkeys." *Journal of Neuroscience,* 14: 2128–2139.

Bates, E., J. Reilly, B. Wulfeck, N. Dronkers, M. Opie, J. Fenson, S. Kriz, R. Jeffries, L. Miller, and K. Herbst. 2001. "Differential effects of unilateral lesions on language production in children and adults." *Brain and Language*, 79: 223–265.

Bates, E., D. Thal, D. Trauner, J. Fenson, D. Aram, J. Eisele, and R. Nass. 1997. "From first words to grammar in children with focal brain injury." *Developmental Neuropsychology*, 13: 275–343.

Bowlby, J. 1969. *Attachment and loss.* New York: Basic Books.

Buonomano, D. V., and M. M. Merzenich. 1998. "Cortical plasticity: From synapses to maps." *Annual Review of Neuroscience*, 21: 149–186.

Desai, A. R., and S. K. McConnell. 2000. "Progressive restriction in fate potential by neural progenitors during cerebral cortical development." *Development*, 127: 2863–2872.

de Schonen, S., J. Mancini, R. Camps, E. Maes, and A. Laurent. 2005. "Early brain lesions and face-processing development." *Developmental Psychobiology*, 46: 184–208.

Frantz, G. D., and S. K. McConnell. 1996. "Restriction of late cerebral cortical progenitors to an upper-layer fate." *Neuron*, 17: 55–61.

Goldman, P. S. 1974. "Functional recovery after lesions of the nervous systems. 3. Developmental processes in neural plasticity: Recovery of function after CNS lesions in infant monkeys." *Neurosciences Research Program Bulletin*, 12: 217–222.

Goldman, P. S., and T. W. Galkin. 1978. "Prenatal removal of frontal association cortex in the fetal rhesus monkey: Anatomical and functional consequences in postnatal life." *Brain Research*, 152: 451–485.

Goldman, P. S., and H. E. Rosvold. 1972. "The effects of selective caudate lesions in infant and juvenile rhesus monkeys." *Brain Research*, 43: 53–66.

Goldman, P. S., H. E. Rosvold, and M. Mishkin. 1970. "Selective sparing of function following prefrontal lobectomy in infant monkeys." *Experimental Neurology*, 29: 221–226.

Harlow, H. F., and M. K. Harlow. 1965. "The affectional systems." In *Behavior of nonhuman primates*, ed. A. M. Schrier, H. F. Harlow, and F. Stollnitz, 287–334. New York: Academic Press.

Hubel, D. H., T. N. Wiesel, and S. LeVay. 1977. "Plasticity of ocular dominance columns in monkey striate cortex." *Philosophical Transactions of the Royal Society of London*, ser. B, *Biological Sciences*, 278: 377–409.

Huttenlocher, P. R. 1990. "Morphometric study of human cerebral cortex development." *Neuropsychologia*, 28: 517–527.

Huttenlocher, P. R., and A. S. Dabholkar. 1997. "Regional differences in synaptogenesis in human cerebral cortex." *Journal of Comparative Neurology*, 387: 167–178.

Johnson, M. H. 2001. "Functional brain development in humans." *Nature Reviews Neuroscience*, 2: 475–483.

———. 2005. "Sensitive periods in functional brain development: Problems and prospects." *Developmental Psychobiology*, 46: 287–292.

Kaas, J. H. 1991. "Plasticity of sensory and motor maps in adult mammals." *Annual Review of Neuroscience*, 14: 137–167.

Kaas, J. H., M. M. Merzenich, and H. P. Killackey. 1983. "The reorganization of somatosensory cortex following peripheral nerve damage in adult and developing mammals." *Annual Review of Neuroscience*, 6: 325–356.

Karmiloff-Smith, A., K. Plunket, M. H. Johnson, J. L. Elman, and E. A. Bates. 1998. "What does it mean to claim that something is 'innate'? Response to Clark, Harris, Lightfoot and Samuels." *Mind and Language*, 13: 588–604.

Keller, E. F. 2001. "Beyond the gene but beneath the skin." In *Cycles of contingency: Developmental systems and evolution*, ed. S. Oyama, P. E. Griffiths, and R. D. Gray, 299–312. Cambridge, MA: MIT Press.

Knudsen, E. I. 2004. "Sensitive periods in the development of the brain and behavior." *Journal of Cognitive Neuroscience*, 16: 1412–1425.

Kolb, B. 1987. "Recovery from early cortical damage in rats. I. Differential behavioral and anatomical effects of frontal lesions at different ages of neural maturation." *Behavioural Brain Research*, 25: 205–220.

Kolb, B., and W. Elliott. 1987. "Recovery from early cortical damage in rats. II. Effects of experience on anatomy and behavior following frontal lesions at 1 or 5 days of age." *Behavioural Brain Research*, 26: 47–56.

Kolb, B., C. Holmes, and I. Q. Whishaw. 1987. "Recovery from early cortical lesions in rats. III. Neonatal removal of posterior parietal cortex has greater behavioral and anatomical effects than similar removals in adulthood." *Behavioural Brain Research*, 26: 119–137.

Kolb, B., and J. A. Tomie. 1988. "Recovery from early cortical damage in rats. IV. Effects of hemidecortication at 1, 5 or 10 days of age on cerebral anatomy and behavior." *Behavioural Brain Research*, 28: 259–274.

Kostovic, I., M. Judas, M. Rados, and P. Hrabac. 2002. "Laminar organization of the human fetal cerebrum revealed by histochemical markers and magnetic resonance imaging." *Cerebral Cortex*, 12: 536–544.

Kostovic, I., and P. Rakic. 1990. "Developmental history of the transient subplate zone in the visual and somatosensory cortex of the macaque monkey and human brain." *Journal of Comparative Neurology*, 297: 441–470.

Lenneberg, E. H. 1967. *Biological foundations of language*. New York: Wiley.

Levine, S. C. 1993. "Effects of early unilateral lesions: Changes over the course of development." In *Developmental time and timing*, ed. G. Turkewitz and D. A. Devenny, 143–165. Hillsdale, NJ: Lawrence Erlbaum Associates.

Levine, S. C., P. Huttenlocher, M. T. Banich, and E. Duda. 1987. "Factors affecting cognitive functioning of hemiplegic children." *Developmental Medicine and Child Neurology*, 29: 27–35.

Levine, S. C., R. Kraus, E. Alexander, L. W. Suriyakham, and P. R. Huttenlocher. 2005. "IQ decline following early unilateral brain injury: A longitudinal study." *Brain and Cognition*, 59: 114–123.

Lorenz, K. 1957. "The conception of instinctive behavior." In *Instinctive behavior*, ed. C. H. Schiller, 129–175. New York: International Universities Press.

Marler, P. 1970. "A comparative approach to vocal learning: Song development in white-crowned sparrows." *Journal of Comparative and Physiological Psychology*, 71(2, pt. 2): 1–25.

McConnell, S. K., and C. E. Kaznowski. 1991. "Cell cycle dependence of laminar determination in developing neocortex." *Science*, 254: 282–285.

Merkle, F. T., and A. Alvarez-Buylla. 2006. "Neural stem cells in mammalian development." *Current Opinion in Cell Biology*, 18: 704–709.

Michel, G. F., and A. N. Tyler. 2005. "Critical period: A history of the transition from questions of when, to what, to how." *Developmental Psychobiology*, 46: 156–162.

Nelson, K. B., and J. K. Lynch. 2004. "Stroke in newborn infants." *Lancet Neurology*, 3: 150–158.

Raja, A. C., G. Josse, L. W. Suriyakham, J. A. Fisher, P. R. Huttenlocher, S. C. Levine, and S. L. Small. 2006. "Regional brain activation after early left and right hemisphere stroke: Relation to cognitive functioning." Organization for Human Brain Mapping Meeting, Florence, Italy, June 11–15.

Reilly, J., M. Losh, U. Bellugi, and B. Wulfeck. 2004. " 'Frog, where are you?' Narratives in children with specific language impairment, early focal brain injury, and Williams syndrome." *Brain and Language*, 88: 229–247.

Reilly, J. S., E. A. Bates, and V. A. Marchman. 1998. "Narrative discourse in children with early focal brain injury." *Brain and Language*, 61: 335–375.

Reilly, J. S., S. C. Levine, R. D. Nass, and J. Stiles. In press. "Brain plasticity: Evidence from children with perinatal brain injury." In *Child neuropsychology*, ed. J. Reed and J. Warner. Oxford: Blackwell Publishing.

Reilly, J. S., and B. B. Wulfeck. 2004. "Issues in plasticity and development: Language in atypical children." *Brain and Language*, 88: 163–166.

Saccuman, M. C., F. Dick, M. Krupa-Kwiatkowski, P. Moses, E. Bates, D. Perani, J. Stiles, and B. Wulfeck. 2006. "Language processing in children and adolescents with early unilateral focal brain lesions: An FMRI study." Organization for Human Brain Mapping Meeting, Florence, Italy, June 11–15.

Soriano, E., and J. A. Del Rio. 2005. "The cells of Cajal-Retzius: Still a mystery one century after." *Neuron*, 46: 389–394.

Stiles, J., P. Moses, K. Roe, N. A. Akshoomoff, D. Trauner, J. Hesselink, E. C. Wong, L. R. Frank, and R. B. Buxton. 2003. "Alternative brain organization after prenatal cerebral injury: Convergent fMRI and cognitive data." *Journal of the International Neuropsychological Society*, 9: 604–622.

Stiles, J., R. D. Nass, S. C. Levine, P. Moses, and J. S. Reilly. In press. "Perinatal stroke: Effects and outcomes." In *Pediatric neuropsychology: Research, theory, and practice*, ed. K. O. Yeates, M. D. Ris, H. G. Taylor, and B. Pennington. New York: Guilford Press.

Stiles, J., B. Paul, and J. Hesselink. 2006. "Spatial cognitive development following early focal brain injury: Evidence for adaptive change in brain and cognition." In *Process of change in brain and cognitive development*, ed. Y. Munakata and M. H. Johnson, 535–561. Attention and Performance 21. Oxford: Oxford University Press.

Stiles, J., J. Reilly, B. Paul, and P. Moses. 2005. "Cognitive development following early brain injury: Evidence for neural adaptation." *Trends in Cognitive Science*, 9: 136–143.

Thomas, M., and A. Karmiloff-Smith. 2002. "Are developmental disorders like cases of adult brain damage? Implications from connectionist modelling." *Behavioral and Brain Sciences*, 25: 727–750; discussion, 750–787.

Uylings, H. B. M. 2006. "Development of the human cortex and the concept of 'critical' or 'sensitive' periods." *Language Learning*, 56: 59–90.

Wiesel, T. N., and D. H. Hubel. 1963a. "Receptive fields of cells in striate cortex of very young, visually inexperienced kittens." *Journal of Neurophysiology*, 26: 994–1002.

———. 1963b. "Single-cell responses in striate cortex of kittens deprived of vision in one eye." *Journal of Neurophysiology*, 26: 1003–1017.

———. 1965. "Comparison of the effects of unilateral and bilateral eye closure on cortical unit responses in kittens." *Journal of Neurophysiology*, 28: 1029–1040.

Zecevic, N., J. P. Bourgeois, and P. Rakic. 1989. "Changes in synaptic density in motor cortex of rhesus monkey during fetal and postnatal life." *Brain Research. Developmental Brain Research*, 50: 11–32.

Glossary

Index

# Glossary

**Actin microfilaments.** Actin microfilaments are present in the apical (top) regions of all cells throughout the neuroepithelium. They are part of the cell's cytoskeleton, and one of their functions is to support the cell's shape.

**Activity-dependent cortical organization.** The conditions under which the emergence of structural and/or functional organization of the cortex is influenced or directed by the activity of the neural system.

**Adenine (A).** *See base.*

**Adhesion differential.** The tendency for some cells to adhere and others to be repelled.

**Agonist.** *See antagonist.*

**Alar plate.** A structure in the dorsal regions of the caudal neural tube that establishes the neurons of the spinal-cord sensory tracts.

**Allele.** One member of a pair of genes. Higher organisms possess paired homologous chromosomes. For each pair of genes on a chromosome, there can be allelic variation. If an individual possesses two copies of the same gene they are considered to be homozygous, and if the two alleles differ they are considered heterozygous.

**Alpha-fetoprotein.** The major blood-serum protein produced in early embryonic life. It normally passes from fetal serum into fetal urine and then into the amniotic fluid, but concentrations outside the infant's body should remain relatively low. Elevated levels in either maternal blood or the amniotic fluid suggest the presence of an open neural tube malformation. When high levels of $\alpha$-fetoprotein are detected, confirmation of the neural tube defect can be achieved through the use of ultrasonography.

**Alternative splicing.** The range of possible edited transcripts that can be formed from the initial nRNA. Editing can involve elimination of introns

393

or combinations of introns and exons. Each variation in splicing produces a different form of mRNA and thus a different protein during mRNA translation.

**Amino acids.** A class of organic molecules that can combine in linear sequences to form proteins.

**Amniotic cavity.** A fluid-filled cavity that initially sits dorsal to the embryonic disc but by the beginning of the second month postconception surrounds and insulates the developing embryo.

**Anencephaly.** A catastrophic loss of forebrain structures that results from failure of the rostral end of the neural tube to close.

**Antagonist.** A substance that acts to negate the action of another substance, for example, a gene product that blocks the activity of other genes. It contrasts with an agonist, which enhances the action of another substance.

**Anterior and posterior neuropores.** Openings at the two ends of the neural tube.

**Anterior visceral endoderm (AVE).** A structure that develops prior to gastrulation and is derived from extraembryonic tissue (and thus is not part of the embryo). The AVE expresses genes that suppress posterior signaling in the epiblast layer of the bilaminar disc, thus providing an early channel for specifying the anterior fate of the overlying epiblast cells.

**Antiapoptotic genes.** Genes that promote cell survival. In mammals, the critical antiapoptotic genes are $Bcl2$ and $Bclx_L$.

**Apical-basal polarity.** Polarized organization in which neuroepithelial cells have asymmetrical organization rather than being uniform in shape and distribution of cellular materials.

**Apoptosis.** A form of programmed cell death that is distinct from necrotic or pathological cell death in both the sequence of events that occur and the regulatory signals that control the sequence. Apoptosis is a complex and highly regulated process that is part of the intrinsic program in all cells. Different sets of genes are known to control the triggering or blockade of the apoptotic sequence. Both organism-intrinsic and extrinsic factors can modulate the apoptotic process. Apoptosis is an important and pervasive process in brain development that serves to control cell numbers, eliminate transient structures, and facilitate neuronal population matching.

**Archicortex.** See *cerebral cortex*.

**Asymmetrical cell division.** A type of cell division that produces two daughter cells that differ both in the cell-intrinsic fate-determining molecules they contain and in their capacity to receive extrinsic signaling from other cells. The asymmetrical division of neural progenitor cells produces a progenitor that reenters the mitotic cycle and a postmitotic neuron that migrates away from the proliferative zone.

**Axons.** Nerve fibers that conduct impulses away from the cell body of a neuron. Neurons extend axonal processes that traverse the cellular matrix of the brain. The growth cone on the leading edge of the axon samples the surrounding space for signaling cues that direct its movement. Eventually extension stops, and connections with other neurons are made.

**Basal ganglia.** A group of structures located in the ventral region of the brain that are crucial for movement and coordination.

**Basal plate.** A structure in the ventral regions of the caudal neural tube that establishes the neurons of the spinal-cord motor system.

**Basal progenitor cells.** *See intermediate progenitor cells.*

**Basal transcription factors.** The six accessory proteins that are produced in all cells and are necessary for gene expression.

**Base.** The component of a nucleotide that contributes to the information sequence of a gene within the DNA or RNA strand. There are four bases in DNA: adenine, guanine, thymine, and cytosine. In RNA, uracil replaces thymine.

**Base pair.** In a DNA molecule, the two nucleotide strands are joined together by the complementary bonding of their bases. Each base in one strand of DNA, pairs and bonds with a complementary base in the second strand. Base compounds form specific, complementary pairs, such that adenine and thymine always form base pairs, and guanine and cytosine always form base pairs.

**Beta-catenin.** Molecules contained in the apical membrane that are part of a Wnt signaling pathway necessary to establish the appropriate orientation of cell cleavage.

**Bilaminar disc.** A two-layered structure derived from the inner cell mass of the blastocyst and present by E13. It is composed of two cell layers. The epiblast-layer cells give rise to the three primary germ-cell layers of the embryo, and the hypoblast layer differentiates into extraembryonic tissues.

**Binocular deprivation.** A condition, either naturally or experimentally induced, in which input to both eyes is blocked.

**Blastocele.** A large cavity in the center of the embryo at the blastocyst stage of development; Also known as the blastocyst cavity.

**Blastocyst.** *See cleavage.*

**Blebs.** Membrane protrusions that occur in the late stages of apoptosis.

**Cadherins.** Molecules contained in the apical membrane that are involved in cell-cell signaling and regulate both cell proliferation and differentiation.

**Cajal-Retzius cells.** A class of neurons that are produced early and migrate initially to the preplate. They later make up a significant proportion of the cells in the marginal zone, the outermost layer of the cortex. They express the protein reelin, which directs the signaling pathway that provides critical positional information to later-developing neurons, essentially providing the stop signal for neuronal migration.

**Cell adhesion molecules (CAMs).** Classes of molecules expressed in the surface of cells (including growth cones) that promote the adhesion of the advancing growth cones to the surrounding cells.

**Cerebellum.** A structure at the base of the brain that is derived from the metencephalic vesicle. The cerebellum plays a critical role in the integration and coordination of sensory and motor output. Recent data suggest the cerebellum also plays an important role in modulating sensory temporal information for a variety of higher cognitive functions including attention, language, and music processing.

**Cerebral cortex.** The outer layer of gray matter that overlies the cerebrum. In mammals it is composed of three regions. The paleocortex is one of two phylogenetically older divisions of the cerebral cortex. It arises from the lateral portion of the early telencephalic vesicle and forms the olfactory cortex. The archicortex is the second phylogenetically older division of the cerebral cortex. It derives from medial regions of the vesicle and gives rise to the hippocampus, an important memory area. The neocortex is the phylogenetically newest cortical region and is unique to mammals. It arises out of the dorsolateral region of the telencephalic vesicle and constitutes by far the largest part of the cerebral cortex. It controls sensation, perception, cognition, and action. The neocortex is also called isocortex.

**Cerebral gray matter.** The gray-matter regions of the brain contain primarily neuronal cell bodies, dendrites, and supporting tissue.

**Cerebral white matter.** The white-matter regions of the brain contain myelinated axons. Myelin is a white, fatty substance that gives these regions their characteristic appearance.

**Cerebrospinal fluid (CSF).** The clear fluid that fills the ventricular system of the brain and the brain and spinal-cord subarachnoid spaces. It is produced in the lateral ventricles, is continuously renewed, and exits via the venous system. It functions to cushion and protect the brain and to transport a variety of ions, molecules, and proteins and also acts to clear waste products.

**Chemoattractants.** Molecules that promote the advancement of growth cones.

**Chemorepellents.** Molecules that direct movement of growth cones away from a region.

**Chordamesoderm.** *See mesoderm.*

**Chorioamnionitis.** An intrauterine infection caused by an infectious agent that originates in the vagina and enters the amniotic fluid. In many cases, the infection is "silent" and is diagnosed only after the birth of the infant. The infection is common in preterm pregnancies, but the incidence declines with increasing gestational age.

**Chorion.** *See placenta.*

**Chromatin.** The DNA and associated histone proteins in the cell nucleus.

**Cilium.** A hairlike projection from the surface of a cell. The movement of the cilium can direct the movement of fluid in the surrounding area.

**Cleavage.** The process by which a fertilized egg undergoes a series of cell divisions. By E5, the process of cleavage produces the blastocyst, which is composed of two cell groups, the inner cell mass and the outer cell mass. The inner cell mass forms the embryo and other extraembryonic structures, such as the amnion and the yolk sac. The outer cell mass, or trophoblast, surrounds the inner cell mass and forms the chorion, which is the embryonic contribution to the placenta.

**Coding problem.** The problem of translating the "information" in sequences of the nucleotides that make up the genes within DNA into the relevant protein sequences that define and support biological structure, function, and development.

**Codons.** Nucleotide triplets within the mRNA that serve to specify the amino-acid sequences in the emerging protein strand.

**Colinearity.** Colinearity occurs when the order of nucleotides in the final transcript is the same as that in the original DNA sequence.

**Connecting stalk.** The embryo's anchor to the tissues that line the wall of the uterus that will later lengthen and form part of the umbilical cord.

**Constructivism.** In developmental psychology, the view that knowledge is constructed by the child based on sensory, perceptual, and motor input and experience with the world.

**Convergent extension.** A process by which the embryo elongates just before the neural tube begins to form. The cells intercalate (interdigitate) to form longer but thinner columns.

**Cortical plate (CP).** A structure that splits the preplate into two subdivisions, the marginal zone and the subplate. It gives rise to the cerebral cortex.

**Corticothalamic pathways.** The major output pathways that send signals from the cortex back to the thalamus.

**Critical period / sensitive period.** Temporally defined periods during which input from the environment is required to establish a particular behavior or can exert influence on the organization and function of a developing neural system.

**Cytosine (C).** *See base.*

**Dendrites.** The projections of a neuron that receive signals from other neurons.

**Diencephalon.** *See secondary brain vesicles.*

**Differentiation (neuronal).** The acquisition of appropriate neurochemical signaling factors and the establishment of connections with other neurons.

**Diffusion tensor imaging.** An MRI technique that provides information about the diffusion properties of molecules in tissue. Within the brain, it provides a measure of white-matter pathway development and/or integrity by measuring the "fractional anisotropy" of the movement of water molecules. In solution, water molecules move isotropically, diffusing equally in all directions, while in the presence of a tissue such as a white-matter fiber tract, movement is anisotropic and exhibits directionality along the tissue. Fractional anisotropy provides a measure of the degree of directionality of movement.

**Domain.** One of the three components of a receptor.

**Dorsal mesoderm.** *See mesoderm.*

**Dorsolateral hinge point.** A region of bending in the elevated portion of each neural fold that forms near the point of contact between the neural plate and the rest of the ectoderm. The cells in the dorsolateral hinge point become wedge shaped, forcing the bending that is necessary to position the two folds near enough to fuse and form the neural tube.

**Double crossover.** A complex form of recombination reported by Sturtevant in which there are two crossover sites between chromosomal strands.

**Double helix.** The description of the structure of DNA originally provided by Watson and Crick in 1953. The term describes two well-defined nucleotide strands that are linked together along their length and coiled into a spiral.

**Ectoderm.** The top germ cell layer of the trilaminar disc. A subset of progenitor cells located along the anterior-posterior midline of the ectodermal layer has the potential to produce the cells of the central nervous system. Progenitor cells in more lateral regions become epidermal cells that give rise to the epidermis, nails, hair, the glandular system, the sensory epithelium of the ear, nose, and eye, and the enamel of the teeth.

**Emboitement.** The literal meaning is "encapsulation." In preformationist theory, the idea that a fully formed adult organism is contained in miniature within each germ cell, and each miniature in turn contains a complete miniature within its germ cells, in an infinite series.

**Embryo.** The unborn young in the early stages of development. In humans the embryonic period extends from implantation through GW8.

**Embryonic stem cells.** Cells that are capable of dividing and can produce all of the cell types in the body.

**Endoderm.** The inner germ layer of the trilaminar disc. The progenitor cells in this layer give rise to the lining of the gastrointestinal tract, the respiratory tract, and the urinary bladder, the body of the thyroid, liver, and pancreas, the tympanic cavity, and the auditory tube.

**Enhancer sites.** Regions of a gene where special transcription factors bind to regulate the expression of the gene.

**Enucleation.** An experimental procedure in which the eye is removed to prevent visual input.

**Epiblast layer.** *See bilaminar disc.*

**Epigenesis.** The theory of inheritance that can be traced back to Aristotle and is based on the idea that form arises through gradual elaboration.

**Epigenetic inheritance.** Heritable changes in gene expression that do not involve change in DNA sequences.

**Epithelium (epithelial cell).** Tissue that is made of closely packed cells arranged in a sheet. They cover the surface of the body and line its cavities. Epithelial cells have an apical-basal organization.

**Euchromatin.** Regions of chromatin that allow more open access to DNA and have many more actively transcribing genes than the more compacted heterochromatin region.

**Excitotoxic injury.** Transynaptic injury caused by the release of an excess of excitatory neurotransmitters or other factors that allow high levels of calcium ions to enter the cell. The high levels of calcium activate a signaling cascade that damages cell components.

**Exencephaly.** A failure of neural tube closure in cerebral regions. In this condition, fetal forebrain development ceases to progress. The mesodermal tissues do not differentiate, and thus the skull fails to form. As a result, the neural tissue is exposed to amniotic fluid.

**Exocytosis.** The process in which the vesicles fuse with the presynaptic membrane and release their neurotransmitter into the space between the pre- and postsynaptic membranes called the synaptic cleft.

**Exons.** Protein-coding nucleotide sequences within a strand of DNA.

**Experience-dependent change.** The systematic changes in measures of neural organization (e.g., synaptic density) that are related to the experience of the individual mature organism. These effects are observed across the lifespan, reflect the specific experience of the individual, and are considered to be the neural basis of learning.

**Experience-expectant change.** The systematic changes in measures of neural organization (e.g., synaptic density) that are related to the experience of the young organism but are thought to reflect the effects of species-typical experience that are critical for the initial establishment of basic aspects of neural organization.

**Explants.** Sections of living tissue that are taken from a donor animal and transferred to a culture medium for growth or transplanted into a host animal.

**Extraembryonic tissue.** Tissue from four supporting structures in mammals. The amniotic cavity is derived from the ectoderm and produces fluid to surround the embryo. The yolk sac is derived from the endoderm and is involved in transport and metabolism of nutrients and in the production of embryonic blood cells. The allantois is derived from the endoderm and serves the maternal-fetal interface of the placenta. The chorion is derived from the mesoderm and forms the fetal contribution to the placenta.

**F-actin.** A filament-shaped protein that is found in high concentrations in filopodia.

**Fetal alcohol syndrome (FAS).** A neurodevelopmental disorder associated with prenatal exposure to alcohol related to maternal consumption. The disorder is characterized by abnormal facial morphology, growth deficiencies, CNS abnormalities, and learning problems.

**Fetus.** The unborn young beyond the embryonic stage. In humans the fetal period extends from GW9 through birth.

**Filopodia.** Fingerlike extensions of the cytoplasm that extend from the leading edge of cells. The filopodia of axonal growth cones are long, thin spikes of membrane on the leading edge of the growth cone that act as sensory receivers sampling the extracellular space for guidance signals in the local environment of the advancing growth cone. They convert the external directional signals into internal signals that direct the movement of the growth cone.

**Flexure.** A bend.

**Floor plate.** A structure formed in posterior regions of the developing nervous system when *Shh* expression induces cells in the medial hinge plate to express Shh. The floor-plate cells establish a second *Shh* signaling center in the most ventral regions of the neural tube.

**Functional magnetic resonance imaging (FMRI).** FMRI is a rapid neural imaging technique that can detect changes in local magnetic-field signal strength associated with increases in blood flow and oxygen extraction that are triggered by neural activity. It thus provides a means of coupling behavior with brain activity.

**G-actin.** The subunits that combine (polymerize) to create the F-actin filaments.

**Gamma-aminobutyric acid (GABA).** The primary inhibitory neurotransmitter.

**Ganglionic eminences (GEs).** During fetal development, structures that serve as important neuronal and glial proliferative regions. They are the source of inhibitory interneurons and glial cells. Later in development, these structures give rise to the basal ganglia. There are three subdivisions of the ganglionic eminences—medial, lateral, and caudal—each giving rise to different populations of neurons and glia.

**Gastrulation.** The process by which relatively undifferentiated embryonic tissue specializes into three primary germ layers: ectoderm, mesoderm, and endoderm.

**Gemmule.** In Darwin's theory of pangenesis, internal factors that are inherited from an organism's parents but are also the source of variability within the organism.

**Gene-environment interaction.** The circumstance where risk from an environmental factor varies according to genotype or where genotype effect varies according to environment.

**Genotype.** The class to which an organism belongs based on its genetic makeup.

**Glial cells.** Neuronal support cells that provide structure to the brain and support for the neurons.

**Glutamate.** The primary excitatory neurotransmitter.

**Growth cone.** A structure that forms at the tip of an axon and establishes contact with the surrounding environment, allowing it to respond to signaling cues in the local environment.

**Guanine (G).** *See base.*

**Gyrencephalic.** Having numerous convolutions.

**Gyri.** Convolutions of the cerebral cortex.

**Gyrification.** The macroscopic transformations that take place in the cerebral mantle and result in cortical folding.

**Gyrification index (GI).** A measure of the degree of cortical folding that is a ratio of the total length of the cortical surface contour to the length of an outer, or superficially imposed, contour.

**Hebbian learning.** The principle that connections between neurons that are simultaneously active are strengthened (i.e., cells that "fire together wire together").

**Heterochromatin.** Highly compact regions of chromatin that limit access to DNA and contain few actively expressed genes. Contrast with euchromatin, which are less compact and contain many more actively transcribing genes.

**Histology.** The microscopic study of cells and tissues.

**Histone core.** The basic component of a nucleosome. It is composed of two copies each of four histone proteins (H2A, H2B, H3, H4). It provides structure and participates in modulating expression of genes in the strands of DNA that wrap around it.

**Holoprosencephaly.** A serious malformation of the brain characterized by failure of the cerebral hemispheres to separate. Alobar holoprosencephaly is a serious malformation of the brain characterized by complete lack of separation between the hemispheres, a single undivided midline ventrical, undifferentiated ventral forebrain structures (e.g., basal ganglia), and absent central fissure and corpus callosum. In severe cases, a large dorsal cyst is common. Semilobar holoprosencephaly is a serious malformation of the brain in which the anterior hemispheres fail to separate, but there is some separation in posterior regions. The corpus callosum is missing in the front but evident in the back of the brain. Lobar holoprosencephaly is the mildest form of holoprosencephaly. Most of the hemispheres are separated except in the most rostral and ventral regions. Most of the corpus callosum is present, though the most posterior segment may be missing.

**Hydrocephalus.** A condition that can develop when the circulation of cerebrospinal fluid is blocked, and fluid builds up in the ventricles and is not reabsorbed. The accumulation of fluids can cause pressure to build in the brain, and that pressure can damage neural tissue.

**Hydrolysis.** The decomposition of a chemical compound by reaction to water.

**Hypoblast layer.** *See bilaminar disc.*

**Hypoxia.** Deficiency in the amount of oxygen reaching tissues.

**Inner cell mass.** *See cleavage.*

**Intercalation.** A process whereby cells become interdigitated.

**Interhemispheric fissure.** One of the earliest fissures to develop, that separates the two cerebral hemispheres. Also called the longitudinal fissure.

**Interkinetic nuclear migration.** Refers to the movement of the nucleus within a cell. During the division of neural progenitor cells the nucleus of a cell begins to move up and then down within the ventricular zone. DNA synthesis occurs as the nucleus reaches the outer reaches of the ventricular zone; cell division occurs upon the return of the nucleus to the vicinity of the lumen.

**Intermediate progenitor cells.** A class of progenitors that are produced by radial glial cells in the ventricular zone but that move to the subventricular zone, where they divide symmetrically. Approximately 10 percent of the intermediate progenitor cells produce two daughter cells that are also progenitors. The remaining 90 percent of cells produce two postmitotic neurons. Intermediate progenitors are thought to produce many of the neurons that form the upper cortical layers. They are also called basal progenitor cells.

**Intermediate zone (IZ).** The region that separates the ventricular zone from the preplate.

**Internal capsule (IC).** The major fiber pathway connecting the cortex with the diencephalon and the brainstem.

**Interneurons.** Neurons that are produced in the ventral proliferative region of the ganglionic eminences and migrate tangentially to the cerebral cortex (but also see Letinic, Zoncu, and Rakic [*Nature*, 2002] for discussion of possible evolutionary differences in proliferative sites in humans). Along with projection neurons, they form the information-processing network of the cerebral cortex.

**Introns.** Non-protein-coding nucleotide sequences within a strand of DNA.

**Ischemia.** Deficiency in the local blood supply.

**Isthmus.** A border region, specifically the border between the cerebellum and the tectum.

**Junctional complex.** An attachment zone between epithelial cells.

**Knockout animal models.** Strains of experimentally altered animals for which a normal gene has been experimentally replaced with a defective, non-functional form of the gene.

**Lamellipodia.** Sheetlike extensions of the cell's cytoskeleton. They allow the cell to adhere to the surrounding surface and promote cell movement. Lamellipodia of axonal growth cones connect the filopodia and promote axon guidance.

**Lateral geniculate nucleus (LGN).** The subdivision of the thalamus that receives visual input from the retina and then projects that information to the primary visual cortex. The LGN is partitioned into eye-specific layers.

**Ligands.** Specific signaling proteins that bind to the extracellular domain of a receptor and transmit signals into the cell.

**Lissencephaly.** The condition of being smooth brained. The cortical surface of a lissencephalic brain lacks gyral and sulcal folding. Lissencephaly is typical of lower mammalian species such as mice and is a sign of serious pathology in humans.

**Lumen.** A hollow center of a tube, as in the case of the cavity formed when the flat three-layered embryonic plate reshapes into a closed cylinder.

**Lysis.** Swelling and rupture of the cell membrane.

**Marginal zone.** A subdivision of the preplate that is located along the pial surface and becomes cortical layer 1. It contains a class of cells, the Cajal-Retzius cells, that provide critical signals to migrating neurons about their future positions in the cortex.

**Median hinge point.** A region of bending in the neural plate at the middle of the spinal column. Signaling from the underlying notochord induces the median hinge point cells to become wedge shaped, thus forming an anchor point for the base of the neural groove.

**Meiosis.** A form of cell division that produces haploid (containing a single set of chromosomes) gamete cells (sperm and egg cells). Most mammalian cells are diploid (containing two sets of chromosomes). During meiosis, the number of chromosomes in the dividing cell is reduced by half. Then, when gametic recombination (fertilization of the egg by the sperm) occurs, the diploid state of the parents is reestablished.

**Meninges.** Membranes that cover and protect the spinal cord and brain.

**Mesencephalon.** *See primary brain vesicles; secondary brain vesicles.*

**Mesendoderm.** The organizer cell lines that migrate earliest form the pharyngeal endoderm and the dorsal mesoderm. The cells that form these two structures constitute the mesendoderm.

**Mesoderm.** The middle germ layer of the trilaminar disc that contains the progenitor cells that have the potential to become muscle, cartilage, and bone. Cells in this layer give rise to the vascular system, the urogenital system, and the spleen. Mesodermal cells also provide important signals for the development of the central nervous system. The prechordal plate mesoderm is the anterior portion of the mesoderm. It plays an important role in specifying cell types in anterior regions of the nervous system. The chordamesoderm is located immediately adjacent and posterior to the prechordal plate and plays a crucial role in specifying a posterior neural fate for cells in the overlying ectodermal layer. The prechordal plate mesoderm and the chordamesoderm together make up the dorsal mesoderm.

**Messenger RNA (mRNA).** A molecule that carries the coded DNA nucleotide sequence from the nucleus of the cell to the cytoplasm, where it is then translated into the amino-acid sequence of proteins. It is the critical intermediary involved in gene expression.

**Metencephalon.** *See secondary brain vesicles.*

**Migration (neuronal).** Neuronal movement away from the proliferative zones to regions of the brain where they will enter into neural circuits.

**Mitochondria.** The small intracellular organelles responsible for energy production and cellular respiration.

**Mitosis.** The process by which the chromosomes in the nucleus of a cell are duplicated to create two complete sets of chromosomes and the nucleus divides to create two nuclei. Mitosis is followed by cytokinesis, when the cell cytoplasm and membrane divide, creating two cells, each containing one nucleus.

**Mitotic cycle.** The cell-division cycle, during which new cells are generated. When cells leave the mitotic cycle, they are no longer capable of dividing.

**Monocular deprivation.** A condition, either naturally or experimentally induced, in which input to one eye is blocked.

**Morphogen.** A diffusible substance that disperses in a graded fashion away from its source, creating a concentration gradient of the substance. The concentration of the diffusible substance is greatest near the source and declines gradually with distance. The specific signal generated by a morphogen is concentration dependent; thus the fate of cells receiving a signal from a morphogen depends on the local concentration of the morphogen.

**Myelencephalon.** *See secondary brain vesicles.*

**Myelin.** The white, fatty substance that surrounds the axons of neurons and serves to enhance the transmission of neuronal signals. Myelin is formed in the CNS by oligodendrocytes and in the peripheral nervous system by Schwann cells. The cell membrane of oligodendroctyes that wraps around the axon is a two-layered structure that contains both proteolipid protein (PLP) and myelin basic protein (MBP).

**Myelination.** The process by which the axons within the brain become surrounded by myelin.

**Nativism.** In developmental psychology, the view that some classes of knowledge, called core knowledge, do not have to be learned. Rather, core knowledge is innately available.

**Naturalists.** Scholars whose primary method of investigation is observation, usually of plants or animals within their natural environment.

**Necrotic cell death.** A form of cell death usually associated with pathology. It is distinct from apoptotic cell death in both the sequence of events that occur and the regulatory processes that control the sequence.

**Neocortex.** *See cerebral cortex.*

**Nerve growth factor (NGF).** A neurotrophic factor identified by Levi-Montalcini and Hamburger. In a variety of in vitro and in vivo studies, they demonstrated that the survival of certain classes of neurons is critically dependent on the availability of NGF.

**Neural crest.** A class of cells that originate in the dorsalmost regions of the developing neural tube along its entire length and form a wide range of structures, including the peripheral nervous system, endocrine-system structures, pigment-producing cells, facial bone and cartilage, smooth muscle, fatty tissue of the head and neck, and connective tissue of the eye, mouth, and skin.

**Neural folds.** Two elevations of tissue that rise up on either side of the midline of the neural plate and extend along the anterior-posterior axis. Later in development, the two folds meet and fuse to form the neural tube.

**Neural groove.** The depression created by the progressive elevation of the neural folds.

**Neural induction.** A complex process of genetic signaling that results in the differential development of a subset of cells in the ectodermal germ layer of the trilaminar disc into the cells that will give rise to the brain and the central nervous system.

**Neural progenitor cells.** A population of cells that generate the cells of the brain and the central nervous system. They are also referred to as neuroepithelial or neuroblast cells.

**Neural tube.** The embryonic structure from which the central nervous system develops.

**Neural tube defects (NTDs).** Common birth defects caused by improper closure of the neural tube during embryonic development that occur at different levels within the nervous system and result in different specific disorders.

**Neuritogenesis.** A process in which neurons extend neuronal processes, specifically axons and dendrites.

**Neuroblasts.** Cells in the neurectodermal layer that produce all the cells that make up the central nervous system. The neural progenitor cells.

**Neuroepithelium.** The cells that make up the neural plate.

**Neurogenesis.** The production of neurons.

**Neuronal cell birthday.** An event in which one daughter cell produced as a result of asymmetrical cell division exits the proliferative cycle and migrates away from the ventricular zone.

**Neurotransmitter.** A type of signaling molecule that is critical in the transmission of signals between neurons.

**Neurotrophic factor.** *See trophic factors.*

**Neurulation.** The set of events that begins in late gastrulation with the formation of the neural plate and culminates with the generation of the primitive nervous-system structure called the neural tube. Neurulation is typically divided into two sets of processes described as primary neurulation and secondary neurulation, which involve different segments of the neural tube.

**NMDA receptor.** NMDA receptor activity plays a critical role in Hebbian learning. NMDA receptors on postsynaptic cells differ from other receptors in that under most conditions, the neurotransmitters cannot bind to and transmit a signal to the postsynaptic cell. However, when the postsynaptic cell is at or near depolarization, the NMDA receptor is "unblocked," allowing the neurotransmitter to bind to the NMDA receptor. The co-occurrence of neurotransmitter release, which is brought about by the activity of the presynaptic cell, and depolarization of the postsynaptic cell allows for concurrent firing of the pre- and postsynaptic cells.

**Node.** A structure on the epiblast surface of the bilaminar disc that forms at the anterior end of the primitive streak. On E16 a depression forms in the node that is called the primitive pit. The primitive pit is the point where migrating cells move out of the epiblast layer to form the more ventral endodermal and mesodermal layers of the trilaminar disc.

**Notochord.** An important embryonic structure that is critical during the formation of the hindbrain and the spinal column.

**Nuclear RNA (nRNA).** The RNA transcript that is first generated from the DNA nucleotide sequence. The nRNA sequence is edited in the cell nucleus to generate the mRNA. The mRNA leaves the nucleus and provides the template for protein synthesis.

**Nucleosome.** The basic unit of chromatin that consists of 146 base pairs of DNA wrapped around a histone core.

**Nucleotide.** The basic molecular unit of the DNA molecule. Each nucleotide contains a base that in combination with the bases of adjacent nucleotides defines the coding sequences of the genes contained within the DNA.

**Ocular dominance columns (ODCs).** Structures in the primary visual cortex that develop early and take the form of eye-specific columns. Along the length of the primary visual pathway from the retina to the thalamus to the primary visual cortex (PVC), inputs from the two eyes remain segregated. That segregation is observed in the input layer of the PVC as eye-specific bands of the cortex.

**Oligodendrocytes.** The cells that provide the myelin sheaths within the central nervous system.

**Organizer.** A set of cells produced during gastrulation that provides the signaling required for the initial specification of neural tissue. The cells of the node and the mesendoderm (which includes the pharyngeal endoderm and the dorsal mesoderm) together constitute the organizer. The concept of the organizer was originally proposed by Spemann in his early studies of amphibians. He suggested that something in the organizer signaled the transformation of ectodermal tissue to neural tissue. Subsequent work by Hemmati-Brivanlou showed that the induction of neural tissue requires blocking of BMP4 proteins that signal ectodermal cells to become epidermal. In the absence of BMP4 proteins, the default developmental pathway for ectodermal cells is to become neural. One important role of organizer cells is the production of BMP4 antagonists. In addition, subsets of cells within the organizer play important roles in specifying the anterior and posterior fates of neural progenitor cells in different regions of the embryo.

**Paleocortex.** *See cerebral cortex.*

**Pangens.** In de Vries's theory of inheritance, the hereditary material of the organism. Pangens are initially located in the nucleus of the cell but pass to the cytoplasm, where they become metabolically active.

**Paracrine factors.** A class of extracellular secreted proteins that is important in the regulation of development.

**Paralogous group.** In a family of genes that have undergone evolutionary duplication, such as the mammalian *HOX* genes, the set of genes that are equivalent. For example, complexes of mammalian *Hox* genes are numbered from 1 to 13 (e.g., *Hoxa1, Hoxa2, . . . Hoxa13*), and there are four complexes (*Hoxa, Hoxb, Hoxc, Hoxd*) created during evolution by duplication. The set of homologous genes from the four complexes (e.g., *Hoxa1, Hoxb1, Hoxd1*) form a paralogue group.

**Periventricular leukomalacia (PVL).** A disorder of the deep, central cerebral white matter that is common among premature infants and is the major neuropathology associated with cerebral palsy.

**Pharyngeal endoderm.** The anterior region of the endodermal germ layer.

**Phenotype.** The class to which an organism belongs based on its physical and behavioral characteristics (height, weight, eye color, movement patterns). Phenotypic traits are not necessarily genetic.

**Placenta.** A transient organ that provides oxygen and nutrients to the mammalian fetus and removes carbon dioxide and other waste products. It has two components. The chorion is contributed by the developing embryo, and the decidua basalis is composed of maternal endometrial tisse. The chorion is composed of extraembryonic tissue derived from the trophoblast and the extraembryonic mesoderm.

**Pleiotropic.** Able to produce multiple effects or affect multiple aspects of developmental outcome.

**Prechordal plate mesoderm.** *See mesoderm.*

**Precursor neurotrophic factors (proNTs).** The initial products of the synthesis of neurotrophic factors that later cleave to form mature neurotrophic factors.

**Preformationism.** A theory of inheritance that can be traced back to Plato and that is based on the idea that the form of the individual is predetermined and inherent in the organism.

**Preplate.** A horizontal monolayer; also called the primordial plexiform layer. It is the first layer to form in the developing neocortex.

**Primary brain vesicles.** The term *vesicle* is a general anatomical term describing a structure that forms a pouch. The primary brain vesicles are the anatomical subdivisions that emerge along the anterior-posterior axis within the anterior region of the neural tube. The most anterior of these embryonic vesicles is called the prosencephalon and is the embryonic precursor of future forebrain structures. The middle vesicle is the mesencephalon and is the precursor of midbrain structures. The most posterior is the rhombencephalon and will become the hindbrain.

**Primary germ layers.** The embryonic layers that compose the trilaminar disc. Each of the three primary germ cell layers contains cells that will give rise to different types of body tissue. *See ectoderm; endoderm; mesoderm.*

**Primary neurulation.** The process by which the primitive embryonic structure that will give rise to the brain and most of the spinal column (to the level of the sacrum in the very low back) is formed. This early structure is derived from neuroectodermal cells.

**Primitive groove.** *See primitive streak.*

**Primitive pit.** *See node.*

**Primitive streak.** A structure that forms on the surface of the epiblast layer of the bilaminar disc. It begins as a midline thickening at the posterior end of the embryo and gradually extends anteriorly. A depression forms in the streak that is referred to as the primitive groove.

**Proapoptotic genes.** Genes that, upon expression, initiate a signaling cascade involving a number of molecules, including caspase-9, which, in turn, signals expression of *caspase-3*. In mammals, critical pro-apoptotic genes are *Bax* and *Bad.*

**Progenitor cells.** Cells that are capable of dividing and can produce other cell types. They differ from embryonic stem cells in that the range of cell types that they can produce is more limited. Progenitor cells can be multipotent or unipotent, whereas stem cells are pluripotent.

**Programmed cell death.** *See apoptosis.*

**Projection neurons.** Neural cells that are initially produced exclusively in the ventricular zone and later in the subventricular zone that, along with interneurons, form the information-processing network of the cerebral cortex.

**Proliferation (neuronal).** The generation of neurons. *See neurogenesis.*

**Promoter region.** The site on a gene where the enzyme necessary for the synthesis of RNA, RNA polymerase, binds to initiate gene transcription.

**Prosencephalon.** *See primary brain vesicles.*

**Protein.** The primary product of gene expression. Proteins are composed of sequences of amino acids and are the principal constituents of cells. They interact to direct the development and functioning of the organism.

**Protein isoforms.** Protein that have only very small differences in their structure. Alternative splicing of tRNA can give rise to protein isoforms.

**Protein synthesis.** The translation of the information in the mRNA into the amino-acid sequences of proteins.

**Protocortex.** A theory of brain development that asserts that early in development, the neocortex is comparatively homogeneous and that the assignment of functional roles for neurons is dependent on input to and activity of neurons.

**Protomap.** A theory of brain development that argues that molecular signaling of neural progenitor cells in the proliferative zone establishes both the positional value and the basic function of neurons within the primary subdivision of the cortex.

**Purinergic signaling.** A form of nonsynaptic neuronal and glial signaling involving adenosine triphosphate (ATP), which is a purine that may be involved in signaling myelin formation. ATP is released along the extent of the axon when neurons fire. Oligodendrocytes and Schwann cells have receptors for ATP. ATP signaling promotes the differentiation of immature oligodendroctyes.

**Purines.** The two nucleotide bases, adenine and guanine, with a double-ring chemical structure.

**Pyrimidines.** The two nucleotide bases, thymine and cytosine, with a single-ring chemical structure.

**Radial glial cells.** An important class of neural progenitor cells that appear with the onset of neurogenesis. Radial glial cells were originally thought to serve only a supporting role in cortical development as a kind of cellular scaffolding that provides support and guidance for new neurons migrating from the ventricular zone to the developing neocortex. Recent work has shown that RG cells are the primary neural progenitor cell line, and the great majority of projection neurons derive either directly or indirectly from RG cells.

**Radial glial-guided locomotion.** The predominant mode of neuronal migration from the ventricular zone, which involves cell movement along an intricate and radially oriented cellular scaffolding composed of radial glial cells.

**Reactive oxygen species (ROS)/reactive nitrogen species (RNS).** ROS and RNS, including oxygen ions, nitrous oxide, free radicals, and peroxides, are produced as a result of normal oxygen and nitrogen metabolism, but the quantities of ROS/RNS can increase to toxic levels under conditions of oxidative and nitrative stress. Both hypoxic-ischemic events and inflammatory conditions associated with infection can trigger these stress reactions, which can damage vulnerable tissues. Immature oligodendrocytes have been shown to be particularly susceptible to the damaging effects of oxidative and nitrative stress reactions.

**Receptors.** Proteins whose structure spans the cell membrane and have three domains: the extracellular domain, the transmembrane domain, and the

cytoplasmic domain. Receptors act to conduct signals originating outside
the cell into the cell.

**Recombination.** A specific mechanism of discontinuous variation, originally
proposed by T. H. Morgan, in which the two chromosomal strands become intertwined, or "cross over," during meiosis, resulting in a systematic
exchange of genetic material.

**Regulatory genes.** A class of genes that are thought to code for repressors
whose function is to control the activity of structural genes.

**Rhombencephalon.** See *primary brain vesicles.*

**Rhombomere.** A transient embryonic structure composed of a parcellated
group of cells that constitutes a separate functional unit within the hindbrain and that serves an important organizational function early in
development.

**Ribosomes.** Structures in the cell cytoplasm that have been described as factories for assembling amino-acid sequences in that they physically support
the mRNA and other molecules involved in protein synthesis and aid in
the formation of bonds between amino acids in the emerging protein.

**RNA polymerase.** The enzyme necessary for the synthesis of RNA.

**RNA synthesis.** A process in which the sequence of nucleotides that make up
the growing RNA strand is generated on the basis of the template provided in the exposed section of DNA.

**RNA transcript.** A copy of a DNA sequence. The initial RNA transcript, nuclear RNA (nRNA), is edited to produce the messenger RNA (mRNA).
The mRNA is transported out of the cell nucleus through small openings
in the nuclear membrane called neural pores and enters the cytoplasm of
the cell. The mRNA transcript is used as a template for producing
proteins.

**Roof plate.** A dorsal midline structure formed by the expression of *BMP4*
and *BMP7*. The roof-plate cells establish a second dorsal signaling center
that begins to express *BMP4*.

**Schwann cells.** The cells that provide the myelin sheaths within the
peripheral nervous system.

**Secondary brain vesicles.** The primary brain vesicles subdivide into the secondary brain vesicles. There are five secondary vesicles. The telencephalon is a division of the prosencephalon from which the cerebral
cortex, the basal ganglia, and the basal forebrain form. The diencephalon
is a division of the prosencephalon from which the thalamus and the hypothalamus develop. The mesencephalon does not further subdivide.
The metencephalon is a division of the rhombencephalon from which
the pons and the cerebellum form. The myelencephalon is a division of
the rhombencephalon from which the medulla forms.

**Secondary neurulation.** The process by which the primitive embryonic structure that will give rise to the most caudal region of the spinal column (including most of the sacral and all of the coccygeal regions) develops. The structures that arise during secondary neurulation are derived from mesodermal rather than ectodermal cells, and the process of tube formation is quite different from that of primary neurulation.

**Sensitive period.** *See critical period.*

**Small nuclear RNA (snRNA).** Short RNA transcripts that combine with proteins called splicing factors to form spliceosomes.

**Somal translocation.** A mode of migration in which neurons traverse relatively small distances to exit the ventricular zone. The cell extends a long process that attaches to the outer surface of the ventricular zone. The cell nucleus then translocates into the cytoplasm in a single smooth and continuous movement. This mode of migration is observed more frequently among the neurons that migrate early and less frequently in mid- to late corticogenesis.

**Somites.** An important but transient set of structures that form out of mesodermal tissue. They are located lateral to the notochord and guide the development of the segmented body plan.

**Special transcription factors.** A class of proteins that is important in the regulation of development. They act in the nucleus of cells to regulate the expression of other genes by binding special regulatory segments of genes, called enhancer sites.

**Spina bifida.** A type of neural tube defect in which the tube fails to close in the most caudal regions. The disorder involves failure of the vertebral arch to close. There are different forms of spina bifida that vary in severity.

**Spina bifida cystica.** A serious neural tube defect that involves either neural tissue or the membranes that surround and protect the spinal cord. Meningomyelocele is a form of spina bifida cystrila in which both neural tissue and the meninges protrude.

**Spina bifida occulta.** The least debilitating of the spinal neural tube defects, in which the vertebral arch is open, but the neural tissue is not directly involved and the neural tube defect is covered with skin.

**Spina bifida with rachischisis.** A form of spina bifida in which the neural tissue underlying the vertebral arch fails to fold and form that section of the neural tube.

**Spliceosomes.** Special complexes that consist of snRNA and a number of proteins called splicing factors. Spliceosomes accumulate at splicing sites on the tRNA transcript and participate in tRNA editing by excising introns and other tRNA sequences and by acting to rejoin the segments of tRNA after editing is complete.

**Splicing factors.** Proteins that combine with snRNA to form spliceosomes.

**Subplate.** A subdivision of the preplate that is a transient embryonic structure but plays a critical role in the early development of brain circuitry.

**Substrate adhesion molecules (SAMs).** Adhesion molecules expressed in the extracellular matrix surrounding cells. SAMs play a role in axon guidance.

**Subventricular zone (SVZ).** A proliferative region immediately adjacent to the ventricular zone. The SVZ begins to form at the onset of neurogenesis and later becomes a major source of neurons that form the upper layers of the cortex. The progenitor cells of the SVZ are produced by radial glial cells of the ventricular zone and are referred to as intermediate, or basal, progenitors.

**Sulci.** Grooves of the brain. Primary sulci are regularly positioned grooves or indentations on the surface of the brain that become increasingly deep with development. Secondary sulci are a network of side branches that form off the primary sulci. Tertiary sulci are a network of side branches that form off the secondary sulci.

**Sulcus limitans.** A structure that contains interneurons and serves as a conduit to relay information between the sensory and motor systems within the spinal cord.

**Symmetrical cell division.** A type of cell division in which each of the daughter cells that is produced is identical to the other daughter and to the parent cell. The symmetrical division of neural progenitor cells increases the pool of cells capable of producing neurons.

**Synapse.** The junction between neurons across which impulses are passed from one neuron to another.

**Synaptic cleft.** The space between the pre- and postsynaptic membranes.

**Synaptic elimination.** The pruning of synaptic connections as a result of cells' failure to establish active connections.

**Synaptic exuberance.** The process by which many more connections are formed between neurons than will be present in the mature system.

**Synaptogenesis.** The formation of synapses between neurons.

**Tangential migration.** A mode of migration in which neurons move across the plane of the developing brain to reach their target locations in the cortical plate.

**Tectum.** Any rooflike structure in the body. In particular, the structure in the dorsal regions of the midbrain.

**Telencephalon.** See *secondary brain vesicles.*

**Thalamocortical pathways.** The primary sensory input pathways that transmit information between the sensory relay nuclei in the thalamus and the cortex.

**Thymine (T).** See *base.*

**Transcription initiation site.** The site on the nucleotide sequence of the gene where DNA transcription begins.

**Transcription termination site.** A region of the gene that serves as a stop signal for DNA transcription.

**Transfer RNA (tRNA).** A class of small RNA molecules found in the cytoplasm of the cell. Each tRNA consists of three nucleotides to which a specific amino acid is attached. The three nucleotides constitute an "anticodon." During mRNA translation, the anticodon of the tRNA pairs with the codon of the mRNA. The associated amino acid is released and incorporated into the growing protein strand.

**Transgenic animal models.** Strains of experimentally altered animals whose genome has been changed by the introduction of genes from an external source.

**Translation initiation site.** A region of the gene that is coded during gene transcription and becomes part of the mRNA transcript. It is the site on the mRNA transcript where mRNA translation begins.

**Translation termination site.** A region of the gene that is coded during gene transcription and becomes part of the mRNA transcript. It is the site on the mRNA transcript where mRNA translation stops.

**Trilaminar disc.** An orderly three-layered structure composed of three primary germ layers that is formed by the end of gastrulation.

**Trophic factors.** Factors that promote cell growth and survival. Neurotrophic factors promote growth and survival of neurons.

**Trophoblast.** *See cleavage.*

**Unit factor.** In Mendel's theory, the material substance that is inherited by an organism from its parents. The unit factors account for both the stability of trait transmission and individual variation.

**Uracil.** *See base.*

**Ventricular zone (VZ).** A region in the center of the neural tube composed of neurectodermal cells. It is one of the primary proliferative zones for the central nervous system in that many of the neurons that form these structures are born in the ventricular zone and migrate out to form neural structures.

**Vertebral arch.** A bony structure that normally encloses the spinal cord on the dorsal side.

**Vesicle.** *See primary brain vesicles.*

**Watershed brain regions.** Brain regions at the distal extreme of the cerebral blood-supply system that receive only minimal perfusion and are thus predisposed to ischemia.

**Wild types.** Forms of organisms obtained in their natural, unaltered state.

**Yolk sac.** An important structure during the early embryonic period that transports and metabolizes serum proteins and macromolecules derived from the mother. It is also the source of red blood cells in the early embryonic period and provides the mechanism for blood circulation.

**Zona limitans intrathalamica (ZLI).** A thin band of cells that separates two regions of the prosencephalon. The regions are defined by the expression of two different transcription factors. The region anterior to the ZLI expresses *Six3*, while the posterior region expresses *Irx3*.

# Index

417